CONCEPTIONS

Fertility, Reproduction and Sexuality

For a full volume listing please see back matter.

CONCEPTIONS

Infertility and Procreative Technologies in India

Aditya Bharadwaj

berghahn
NEW YORK • OXFORD
www.berghahnbooks.com

First published in 2016 by

Berghahn Books

www.BerghahnBooks.com

Library of Congress Cataloging-in-Publication Data

Names: Bharadwaj, Aditya, - author.
Title: Conceptions : infertility and procreative technologies in India / Aditya Bharadwaj.
Other titles: Fertility, reproduction, and sexuality ; v. 34.
Description: New York : Berghahn Books, 2016. | Series: Fertility, reproduction and sexuality ; volume 34 | Includes bibliographical references and index.
Identifiers: LCCN 2016021769| ISBN 9781785332302 (hardback : alk. paper) | ISBN 9781785332319 (ebook)
Subjects: | MESH: Reproductive Techniques, Assisted--psychology | Infertility--psychology | Sociological Factors | India
Classification: LCC RG133.5 | NLM WQ 208 | DDC 618.1/78060954--dc23 LC record available at https://lccn.loc.gov/2016021769

British Library Cataloguing in Publication Data

A catalogue record for this book is available from the British Library.

ISBN 978-1-78533-230-2 (hardback)
ISBN 978-1-78533-231-9 (ebook)

for my parents who made it all possible

Contents

List of Tables and Figures

Figures

Tables

Preface

Test-Tube Conceptions

This book has long been in the making. In India, assisted conception, especially in vitro fertilisation (IVF), became normalised as test-tube babymaking in the early 1980s. My first encounter with the phrase 'test-tube baby' dates back to 1986 when the Indian media heralded the birth of India's so-called first scientifically documented test-tube baby with much fanfare. I was in school in New Delhi and living with my family. I felt an instantaneous connection between the big news of the day and the cover of a *TIME Magazine* from 1978 gathering dust in my father's bookcase that featured a large test tube with a human embryo floating in translucent liquid. My school friends and I were convinced that babies could now be made in glass tubes, a scientific possibility that fitted beautifully into our science fiction world of *Star Wars*. While our childish imaginations had simplistically accepted the possibility of making babies in tubes, in actual fact, this imagination had percolated down much further. Fifteen years ago, one of my interview respondents, for instance, recalled his family's worries on learning of their son and daughter-in law's decision to have a test-tube baby. It took nothing short of a visit to his hometown with his visibly pregnant wife to allay his family's fears that the baby was not incubating in a large tube elsewhere.

A lot has changed in India since then. The test-tube baby breakthrough in the India of my childhood occurred in a radically different world: the Cold War was far from over, the Berlin Wall was intact and geopolitically the world was bipolar. In this world order, knowledge, wealth and power flowed from the developed North/West to the developing South/East. Science fiction babies conceived in test tubes could emerge only in global locales like the United

Kingdom and, as the book will later show, competing claims from a former colony would remain patently untenable until an economically and ideologically 'liberalised' India of the late 1990s would begin to assert itself as the locus of knowledge production and wealth generation.

The economic liberalisation and opening up of the Indian economy in 1991 to the ebbs of global market forces and flows of international capital would author another significant shift. India would finally emerge from the shadow of its colonial past and begin a painfully slow drift towards the American model of economic capitalisation and cultural expansion. However, in the 1980s of my childhood and teenage years, British cultural influence was everywhere: from BBC soap operas on television and English curriculum in schools to fashion trends and Britpop animating the lives of middle-class teens. As the test-tube saga unfolded in India, I remember vividly a popular dirty joke doing the rounds in my all-boys Catholic school. The joke, 'spare the rod spoil the child', was inspired by the lowbrow, but popular, British show *Benny Hill* and the Rugby Jokes compendiums. The senior boys in my school were particularly tickled by the clinical and non-sexual modality of test-tube conception. Within a decade, however, Britain would be dislodged as the core cultural reference point, both high and low, amongst the English-speaking Indian middle classes, and a more mainstream American sensibility would emerge. In this changing world, still an ongoing process, 'mates' would become 'dudes', British slapstick would give way to American sitcom and the political establishment would undergo a post-Cold War thaw, warming up to the United States. The privileged middle-class childhood I recall here, like the test-tube conceptions, existed in a parallel universe from which millions of poor Indians were shut out. Larger shifts in India's global standing and relations with Britain and the United States have little impact on their everyday lives, except perhaps to make it that much harder to survive in booming neo-India. To this day they could never even dream of accessing these conception technologies, except when it is their body parts that are bought and contracted to bring forth new life for the local and global elites.

Throughout the 1990s my encounters with the world of the infertile and test-tube babies were confined to mass media accounts. Media attention, if anything, had become more persistent, and by 1995 I had begun contemplating researching assisted conception in contemporary India. In 1996 I was in the 'field' armed with a close reading of feminist and anthropological research with a distinctive

Euro-American focus. Rather disappointingly, this body of scholarship was largely silent on the issue of reproductive technologies, at least the conception variety, in the so-called Global South. The reality in India, however, was very different. In a country of one billion people and growing, test-tube baby clinics were everywhere and this needed explaining. Additionally, the figure of the test tube, a quintessential scientific signifier, in the making of babies fascinated me. Much to my disappointment I later discovered that embryology laboratories in India, as in the Euro-American countries, used Petri dishes, not test tubes, to mix gametes and culture embryos. Yet, test tubes were everywhere, from popular imagination to media renditions.

The genealogy of test-tube babymaking is rooted in a very specific kind of (science) fictional imagination. The test tube came to signify three significant elements: first, the test tube signified the humbling of nature, an ideological project that ran unabated in European (and later American) philosophical self-fashioning from Biblical times through the Age of Reason and the hyper modernity of the twentieth century. The replacing of women's fallopian tubes with test tubes served as another landmark on the long perilous journey to humble nature with reason. For a host of complex gendered genealogies, both women and reproduction were deemed close enough to nature to become prime sites for such ideologically driven interventions. Second, the use of the test tube signified the laboratory as a confined and demarcated space, a theatre reserved for performing and witnessing dramatic scientific spectacles and breakthroughs. This was a different order of confinement from the birthing subject forced to convulse in lying-in hospitals in the Victorian Age. Here the gaze penetrated beyond the surface in pursuit of knowledge. While science aimed to control the whole body, it focused on what could be cultured, or nurtured, in metaphoric test tubes: a technical assisting of conception and hitherto unseen intervention into the reproductive anatomy of the female subject. Third, as a metaphoric postulation, the test tube came to symbolise progress and became the crucible of gestating future itself. The future of reproduction and futuristic technology could be actualised both in and through the figure of the humble test tube.

The emergence of test-tube babymaking was greeted with its fair share of moral panic in its Euro-American formations. For example, long before accusations of playing God became routine in Britain in the 1970s and feminist fiction celebrating the liberating potential of test-tube conception, as well as radical feminist critiques of the early 1980s, became commonplace, popular culture in the United States sensationalised test-tube conception as deviant and immoral. The 1948 Hollywood production, *Test-tube Babies*, depicts the process as unnatural and immoral – a by-product of illicit sexuality. The racy movie poster presented the lurid thriller as a cautionary narrative on the perils of a promiscuous life. The poster imagery was equally compelling: a sketch of a naked blond woman hugging an enormous test tube with a human foetus floating in green liquid, a common technique employed by Disney and Marvel to depict scum. I am able to make these partial connections because bootlegged avatars of both these comic materials were freely available to middle-class kids in India when I was a child. This occurred despite mixed economy rhetoric that sought to protect subject citizens from corrupting capitalist influences, especially the kind emanating from the United States (India's answer to the Marvel superheroes for instance took the form of indigenous comic books featuring many of India's mythological heroes). To be fair, the barriers to information and consumption in India at the time were driven more by postcolonial socialist policies, predicated on the rhetoric of self-reliance and self-sufficiency, than by ideological dogma seeking to outlaw pernicious Western influences. Under the mixed economy model, which championed a 'healthy' mix of the best of capitalist and socialist ideology, there were occasional flashes of images and artefacts from the Western hemisphere. But these were scarce enough to create the fantasy body of a free, abundant West where unbridled consumption paved the way to ultimate success and happiness. Test-tube babies were part of this imagined success story of the West. The *TIME Magazine* cover announcing 'the test-tube baby birth watch in Britain' offered a tantalising glimpse into the fantastic world of an inaccessible 'other', desirable partly because of its inaccessibility. While scientific and technological imports from the Soviet Union, and to a much lesser extent from elsewhere in the West, were commonplace, these were almost always indigenised or absorbed within the folds of public sector suzerainty, while ensuring that private enterprise was not entirely stifled. This public–private sector amalgam remained the defining feature of health care in India until the new century when a veritable explosion of private corporate health care nudged aside the family physician and high street surgeries as the first port of call for the well-off middle classes. It is perhaps surprising that test-tube babymaking in India was perfected in the public sector in the early 1980s and was entirely taken over by the private sector in the 1990s. To this day 'babymaking' thrives in private clinics and super speciality units in large private hospitals. The scientific ability to conceive test-tube babies was an ironic gift from the Indian state, obsessed with controlling the fecundity of its citizens. Placed in its proper international context, this obsession was largely a feature of pressure emanating from the United States Agency for International Development, the World Bank, the United Nations and the Ford Foundation. Post-independence India's aid package, and most notably U.S.-sponsored food aid, was conditional on India's commitment to aggressive population control policies. The ideological import of the Malthusian 'development' discourse from the capitalist West melded effortlessly with the Soviet inspired five-year plans that India embraced to consolidate its postcolonial economic goal of self-sufficiency. It is in this 'mix' – of state controlled planned development – that India's population control policy was to become a brutal reality and scar innumerable lives.

These postcolonial developments also heralded a unique new chapter in the story of India's tryst with modernity. The mixed message of mixed economy championed agriculture and industrial development as potent signifiers of independent India's janus faced development: traditional yet modern. This mix of traditional and modern, once again imagined as the best of both, would touch every aspect of Indian reality from popular culture and art to state sponsored investments in science and technology. This mix of capitalist and socialist ideologies, together with traditional and modern normativity, would allow India to re-reinvent itself as ancient and yet modern. Test-tube, hereafter 'assisted', conception is one such site where an imagination of old/traditional, new/modern and now increasingly local/global continues to reproduce a peculiarly Indian modernity.

India continues to change, as it has done for centuries. New conceptions do not displace older ones but rather reproduce them and bring forth the reproduced difference as new but encored in temporal fractals of the past, present and the future. This book is an effort to unpick some of these dimensions in order to better understand the pursuit of conception in India today. It has been a long personal journey. I grew up with the test-tube baby saga in India and have had the rare privilege to witness its rise for more than fifteen years. To collate and collapse this experience between the covers of a book is next to impossible. This monograph is not intended to be a definitive account but rather a mere point of departure. Many loose threads remain and many more will be interwoven by a new generation of scholars hard at work as I complete this account. It is my sincere hope that this book will serve as a comfortable pit stop for those on an intellectual or personal journey toward conception.

Aditya Bharadwaj
Geneva, 2015

Acknowledgements

I am deeply indebted to numerous people who generously supported me on this long and sometimes difficult journey of exploration and discovery, and to more than one hundred couples and individual women, clinicians, scientists and clinical staff spread across more than thirty IVF units throughout India for generously sharing their life stories and everyday tribulations on the road to conception.

In Britain, where this journey of exploration began in the late 1990s, I remain indebted to Jackie West at the University of Bristol. Her unflinching support and steadfast encouragement gave me the courage to undertake this journey. I am also indebted to Theo Nichols, Harriet Bradley and Rohit Barot for their wisdom, scholarly insights and above all unwavering friendship and support. I also wish to thank my dear friend Ranji Devadason. The groundbreaking work of Sarah Franklin has been a constant companion. I wish to thank her for her helpful comments, feedback and ongoing conversations. Bob Simpson and Michal Nahman remain a constant source of intellectual stimulation.

At Cardiff University I wish to thank Paul Atkinson for three memorable years of scholarship, reading, writing and life shaping conversations. I also wish to thank my dear friend and colleague Katie Featherstone for intellectual companionship and friendship. I also wish to acknowledge Gabrielle Ivinson, Renata Kowalik and Daniela Plitz for enriching my intellectual and social life in Cardiff.

At the University of Edinburgh I wish to thank Donald Mackenzie and Lynn Jamieson for their incredible support as well as Janet Carsten for her uplifting intellectual presence.

In the United States I wish to thank several colleagues and friends for being a limitless source of inspiration and intellectual stimulation. The pioneering work of Marcia Inhorn has been a true inspiration.

I wish to salute her for establishing infertility and the burgeoning rise of assisted conception technologies in the developing world as a cutting edge concern in our discipline. I also wish to thank Charis Thompson for providing a significant point of departure for this book. Her scholarship is simply mesmerising. I thank Elizabeth Roberts, my co-traveller on the anthropological road to understanding assisted conception, as well as Lawrence Cohen for keeping the conversation going for nearly fifteen years. I thank Rayna Rapp and Margaret Lock for illuminating my path with their brilliance and wisdom. I wish to salute the pioneering work of Delhi based SAMA and their unwavering commitment to women's health and rights.

In Switzerland I wish to thank my amazing new 'intellectual family' at the department of Anthropology and Sociology at the Graduate Institute for International and Development Studies. In particular I wish to thank Isabelle Milbert, Alasseandro Monsuti, Vinh-Kim Nguyen and Shalini Randeria for their unstinting support. An extra special thank you to my brilliant doctoral students – Gabriela Hertig, Amishi Panwar, Alanna Armitage, Lauren Riggs. It is a true privilege to participate in your adventurous search for answers. And a warm thank you to Nayantara Sheron. It is a pleasure to work and share ideas with you.

At Berghahn Books I wish to thank Marion Berghahn, Dhara Patel and Caroline Kuhtz for their support for this project. I also wish to salute the pioneering vision of Soraya Tremayne for conceiving the *Fertility, Reproduction and Sexuality* Book Series and Marcia Inhorn for nurturing this groundbreaking initiative. I would like to thank the anonymous referees for their generous and thought-provoking ideas. The manuscript has emerged stronger thanks to their helpful suggestions. I also wish to thank Bonnie Rose Schulman for expertly proofreading the manuscript.

My life has been immeasurably enriched by the work of Veena Das. It is from her that I continue to learn the invaluable lesson in 'wording the world' in the innocuous everyday rough and tumble of life! I also wish to thank my family for their patience and unceasing support. Dilip, Meenakshi, Ratna, Shivam, Siya, Tara and Suyash, thank you for nourishing and enriching my life. I dedicate this book to the loving memory of my parents who supported me throughout this research. Thanks *Ma* and *Bappi* for introducing me to this wondrous world and for embedding in me the passion for learning. Thank you for suffusing my life with unconditional love. I miss you!

I wish to acknowledge publishers for granting permission to extract, extend, rephrase and reproduce following chapters: Aditya Bharadwaj, 'Conception Politics: Medical Egos, Media Spotlights, and the Contest Over Test-tube First in India', in Marcia C. Inhorn and Frank van Balen (eds), *Infertility Around the Globe: New Thinking on Childlessness, Gender, and Reproductive Technologies*, by the Regents of the University of California, published by the University of California Press, 2002; Aditya Bharadwaj, 'The Other Mother: Supplementary Wombs, Surrogate State and ARTs in India', in M. Knecht, M. Klotz, and S. Beck (eds), *Reproductive Technologies as Global Form: Ethnographies of Knowledge, Practice, and Transnational Encounters*, Campus Verlag, 2012.

INTRODUCTION

CONCEPTUALISING CONCEPTIONS

Assisted conception has become a visible part of contemporary Indian reality.[1] Popular culture, print and electronic media, and the expansion of in vitro fertilisation (IVF) clinics in many Indian cities and towns have together popularised and normalised the idea of 'test-tube babies' in a country of more than one billion people. Though traditionally long considered a stigmatised condition, infertility and its cultural (biomedical) management has never before in the history of the modern Indian nation been so vocally and publicly articulated.

The primary aim of this book is to show that infertility and assisted reproductive technologies in India lie at the confluence of multiple cultural conceptions. It addresses how assisted conception is understood by both the infertile and their clinicians by placing this encounter in the broader cultural context in which these technologies are received, used and promoted. The book's title, *Conceptions,* invites attention to cultural conceptions that lie behind the struggles of the protagonists (patients/clinicians) who feature in this research. The term 'conceptions', however, appears problematic to a listener trained in filtering semantics in a classic positivist/empiricist truth-seeking tradition. It sounds pejorative because it renders assertions deemed conceptions as false, untrue and subjective, pointing to a flawed understanding of 'facts', which modern science deems otherwise. An anatomical exploration of the term, on the other hand, yields a rich, multifarious body of paradigmatically encrusted meaning. According to the *Oxford Dictionary* the term 'conception' means:

1. The act or an instance of conceiving; the process of being conceived.

2. An idea or plan, esp. as being new or daring.
3. Understanding, ability to imagine.

This polytonality of meaning unpicks the many cultural processes shaping the very notion of 'conception'. The usage of the term goes deeper than establishing a mere correspondence between the biological act of conception and its medically assisted version. In shaping the overall project of understanding infertility and assisted conception in India, this book on one level draws on the term to contain and problematise the biological act of conception, assisted by the modern biomedical edifice, by showing how the two are in the 'process of being conceived' by biomedical experts and infertile patients. On another level, the book deals with social conceptions about infertility and its biomedical management, focusing on how they are understood not only as 'new daring ideas', as they emerge in media discourses and on the politico-commercial face of biomedical expertise, but also as an ancient 'imagination' of infertility management, a cultural frame that resonates with contemporary clinical, as well as social, infertility experience. It is to these conceptions that the anthropological project of understanding the finer relationships between these myriad strands attaches itself.

In other words the book deals with 'conceptions' deemed old and new, seemingly modern and traditional, purportedly scientific and religious, noticeably biological and technological. Conceptions are multiple, some manifestly prominent and others playing a role which is seemingly peripheral. This account reinforces the idea that conceptions seldom provide coherence, especially analytical coherence. That is, some conceptions predominate; others trail; still others seem to be rank outliers disturbing the possibility of narrative coherence. In this sense, this book is also about the incoherence implicit in conceptions jostling for attention. But together these conceptions reveal something important about infertility and assisted conception in India: the destruction of certainty in medically managing conception and the anthropological ability to narrate these complexities.

At the outset I outline four dominant themes that inform my analysis and understanding of infertility and procreative modernity in contemporary India. The first of these undercurrents is located in debates surrounding conceptive technologies in the Euro-American cosmogony. In particular I isolate the ideology of 'nature' as central to the Euro-American worldview – as both a historic project and a contemporary belief – which social science debates endeavour to unpack and problematise. I grapple with the social science critique of nature's place in the so-called Western ideological corpus to better contrast global articulations, such as those in India, where assisted conception is less preoccupied with the figure of nature. Second, if the nature/culture binary underscores much of the historical and contemporary engagement with reproduction and its biotechnological management in the Euro-American formations, an equally entrenched binary of tradition/modern demands critical scrutiny in the Indian context. As the book shows, the twin conceptions of 'tradition' and 'modernity' continue to offer a fascinating conceptual insight into the bourgeoning growth of assisted conception in India. Third, the cultural production of infertility and assisted conception can no longer be understood as a solely Euro-American concern. On the contrary, assisted conception in the new century is strongly positioned at the intersection of the local and global. For example, the transnational movement of Euro-Americans in search of conception to India and beyond has demonstrated the true global reach of assisted reproductive technologies. Lastly, as observed in the preface, this book has long been in the making, and disparate ethnographic encounters and representational quandaries have shaped it in very specific ways. It is to these encounters and representations I return briefly as I narrate facets of assisted conception in India today.

Nature/Culture: Assisted Conception in Euro-American 'Feminist Cosmogony'

The concept of nature stands as an important theme, foregrounding both feminist concerns vis-à-vis the impact of new reproductive technologies on Western women and social-anthropological debates on its implications for ideas of kinship and relatedness. Feminist cartography has long charted the cultural genealogy of nature in Western civilisation. The pre- and post-Enlightenment engagement with nature in Europe emerges as rooted in a cultural conception of man's superiority to nature – a maxim enshrined in the Book of Genesis: 'Fill the earth and subdue it, and have dominion over the fish of the sea and over the birds of the air and over every living thing' (Genesis 1:28).

This ancient belief of man's right to dominate nature receives a further fillip in the work of Enlightenment scholars who propounded a philosophical view of the universe as mechanistic, following predictable laws; those who could liberate themselves from the fetters of medieval superstition could discover through science and manipulate through technology (Davis-Floyd 1990). According to Carolyn Merchant (1983), during the seventeenth-century period of rapid commercial expansion within Europe, the machine came to replace the organism as the underlying metaphor for the organisation of man's universe. Prior to this idea, the earth had been viewed as a living organism infused with a female 'world-soul'. Merchant further argues that philosophers like Descartes, Bacon and Hobbes

> transformed the body of the world and its female soul … into … a mechanical system of dead corpuscles, set into motion by the creator, so that each obeyed the law of inertia and moved only by external contact with another moving body … because nature was now viewed as a system of dead, inert particles *moved by external rather than inherent forces*, the mechanical framework itself could legitimate the manipulation of nature. (Merchant 1983: 193; emphasis added)

By the seventeenth century – the beginning of modern science – Descartes had effected a conceptual separation between mind and body upon which the metaphor of body as machine came to be predicated (Burkitt 1999). Since the body was viewed as an appendage of the mechanistic natural realm, it came to be viewed (medically) as a mere mechanism that could be 'taken apart and put back together' (Kleinman 1995: 36). Some feminists argued that the man who established the idea of the body as a machine firmly established the male body as the prototype of this machine (Davis-Floyd 1990; Davis-Floyd and Dumit 1998; Rothman 1982). This is seen as a significant departure from the ideas propounded in medical texts from the ancient Greeks up until the eighteenth century that described male and female bodies as fundamentally similar. Women had hitherto been conceptualised as embodying the same genitals as men inside their bodies, thus relegating women to 'a lesser version of the male body' (Laqueur 1990; Oudshoorn 1999). Merchant (1983) further argued that any deviation from the male prototype became valid grounds for viewing female biology as abnormal and defective and as untenable as nature itself, thus in need of man's manipulation. Robbie E. Davis-Floyd (1990) similarly concludes that the demise of the midwife and the rise of male-attended mechanically manipulated birth followed close on the heels of the wide cultural acceptance of the female body as a defective machine.

This cultural imagination that placed the female and nature along the same continuum had in fact received critical anthropological attention before Merchant's (1983) groundbreaking *The Death of Nature: Women, Ecology, and the Scientific Revolution* (MacCormack and

Strathern 1980; Rosaldo and Lamphere 1974).[2] Carol MacCormack (1980) questioned assumed links between nature and women as inherently given and, together with a group of scholars, MacCormack and Marilyn Strathern (1980) persuasively critiqued 'universalistic' visions of natural and cultural that located femaleness in biology (nature) and maleness in the social domain (culture). These early feminist and anthropological critiques profoundly influenced the social scientific view of biomedicine and subsequent feminist accounts of reproductive health and technologies. Feminists now began to question the 'othering of women' (Oudshoorn 1999) as a special category of 'patients' within the medical domain from the eighteenth century to the biomedical gynaecological discourses of the nineteenth and twentieth centuries (e.g. Davis-Floyd 1990, 1992, 1994; Martin 1987; Moscucci 1990; Oudshoorn 1994). With biomedicine firmly established as a fundamental source of male assumptions about women's bodies as being closer to nature, and therefore as legitimate objects of scientific study (Oudshoorn 1999), feminists began to evaluate critically new forms of 'biomedicalisations' of the reproductive process (Clarke and Olesen 1999).

The 'new' technical possibilities of bypassing infertility only accentuated feminist disquiet over the increasing medicalisation of birth and the implicit metaphoric postulations of manipulating unpredictable nature (women) through cultural (male) knowledge and artefacts. Whereas the earliest polemical accounts, like Shulamith Firestone's (1971) *The Dialectic of Sex* and Marge Piercy's *Women on the Edge of Time* (1979), viewed technologies of procreation as liberating women, the radical feminist challenge of the early 1980s – spearheaded by Arditti et al.'s (1984) *Test Tube Women: What Future for Motherhood*, Andrea Dworkin's (1983) *Right-Wing Women* and Gena Corea's influential *The Mother Machine: Reproductive Technologies from Artificial Insemination to Artificial Wombs* (1985b) and *Man-Made Women: How The New Reproductive Technologies Affect Women* (1987) – critiqued the new reproductive technologies as instruments of oppression where dominant male scientific enterprise dehumanised, repressed and systematically objectified women.

Subsequent research was less conspiratorial in tone but critically expanded on these earlier concerns, in particular the works of Klein (1989), Klein and Rowland (1988), Lasker and Borg (1989), Spallone (1989), Spallone and Steinberg (1987), Stanworth (1987b). These scholars were now beginning to argue that a 'particular feminist reading [mainly the radical feminist challenge] which sees in these technologies an unmitigated attack on women was inadequate' (Stanworth 1987b: 3). These feminists raised questions about the experimental nature of reproductive technologies and the fear of turning women's bodies into 'experimental sites' (Klein and Rowland 1988).

In the 1990s, however, there emerged a body of feminist scholarship that negotiated with infertility and assisted conception as something to be understood critically and accommodated rather than overtly rejected (e.g. Birke et al. 1990; Cussins 1996; Franklin 1997; Franklin and Ragoné 1998; McNeil et al. 1990; Ragoné 1994; Sandelowski 1990, 1991; Strathern 1992b). Research focused increasingly on the 'lived worlds of infertility and reproductive medicine' (Cussins 2000), though the adverse effects of technologies on women were not entirely ignored and 'the ideological hegemony of the technocratic paradigm as potential future-shaper' was critically revisited (Davis-Floyd 1994: 1125; Davis-Floyd and Dumit 1998). The biomedical perspective on infertility, like that on other biological processes, was therefore seen as illustrative of the 'reflexivity of values in medicine and society', replicating cultural norms in biomedical ideologies about the nature and treatment of disease (Becker and Nachtigall 1994). Scholars like Emily Martin attracted criticism from within this new feminist terrain. For example, Naomi Pfeffer (1993: 176) questioned Martin's interview schedule that excluded infertile women and their experiences, thus conveying the impression that 'all women who live in Baltimore, USA … inhabit fertile bodies'. Arthur L. Greil (1994), on the other hand, critiqued Martin and Davis-Floyd for treating women's responses to medical definitions as an 'epiphenomenona' without giving due attention to women's creativity and agency in working within the medical framework to achieve their own ends, like the infertile women in his study, who transformed the medical model without accepting or rejecting it to better meet their own goals. Sarah Franklin (1997: 165) similarly showed, in the case of women undergoing IVF, that despite the cost and pain, women endorsed the technique and felt that it had 'made something of them' as women. These scholarly negotiations with the new technologies of conception were born partly out of an interest in examining the lived worlds of infertility and reproductive medicine. Feminists now 'granted the technologies a much less monolithic, oppositional and inhuman role' (Cussins 2000: 55–56) in favour of 'a much more mediating and active role than their predecessors had' (Thompson 2005).

These shifts within the feminist terrain concealed a broader tension that Stanworth (1987b: 4) earlier outlined as central to the feminist concern, where 'on the one hand, medical and scientific advances offered women a greater chance to decide if, when and under what conditions to mother, while on the other, they increased the potential for others to exercise an even greater control over women's lives'. Charis Thompson (2005) echoes this dilemma in a comprehensive review of the growth of feminist thinking in relation to infertility and assisted conception. In charting the evolution of this feminist discourse, she isolates two broad phases – phase I from 1984 to 1991 and phase II from 1992 to 1999 – while arguing that a paradoxical tension in feminist engagement with infertility and reproductive technologies lies between empathising with infertile women and their need to seek treatment and recognising the risk that in doing so they perpetuate already entrenched gendered roles and stratifications (Thompson 2005).

This feminist quandary is in a sense produced in relation to the dominant 'technocratic imperative' permeating the Euro-American[3] social matrix:

> *If it can be done, it must be tried … if it can be tried, then I must try it.* In other words, the existence of new reproductive technologies (NRTs) opens up new potentials for reproduction; once they are open, because they exist, they cannot be ignored. At the same time, options that arise out of a more organic or holistic worldview … are rendered invisible in the face of the dazzling potentials of the NRTs. (Davis-Floyd and Dumit 1998: 7)

Franklin's (1997) research similarly suggests that women express two primary aims in relation to IVF: if they succeed, they achieve the ultimate goal of a take-home baby, and if they fail, at least they know they have tried everything. 'The pair of alternate resolutions' according to Franklin (1997: 107) 'was seen to guarantee success one way or the other, a positive outcome was assured'. This 'technocratic imperative' ironically re-emphasises the Euro-American distrust of nature on one level. Davis-Floyd and Dumit (1998: 9) succinctly articulate this distrust, writing that 'because we so deeply trust technology, we cannot trust nature anymore. Natural reproduction, when successful, becomes a special category: lucky'.

Parallel to these debates, nature itself had become a subject of intense social scientific examination. While Thomas Kuhn (1970) unprecedentedly problematised the working of science, many scholars questioned the very idea of an untainted 'nature' waiting to be scientifically uncovered. These scholars showed how natural reality is actively constructed as an object of scientific study (Gilbert and Mulkay 1984; Latour 1987; Latour and Woolgar 1979). Correspondingly, nature and the life sciences included under the rubric of biology and biomedicine came to be viewed by feminists as 'socially, historically, culturally and economically constructed' (Clarke and Olesen 1999: 9). Feminist anthropologists like Strathern (1992a) were quick to point how different historical periods in England had defined and debated nature differently. Postmodern scholarship expressed this new state of nature by questioning 'what remains of the natural when nature is cultural – a product of discourse – and when what had been the territory of the natural is taken over by the intervention of human engineering' (Robertson et al. 1996). From within the disciplinary boundaries of sociology, scholars posed similar but more specific questions about how to think about nature. They emphasised paying critical attention to the issue and shied away from providing grand narratives in reply (Haimes and Williams 1998). On the other hand, anthropologist Paul Rabinow (1992) predicted a future whereby 'nature will be known and remade through technique and will finally become artificial', just as culture would become natural.

While scholars like Merchant placed the emergence of medicine in the context of rapidly expanding industrialism in Europe, which displaced the organism in favour of the 'machine metaphor', postmodern scholarship scrutinised biomedicine in the context of emerging technocratic culture within (late/post) industrial society. Similarly, if the industrial technology was geared to produce a particular kind of mechanistic rationality, which looked at the organic in terms of the inorganic (machine), then the newly emerging technocratic culture produced a rationality that juxtaposed the organic and the inorganic. It has thus become

> routinely thinkable in the post-industrialism of the late twentieth century – or at least presentable in Euro-American media – to make play with juxtaposing images of the organic and inorganic. We are not just supposed to think that machines are like bodies, but that there are aspects of machines that function no differently from parts of the human body even as human beings may embody technological devices within themselves. (Strathern 1992b: 2–3)

This positioning of the organic in relation to the inorganic (or non-human) heralded the birth of 'juxtapositions' (Strathern 1992b), 'hybrids' (Latour 1993) and 'cyborgs' (Haraway 1990, 1991). Haraway's pronouncements that 'we are all cyborgs now', 'cybernetic organisms', 'a fusion of the organic and the technical', 'shocked into being from the force of the implosion of the natural and the artificial' (Haraway 1999: 42–43) further disrupted the idea of 'natural reproduction'. The cyborg metaphor re-emphasised the mediation of reproduction by different kinds of 'technoscientific interventions' (Davis-Floyd and Dumit 1998: 11); it has touched all aspects of assisted conception. Semen, a bodily fluid, technologically processed by semen banks, became 'technosemen', a cyborg (Schmidt and Moore 1998). In vitro fertilisation similarly came to be seen as a 'hybrid of human and machines, of physical practices and textual practices' combining 'old and new reproductive technologies', a cyborg that allowed a retrospective glance at the 'constructed nature of conception' (Mentor 1998: 69–70). The disjunction between the metaphors of the body as machine and the body as cyborg also rendered late twentieth-century engagement with technologies like IVF 'fundamentally schizophrenic and ambivalent' (Mentor 1998). The issue at hand, therefore, is no longer one of critiquing metaphors of bodies working like machines but of machines working both with and within bodies, and while 'natural conception/birth' is still desirable, feminists are equally alert to women's growing unease with leaving 'reproduction' to the caprices of 'nature' (Mentor 1998).

The cyborg metaphor not only problematised the process of 'natural conception' but, more significantly, 'what was now to count as natural' and its implications for the ideas of kinship and relatedness. Thompson (2001) however tempered the discussion by describing the imagined implosions of nature and culture as counterproductive. Instead Thompson (2001: 198) showed the 'productive negotiations of boundaries and explanatory relations between cultural and natural concepts' in a specific area of contemporary infertility clinic in the United States. In fact, anthropologists had been arguing for some time that the twentieth-century conception of nature was inherently biological (Ingold 1986). As a consequence, the idea of natural kinship became biologised, and the meaning of what was natural became more specific (Strathern 1992b). The Euro-American 'reproductive model', according to Strathern, is premised on suppositions about the connections between natural facts and social constructions. Strathern's (1999: 23) remarks that the 'social recognition of parenthood must follow the biological fact', that the act of having sex, transmitting genes and setting into motion the biological development of the embryo followed by the foetus represents a modern, twentieth-century view. Technologically, however, assisted biological parenthood does not replicate exactly the old concept of natural kinship, but it does introduce a contrast between artificial and natural process, where assisted conception creates the 'biological parent as a separate category' (Strathern 1992b: 19–20). The connections between the natural and the social aspects of kinship are therefore rendered variable, with assisted conception offering different ways of configuring biological kinship, i.e. of other ways of 'doing' kinship that configure the mixture of nature and culture differently (Cussins 1998a: 43–63). The twentieth-century 'natural parent' – one who embodied the genetic and social 'kin' credentials – is dispersed either by enabling fertilisation outside the body or by involving donated 'third party' gametes. Franklin (1997: 7) thus speaks of the late twentieth-century British kinship dilemma, 'which is the question of how to make sense of new forms of technological assistance to conception which create new "relativities" in the space where certain relations once stood'. Franklin has two concerns: first about the relationship between 'traditional' kinship idioms of relatedness and the new forms of connectivity put in place by assisted conception; and second about the 'relationship with science and technology', which is rapidly complicating the Euro-American understanding of the self.

The anthropological focus thus rests on 'the emphasis Euro-Americans give to personal and kin identity via the facts of biology, and thus the cultural nexus between conception, sexual connection and individuality that is simultaneously reinforced and bypassed by the new reproductive technologies' (Strathern 1999: 25). Nature, so assisted, is compromised in one significant way; it is no longer a domain from which intervention is absent and 'what is taken as given, is no longer given by nature' but is 'visibly circumscribed by technological capability' (Strathern 1992b). Strathern placed this loss of nature into the wider 'enterprise culture' of the late twentieth century, where 'prescriptive consumerism' derives satisfaction from meeting the desire to consume. In this Euro-American context, where life is being increasingly 'enterprised-up', Strathern (1992b) discerns a subtle shift in the idea of naturalness as related to conception from being 'part of the workings of physiology to attributing it to parental desire'. Desire in the enterprise culture becomes choice, both in the consumerist sense and as a 'natural' desire to be a parent. This technological assistance is considered natural in that 'as long as some element of the entire process of childbirth can be claimed as natural [e.g. a couple's own gametes, or the womb as a natural space], technological intervention appears enabling [and transforms assistance to mean that] nature sometimes needs a helping hand' (Strathern 1992b: 56–57). This is a potent sign of the postmodern age for some feminists, where the Euro-Americans have 'moved so far into the cyborg realm that only those technological transfusions [called] "assisted reproduction" – safe, monitored, controlled – are considered "natural"' (Davis-Floyd and Dumit 1998: 9). However, while the natural became biological in the twentieth century in very particular ways, paradoxically this biological also became inherently 'relative' (Franklin 2013). This biological relativity compelled yet another dissolution of the biological and the technical as IVF not only relatively 'denaturalized' biology but also 'cultured up' the biological exponentially (Franklin 2013: 4).

Hence, central to the biomedicalisation of infertility is the concept of nature, as an ideal to be both opposed and embraced. While cyborgification has broken down and juxtaposed the nature/culture binary, as a process of cultural change, it appears to have turned the 'cyborg experience' into one that responds to (and improves) natural processes and redefines them as 'relatively' cultural. Arthur Kleinman (1995) argues that 'biomedicine instantiates the Western tradition's idea of progress', to which one can add Franklin's (1997: 166) contention that the interplay between reproduction and technology deploys two of the most powerful Euro-American symbols of future possibility: children and scientific progress. It is in this respect that the cyborg conception and eventual birth instantiates the idea of progress and continuity with the future. Establishing this connection has displaced and reconfigured certain core cultural ideas about nature in the Euro-American worldview, and it is this that much of the feminist and social-anthropological scholarship continues to debate.

This vast body of Western literature and debates – and others – relate to this book in three crucial ways. First, despite the manifestly different cultural context in which technologies of conception are embedded in India, the selective use of some substantive ideas in this literature helps to locate globalising fertility techniques in specific cultural concerns. After all, the very idea of 'nature' with a distinctive Euro-American provenance remains implicit and embedded in globalising technologies, like IVF, that reconfigure in different cultural contexts. Second, distinct from the Euro-American experience, the idea of nature in India – *prakriti* – is in some ways equivalent to the divine unknown and unknowable. It is enchantment par excellence, and any human effort to reveal and unravel it only serves to further deepen its 'unknowability.' Nature in this respect becomes a shrouded presence on the margins of human cognition. Nature in this schema is also ontologically multiple: actual, self, real. The continual search for one's true nature has underscored meditative struggles in India for millennia. In brief, nature in India can be imagined as pure philosophical wonder dressed up as context sensitive explanation. The ethnographic context will later show how, as a shrouded, unnamed entity, nature remains present as a quasi-divine object in the narratives and theodices of patients and clinicians. That said, it is important to stress that I do not use the notion of *prakriti* as an analytical trope to understand 'Indian encounters' with assisted conception. The category cannot be made to dovetail a notion of Indian reality any more than the idea of nature explains the entirety of the Euro-American experience. In explicating these conceptual possibilities, I merely gesture towards echoes of these cosmogenic constructs that remain tantalisingly familiar and yet incoherent enough to not map seamlessly onto ideas of 'Indian' or 'Euro-American'. Third, unlike Euro-Americans, their Indian counterparts seldom relate to the category of nature – at least in the Hindu cosmology – as a domain from which human intervention is absent. In this cosmogony, to be nature (*prakriti*) is to remain in a symbiotic relationship with the human and subject to human industry and action. To be brief, according to Hindu tradition, there are four *pursharthas* (forms of human action): *dharma* (righteous/virtuous conduct), *artha* (generation of wealth), *kama* (pleasure, desire and regeneration) and *moksha* (liberation from worldly cycles of birth and death). Manifestly the *purush* (man) / *prakriti* (nature) symbiosis is encoded with a distinct patriarchal bias. At a meta-level, this union underscores a primordial, epochal procreative theory of creation wherein the heteronormative male and female principals come together to reproduce and elicit change and difference. In practical terms this amounts to nature being made/extended/modified through human action just as human action is shaped/curtailed/facilitated by a dynamic nature. At a philosophical level, this symbiosis also symbolises man's attachment to *prakriti* through intervention and domination. Hence, as with all living things, growth, change and movement are inevitable. The only impediments and obstacles in this worldview are the torturous growth pains that mortal resistance to change brings. It is to these changing conceptions that we now turn.

Spliced/Betwixt: Conceptualising Modernity and Traditions in India

As counterparts, modernity and tradition are key to understanding the burgeoning spread of assisted conception technologies and the social implications of infertility and childlessness in India. In so arguing, the book does not allude to the emergence of a 'new modernity' but rather attempts a conceptual incision into the disrupted reproductive terrain. It examines the 'spliced' nature of Indian modernity where the improvised domains of traditional and modern symbiotically sustain, contain and enable the other. The result enables a relationship with the past, present and reproduced future.

Much ink has been spilt on the question of modernity and its multiple, mutating global contours. Whether conceptually demarcated as 'modernity and other traditions' (Friedman 2002), modernity and capitalist hegemony (Comaroff and Comaroff 1997) or simply rampant 'modernity at large' (Appadurai 1996), conceptual notions of the modern can be gainfully captured as being 'co-produced' by the global circulation of capital and capitalist economy. However, the point I wish to make vis-à-vis India is much simpler. At its most elementary, in India today, to be modern is to be anchored in the spatial configuration of the new and in the temporal dimension of the now. In this worldview, tradition, far from being antithetical to the spatial and temporal project of the 'new-now', produces exceptional and contingent modernities that (re)animate the 'then' in the here and now. In this variant of the modern episteme, the Weberian 'calculating spirit' (*Rechnenhaftigkeit*) routinely miscalculates and subrogates 'the disenchantment of the world' (*Entzauberung der Welt*) with an enchanted, instrumental rationality adept at worshipping at the altar of charismatic authority. This peculiarly modernist thought experiment shaped, in large part, postcolonial politics, state and institutions, cultural production, both 'high' and 'low', as well as scientific and technological advances. Lawrence Cohen's (2004: 166) insightful commentary on the elite and state planning reproducing colonial and nationalist structuring of 'masses: … subjects capable of passion but not reason' further illustrates this modernist conundrum. The contradiction according to Cohen is as follows: the Weberian, ascetic modernisation (instantiated by the state-sponsored population control policies), is 'organised around a transformation of reason and will in the production of ascetic moderns, but it takes as its material for transformation a population it constitutes as radically disjunct from reason itself'. The sterilisation operation for Cohen (2004: 166) has a redemptive quality that civilises the masses and produces a body that becomes 'as if it had undergone a transformation of reason' and has become 'inhabited by an ascetic will'.

Paradoxically, the elite state-sponsored discourse, which occupied the space vacated by the colonial modernist self-fashioning, routinely projects similar passions onto the bodies of its citizens. Nation-building in India has always been drive by passion. The passions rage and range from the Nehruvian kind (cf. Roy 2007), to ones shaped by the reaction to the manufactured state of emergency (Tarlo 2003) or reanimated under the impulse of neoliberalisation (Gupta and Sivaramakrishnan 2010; Patnaik 2014) and religious chauvinism (Reddy 2011; Sharma 2006). It appears that postcolonial India has knowingly or unknowingly renounced reason in favour of a passionate embrace of reason. This reasoned modernity is delivering growth, wealth and prosperity while at the same time deepening social poverty, social exclusion and social suffering. Governance in the passionate mode is almost always contingent and tacit rather than rational and calculating. Manifestly, the rational bureaucratic trope, a Weberian ideal type, appears to typify the Indian civil services or its colloquial variant *babu raj*. However, in the 'rough-and-tumble of everyday life', the 'illegibility' of the state (Das 2004: 251) produces as much a descent into unreason and chaos as the passionate masses it seeks to control. In this sense I argue that India's modernist journey is marked by passionate reason: the passion on occasions delivers all that is good and desirable, and reason accentuates millennia old inequalities and uncertainties.

Technologies, such as IVF, that are routinely used to assist conception are not transferred into cultural voids. Rather, local considerations, be they cultural, social, economic or political, shape and sometimes curtail the way in which these Western-generated technologies are both offered to and received by non-Western subjects (Inhorn 2003). In the Indian context, this essentially translates into grappling with complex notions of tradition and modernity. In fact, anthropologists often encounter creative tensions between these concepts and essentialist imaginations of India as standing at the confluence of Western philosophical paradigms and its own perceived normative traditions (Dumont and Pocock 1957). What kind of anthropological response can therefore adequately unpack and explain the interplay between imagined traditions and the supposed modernities in a rapidly globalising India? Let me attempt to step tentatively out of this conceptual problem.

Anyone who has had sustained contact with the contemporary Hindu worldview would notice its unique ability to continuously engage its cultural past. The so-called 'Western' and 'modern' in this worldview emerge embedded in the traditional, a process that connects the imagined past to the present, and the present to an imagination of the future. Milton Singer (1972: 385) tried to explain this as early as 1972, by arguing that 'the traditionalism of Indian civilisation lies elsewhere – in its capacity to incorporate innovations into an expanding and changing structure of culture and society. This capacity is reflected in a series of adaptive mechanisms and processes for dealing with the novel, the foreign, the strange'. In this scheme, therefore, nothing is excluded, making cultural transformation less painful. Hindu epics and deities are invoked in everyday Indian parlance and news media analyses. Objects like nuclear bombs get construed as *brahmastra*, the deadly weapon of Brahma the creator. Similarly, aircrafts are recapitulated as the *pushpak vimana* (aircraft) on which the Hindu God and mythological hero Rama flew back with his wife Sita after killing the demon Ravana, and guided missiles are imagined as Arjuna and Rama's arrows that struck with lethal accuracy in the great wars of the Hindu epics *Mahabharata* and *Ramayana*. A close family friend once referred to (one of the protagonists) Vyasa's rendition of *Mahabharata* (or the Epic Battle) to the blind king Dhritrashtra miles away from the battlefield in the city of Hastinapur, as an ancient form of live television broadcast, a phenomenon that has become an integral part of contemporary Indian culture. Attipate Krishnaswami Ramanujan has likewise shown that new ways of thought and behaviour do not replace, but live alongside, 'older religious ways'. Thus he goes on to assert that computers and typewriters receive *ayudhapuja* (worship of weapons) as weapons of war did once (Ramanujan 1989: 57). Interestingly, this cultural reasoning did not take long to assimilate issues like IVF and surrogacy. Thus, an article entitled 'Sages Knew the Use of IVF' made an appearance in the English daily newspaper *The Statesman*, on 16 January 1995. Similarly the recent advances in embryonic stem cells in India have led scientists like Dr B.G. Matapurkar, who researched adult stem cells in Delhi's Maulana Azad Medical College, to argue that *Adi Parva* of Mahabharata gives clear indication that the Kauravas (one of the protagonist clans) were born from stem cells. Not surprisingly, an article appearing in the Indian English-language magazine *The Week*, on 16 September 2001, carried the following banner headline: 'Stem Cells: A Lost Science of India?' (Bharadwaj 2005). More recently, Prime Minister Narendra

Modi courted controversy by suggesting that plastic surgery and genetic science explain the creation of the Hindu deity Ganesha and mythological hero Karna, according to the *Indian Express* (27 October 2014: 1) in an article entitled 'PM Takes Leaf from Batra Book: Mahabharat Genetics, Lord Ganesha Surgery'.

Archaeology of these developments yields historic echoes that Gyan Prakash archives in his portrayal of the intimate relationship between science, colonialism and the rise of a peculiarly Indian modernity. In the context of colonial science, a prime instrument of the empire, Prakash (1999) shows how the rise of science came to inspire many of the colonised to seek equivalent precedent for scientific thought in India's own intellectual history, creating a form of knowledge that combined Western ideas with Hindu cultural and religious understanding. Thus the very act of displacing the coloniser/colonised binary equated Hindu culture with Western culture and suggested science as the heritage of all Indians (Prakash 1999: 8–9).

However, I do not suggest that this rich historic context adequately explains parallels between the past and the present. Nor do I seek to minimise these occurrences or suggest that Hindu reasoning reduces everything to an antediluvian past. On the contrary, this continuous relationship with the past feeds into daily conversations, acts and attitudes towards the rapidly changing surroundings. There is never a conscious attempt to refer back to these sources, but they crop up either in the act of explaining life and its complexities or cynically furthering political or pseudointellectual agendas. This is a cultural process that is ever present in its apparent social absence. Marilyn Strathern (1992b), in the preface to *Reproducing the Future*, lucidly alludes to how people everywhere express even the most general thoughts in specific and particular forms by making their ideas available to one another. As 'a consequence they are always borrowing, if only from themselves. It is this (cultural) facility that enables us to at once give shape to and provide ourselves with starting points for fresh thoughts' (Strathern 1992b: vii). Thus I argue that, by drawing on and borrowing from the past to make sense of the present, these cultural agents – seen in the examples above – are not trying to establish a truthful and objective narration of the past in relation to the present. Rather, they are trying to assume the 'other' in the image of the 'self', setting into motion the start of a new thought, a new cultural imagination. Whether this produces innocuous and innocent affect or orchestrates certain expedient consequences remains deeply rooted in context.

This process of juxtaposing 'traditional self' with the 'modern other' is best understood in terms of what Veena Das (1999) calls the double entrenchment of tradition in India. She argues that tradition is first entrenched in institutions that may be considered traditional (such as caste or religion) and second in institutions that may be considered modern (such as the bureaucracy and the law). She further argues that:

> An untainted traditional telos is as unavailable in contemporary Indian society as a modern institution, such as a law court, [to this we can now add IVF clinics] which has not been coloured by its location. It is this double articulation which makes institutions such as caste or the religious community into new, original entities; this is not a matter of aggregation by which new features are added to old ones. When, for instance, Gandhi used *satyagraha* [literally 'insistence on truth'] as a form of non-violent resistance to the British Raj, he transformed a traditional concept into a new concept. (Das 1999: 53)

This is not to suggest that India faces a 'mistaken modernity' (D. Gupta 2000)[4] or that traditions are in any narrow sense 'invented' (Hobsbawm and Ranger 1983), for as Fuller (2003: 163) points out, 'even an invented tradition, if it is to have any resonance, must connect with a "collective memory", so that it cannot be entirely new and discontinuous'. In other words, when both the traditional and the modern are continually re-made, traditions are reanimated to become new concepts; modern institutions in turn – when placed in the context of these 'sense-making', 'meaning-giving' improvisations, reformulations and reconfigurations of traditional concepts – stand transformed as they get absorbed and further enmeshed in the changing context.

The presence of biomedicine, encompassing assisted conception as a biotechnological means of bypassing infertility, is a fine example of a modern institution in contemporary India which is 'coloured by its location'. Clinical engagement with infertility provides an insight into how people inhabit several domains simultaneously and how they move, extend and reconfigure ideas from these domains to create newer ones. These newer juxtaposed domains (traditional/modern) allow for an imagination of how things really are (Strathern 1992b). This raises two main issues: first, the traditional Hindu cosmological framework that produces beliefs and norms about human fertility/infertility and how these ideas produce the experience of stigma and social suffering in the face of infertility (Bharadwaj 2003); and second, the modern institution of biomedicine, which is uniquely coloured by its existential location in the wider context of Hindu traditions and whose selective transference enables clinicians and patients to make sense of issues such as the success and failure of assisted conceptive techniques (Bharadwaj 2006). This book focuses on both issues to purport one possible explanation of how seemingly modern and traditional entities in India permeate each other and produce a culture-specific engagement with assisted conception. In the words of Gyan Prakash (1999: 234), Indian modernity cannot be viewed as a simple 'victory of capital over community, modernity over tradition, West over non-West'; none of these neat oppositions dissolve each other; one (modern) does not negate the other (tradition) but rather 'one enables the other's reformulation'. However, it is essential to add a small footnote to Prakash's observation. It is the context-sensitive nature of this precise reformulation that makes, remakes and populates the many differing traditions and competing modernities in India. The resulting image remains shaky, partial and prone to mutations brought about by political, economic and social forces. In this respect, while Parts I and II in this book may appear as straightforward renditions of institutions and the concepts of traditional and modern/secular respectively, Parts III and IV shed light on how seemingly modern and traditional entities permeate each other and produce a culture-specific engagement with assisted conception. Though overtly heuristic and simplistic, this division nevertheless draws our attention to aspects of contemporary Indian reality that have an outward appearance of being modern (and even secular) but remain steeped in traditional concerns at different levels. These traditional concerns, on the other hand, when viewed in the context of modern institutions, reanimate themselves as new concepts that have an outward appearance of being traditional (some may even argue primordial) but are in fact curious new ways of making sense of events within a specific cultural context.

Local/ Global: Infertility and Assisted Conception around the Globe

Acknowledging IVF as a global phenomenon, Strathern (1999) contends that 'diverse locations will find diverse reasons for its use'. Unfortunately, these diverse locations received very little social scientific attention up until the beginning of the twenty-first century. This impasse in the feminist and social-anthropological writings would have persisted uninterrupted had Marcia C. Inhorn's (1994a,

1996a) groundbreaking research in Egypt not broken the silence on the need to examine infertility in non-Western cultural settings and its links with rapidly globalising technologies of conception. The Egyptian example laid bare a bias, within both academic research and the international health community, which views unchecked fertility leading to overpopulation as a predominant attribute of the developing world (Inhorn and Buss 1994). An exclusive focus, in Western feminist scholarship, on the problems of 'affluent Western women' gives the impression that infertility is 'an exclusively Western, bourgeois concern' and in this respect these feminist social scientific endeavours are 'particularly guilty of wearing cross-cultural blinders' (Inhorn 1994a: 26). Thus the 'feminist silence on the plight of non-Western infertile women' and the idea of helping 'infertile subpopulations in high-fertility non-Western settings' has never been a high priority within academia and in the international population circles (Inhorn and van Balen 2002).

Inhorn's (1996b) work drew attention to the silent but swift expansion of high-tech conception in the 'so-called overpopulated' Middle East and North Africa region of the world, deemed to be less developed. Inhorn (1994a: 29) showed how many infertile poor Egyptian women were 'peripatetic pilgrims', travelling to sacred sites, physicians, pharmacists and healers in their 'quest for conception'. She examined their encounters with the 'new' world of 'new reproductive technologies' by focusing on the 'local moral worlds' (Kleinman 1992) of these women, who were often forced to grapple with difficult decisions given that the centrality of Islam in their lives often guided their 'therapeutic praxis' (Inhorn 1994a). By 2003, Inhorn had published a definitive account on the spread of IVF in Egypt (Inhorn 2002, 2003). Other global studies followed, notably on Iran (Tremayne 2006, 2009) and Lebanon (Clarke 2008), and Inhorn embarked on new research covering diverse locales in the Middle East and North Africa (Inhorn 2007, 2012, 2015; Inhorn and Birenbaum-Carmeli 2009). Susan Kahn's (2000) insightful account entitled *Reproducing Jews* spearheaded a wave of new ethnographic engagements with assisted conception in Israel (Birenbaum-Carmeli 2004; Goldberg 2009; Kahn 2002, 2006; Nahman 2008, 2013). In her Ecuadorian ethnography of assisted conception, Elizabeth Roberts (2006, 2007, 2009, 2012) describes a fascinating contemporary example embedded in South America. Lisa Handwerker (2002) focuses on the politics of making 'modern babies' in China.

While Inhorn's contribution is pathbreaking in that it was the first to examine assisted conception in a non-Western setting, her work on the gendered experience of infertility and ethnomedical healing complements a steady trickle of research on infertility emerging from various non-Western sites. Pamela Feldman-Savelsberg (1994, 1999, 2002) studied infertility in the Cameroon Grassfields, where 'violent imagery of plundered kitchens, cannibalistic witchcraft and theft permeates Bangangté women's accounts of infertility and child loss' (Feldman-Savelsberg 1994: 463). Ulla Larsen's African studies explore differentials in infertility in the Cameroon and Nigeria (Larsen 1995) and childlessness, subfertility and infertility in Tanzania (Larsen 1996). Johanne Sundby's account of infertility in Gambia explores traditional health care practices involving healers and spiritual leaders, who are often invoked as the first line of treatment in place of 'modern health care' (Sundby 1997) and more recent research problematising infertility and health care in Sub-Saharan Africa (Sundby 2002). Trudie Gerrits' (1997) research into infertility amongst a matrilineal ethnic group in Macua, Mozambique, similarly found that infertile women adopt various strategies to have children; of these, the predominant recourse was visiting traditional healers as against modern hospital-based medication. Tola Olu Pearce's (1999) study amongst the Yoruba of southwestern Nigeria explored cultural perceptions of infertile and childless women. Pimpawun Boonmongkon's (2000) research looking at infertility over the life course of Thai women and Melissa J. Pashigian's (2000) study on infertility in North Vietnam, together with her insightful account of infertility and relatedness in Vietnam (Pashigian 2009), provide refreshing perspectives from the Far East.

From within the South Asian subcontinent scholars have begun to examine the neglected topic of infertility. Bhatti et al. (1999) addresses the treatment-seeking quest of infertile women in squatter settlements of Karachi, Pakistan, whereas Papreen Nahar and her colleagues examine the lived experience of infertility amongst the urban slum populations and rural settings in Bangladesh (Nahar et al. 2000; Nahar and van der Geest 2014). Robert Simpson (2004) focused on the cultural and ethical framing of new genetics and reproductive technologies in Sri Lanka. Within India, Deborah L. Neff (1994) examined how amongst the Nayars of Kerala, the construction of infertility is traced matrilineally. Additional studies explore the psychosocial consequences of childlessness in the Ranga Reddy district of Andhra Pradesh (Unisa 1999), treatment-seeking behaviour amongst the urban slum populations in Mumbai, as well as amongst disadvantaged rural and urban populations (Ganguly and Unisa 2010; Kumar 2007; Mulgaonkar 2000), and the experience of stigma amongst married childless women in South India (Riessman 2000, 2002). Jyotsna Agnihotri Gupta (2000) coalesced years of feminist activism in her comparative Indo-Dutch account examining a range of technologies from contraceptive, assisted, genetic to prenatal and diagnostic. More recently an independent Delhi-based resource group and organisation, SAMA (2007, 2010), has made major contributions through research, international consultations and advocacy to the debate on the spread of assisted reproductive technologies in India.

While these studies point to the emergence of rapidly accumulating new cross-cultural insights into infertility, the spread of high technology assisted conception to so-called Third World sites remains poorly understood (Van Balen and Gerrits 2001). Even when freely available, these interventions are too expensive despite repeated calls for cheaper and affordable IVF in the developing world (Malpani and Malpani 2002; Ombelet 2011; Ombelet and Campo 2007). More importantly, the global spread of assisted conception technologies, notwithstanding the experience of modern biomedicine for many infertile people, remains restricted to outdated and dangerous gynaecological interventions like dilatation, curettage and thermocauterisation of the cervix (Inhorn and Buss 1993; Sundby and Jacobus 2001; Unnithan-Kumar 2004). Consequently, the focus remains on poorly trained medical personnel and under-resourced medical facilities that often have as severe an iatrogeneous impact on reproductive health as do some traditional medications (Mogobe 2000). Critics from within Third World sites have also questioned the transfer of assisted conception to so-called 'poor resource countries'. Friday E. Okonofua (1996), professor of obstetrics and gynaecology, for instance argues that two attempts to set up IVF clinics in his native Nigeria demonstrated a lack of necessary infrastructure and funding, despite the availability of professional expertise. In addition, he argues that costly reproductive technologies divert money from high priority health problems to benefit a small segment of the infertile population (who can presumably afford it). Whether to invest in advanced medical technologies in the face of gruelling poverty and primary health concerns is a common dilemma for developing countries grappling with limited resources (ICMR 2000). Perhaps for this reason, treating infertility by undertaking technologies such as IVF is rarely a part of state population programmes in developing countries like Egypt and India, where conception technologies remain confined to the private sector (Inhorn and Bharadwaj 2007).

Globally, infertility is thought to impact 15 per cent of couples of childbearing age (Birenbaum-Carmeli and Inhorn 2009; Vayena, Rowe and Peterson 2002). In India, the exact magnitude of infertility, its epidemiological profile and the true extent of medically assisted conception technologies remains ambiguous. Most experts, clinicians on the frontline offering assisted conception, officials and Ministry of Health and Family Welfare (MHFW) and Indian Council of Medical Research (ICMR) bureaucrats contacted between 1996 and 2010 estimated that 10 to 12 per cent of ever-married couples in India were infertile – i.e. between 10 to 12 million couples. On persistent probing, these experts could not reveal the source of this data. Existing literature often provides dated and partial information. A study based on the 1981 census data for instance analyses the pattern of childlessness among ever-married women in India and finds only 5.6 per cent of women childless (Vemuri and Manohar 1986). Another source draws on the National Family Health Survey (NFHS), India, data and puts the incidence of childlessness at 2.4 percent of currently married women over forty years old (Jejeebhoy 1998). A close reading of the NFHS (1992–1993) data suggests that 3.8 per cent of currently married women [N=84678] are listed as 'declared infecund', who have no living children. These figures, however, do not indicate the causes of childlessness or even the type of 'infecundity', i.e. primary or secondary, thus making these data sources problematic. Usha Ram's (2006) study, based on the 2001, 1991 and 1981 censuses of India and the 1998–1999 NFHS surveys, found the general childlessness rate for India to be between 10 and 20 per cent. The study reveals that 'the analysis of zero parity women from the census show that 13 [per cent] of ever-married Indian women aged 15–49 were childless in 1981, which increased to nearly 16 [per cent] in 2001' (Ram 2006: iii). More recent accounts cite extrapolated estimates from World Health Organisation (WHO) figures. The ICMR projects 3 per cent primary and 8 per cent secondary infertility, basing its research on WHO figures 'guesstimating' that 13–19 million couples face infertility in India (Widge and Cleland 2009). Little is also known about the exact causes of infertility in India. A recent twelve-state survey by the National Institute for Research in Reproductive Health found that lifestyle-related infertility amongst couples differed in districts as diverse as Thane, Maharashtra (10.6 per cent), Muzzafar Nagar, Uttar Pradesh (15.1) and Maldah, West Bengal (18.1) (Iyer 2013). This emerging data notwithstanding, one of the main causes of infertility in India remains reproductive tract infections and untreated sexually transmitted diseases. Both of these conditions are commonly held responsible for primary and secondary infertility (Aggarwal et al. 1999; Bang and Bang 1989, 1994; Bhujwala et al. 1988; Chhabra and Fali 1992; Jejeebhoy, Koeing and Elias 2003; Kushtagi et al. 1991; Nandan et al. 2001; Oomman 2000; Parashari et al. 1994). A high level of male factor infertility is now acknowledged as significant. The main causes of infertility amongst Indian men range from traditional tobacco chewing (Kumar and Gautam 2006), genetics (Singh et al. 2005) and chromosomal abnormalities (Mahanta et al. 2011), to environmental estrogens (Rozati et al. 2002) and sexually transmitted diseases and infections (Chaudhuri and Iyengar 1994; Joyee et al. 2007). Genital tuberculosis is also considered a major etiologic cause of infertility in Indian women (Dey 2015; Gupta et al. 2007; Parikh et al. 1997).

There remains a paucity of data on infertility in India, notwithstanding the substantial growth of assisted conception within private health care. In India today, assisted conception is a visible, viable and thriving industry. Gynaecologists and scientists are increasingly moving into this new, more lucrative and prestigious speciality area, making it nearly impossible to count the number of clinics in operation. This researcher for instance could locate more than sixty established clinics (of which some forty could be contacted) offering a range of services such as IVF, embryo freezing and intracytoplasmic sperm injection (ICSI). In the late 1990s alone there was hearsay evidence emanating from my informants that twice as many clinics were in the process of being established. Some unconfirmed estimates go so far as to suggest that there are more IVF clinics in India than in all of Western Europe (some media reports put the total at upwards of 500 clinics). Similarly, Jones et al. estimate that there are over 500 IVF clinics in India (Jones et al. 2007, 2010). In 2013, a high-ranking ICMR official in a newspaper interview argued that the council had identified over 1,100 IVF clinics from public sources (Tikku 2013). Similarly, the British *Daily Mail* made an unsubstantiated claim that there are currently 3,000 fertility clinics in India (Bhalla and Thapliyal 2013). Despite a centralised registry of assisted reproductive technology (ART) clinics in India listing 385 clinics, wild speculations abound ranging from fifty new clinics every year to more than 30,000 functioning ART facilities in India (Sarojini et al. 2011).

India's booming 'medical tourism' industry is probably one of the prime signifiers of India's rise to global prominence in the new century (Bochaton and Lefebvre 2009; Lefebvre 2010). With an economy projected to grow despite the global downturn, India is expanding its private sector health and corporate hospital care at an unprecedented level (Drummer and Cook 2008; Lefebvre 2010). In the same way that it is seen as key in the global search for human organs (Cohen 2001; Das 2000; Scheper-Hughes 2000), surrogate wombs (Pande 2010a, 2010b; Vora 2009) and clinical application of human embryonic stem cells (Bharadwaj 2008, 2010b, 2013a, 2013b, 2013c; Bharadwaj and Glasner 2009), India has become a global destination for cheap IVF and fertility hormones and an abundant source of gamete and embryo supply.

The reproductive segment of the Indian medical tourism market was valued at over $450 million per annum, and the ICMR predicted that this would become a 6-billion-dollar market by 2008 (Smerdon 2009). No current assessments indicate whether this whopping figure has now been reached or surpassed. With no regulatory mechanism in place to control the development, spread and application of these technologies – other than ICMR-sponsored guidelines pending ratification by the Indian parliament – the resulting picture is blurry. For example, there are no mechanisms in place to enumerate data on IVF cycles and document their success rate. Individual clinics are left to self-regulate under the auspices of ICMR-sponsored guidelines, which are legally unenforceable. When individually contacted, clinics were reluctant to provide information on IVF and ICSI success rates. This reluctance is born out of an absence of any regulating mechanisms like the Human Fertilisation and Embryology Authority (HFEA) in Britain. The clinics either did not maintain any records or simply 'constructed them', as some gynaecologists in Delhi informed me. One clinician even confessed that she had destroyed most of her records for better income tax management since the tax authorities routinely harassed her by demanding access to patient records (to enumerate IVF cycles) to determine her total income per patient. The clinician in question had instead instituted what she considered to be an ingenious system of selectively documenting IVF cycles to reflect her income tax returns!

This book is positioned against this vast local and global backdrop of accumulating insights into the culture of infertility and assisted conception technologies. From Euro-American countries and Israel to numerous sites in the Muslim Middle East, Africa, South-East Asia, China and Latin America, the global spread of assisted conception is truly breathtaking. More than thirty-five years since IVF was pioneered and more than five million IVF babies later (Franklin 2013), this monograph seeks to add a critical Indian chapter to this expanding cultural universe of biotechnological interventions into an ever-increasing number of lives facing reproductive disruption around the globe. Given the enormity of the task, the research has sought to isolate certain key facets of the cultural response to this vast and complex reality. It is to these ethnographic complexities that I finally turn.

Encounters/Representations: The Ethnographic Immersion

Social research on 'post-writing cultures' must contend with the idea that 'ethnographic truths are inherently *partial* – committed and incomplete' (Clifford and Marcus 1986: 7). The genre of authoritative truthful accounts is dead. In the Indian context this means that, unlike the 'social scientists who came into the world of knowledge as part of the anti-colonial, nationalist enterprise, the new generation of social scientists in India have to live with a destruction of certainty as the only condition for the production of knowledge about Indian society' (Das 1999: 54). As Das contends, social scientists cannot represent India as if India were absent and silent, but rather can only insert their voice within a plurality of voices. This book is a small step in this direction – an account of infertility and assisted conception in India that remains somewhat underexplored within the discipline of anthropology.

Multi-sited Epistemology

Ethnographically I remain entrenched in multi-sited terrain, a relationship I describe in detail elsewhere (Bharadwaj and Glasner 2009). Although my ethnographic immersion across sites and spaces for more than fifteen years has been rewarding, it inspires me to consider and reconsider my role as ethnographer – as one who is at best providing a partial account in this making of worlds. At its broadest, a multi-sited ethnography inhabits and strings together disparate sites. According to George E. Marcus (1995: 105), '[M] ulti-sited research is designed around chains, paths, threads, conjunctions, or juxtapositions of locations in which the ethnographer establishes some form of literal, physical presence, with an explicit, posited logic of association or connection among sites that in fact defines the argument of the ethnography'. The aim of such multi-sited ethnographic study is not holistic representation or portrayal of a totality, but rather an acknowledgement that the subject is dispersed across several different locales. Methodologically, therefore, the research follows a thread – albeit a bit tangled – connecting different 'sites' that both locate and animate the 'life worlds' of the infertile, their daily struggles and the clinical enterprise of assisting conception. In connecting these locales, a connection of another kind is established, one masked by the use of generic term 'critical sociology', which encapsulates an active engagement with feminist theory, cultural studies and science studies, enmeshed into the anthropological voice to complement this multi-sited journey.

The mode of constructing this multi-sited ethnographic account can best be summed up in what Marcus (1995) alludes to as a process wherein an ethnographer's main aim is to 'follow the metaphor'. Citing Emily Martin's (1994) work on immunity in America, amongst others, Marcus (1995) posits that 'when the thing traced is within the realm of discourse and modes of thought, then the circulation of signs, symbols, and metaphors guides the design of ethnography'. He further argues that such an approach involves tracing social correlates and grounding associations that are at their most vocal and alive in language usage and print or visual media. In Marcus's estimation, 'the most fully achieved multi-sited ethnography is in this mode'.

In understanding the presence of infertility and assisted conception in India, I attempt to chart a similar route, tracing the 'metaphor of conception' through multiple sites, from ancient textual sources to 'modern' technologies of procreation, infertile couples, their families and their engagement with clinical conception, medical practitioners and their representation in mass media, and state policies on health and health care in the private sector. What emerges is a web of connections that conjures a crucial part of the still foggy bigger picture. Clearly, 'this gives the ethnography a fragmented character and invites further reflection on the picture of anthropology as it addresses the questions posed by new technologies' (Das 2000: 284).

Parasitic Location

The methodological contours of ethnographic practice, as an activity of discovery, learning and representation, and the existential predicament of the ethnographer can be best described, following Michel Serres (2007), as inherently 'parasitic'. The parasite according to Serres (2007: 79) is 'the essence of relation'. The parasite, both as biogenetic substance and social actor, thrives on the host. For Serres (2007: 182) it is a simple relationship, irreversible like a river's flow: one feeds on another and gives nothing in return.

This 'elementary relation', like white noise, feeds on sound, sign and information without reciprocation (Serres reminds us that in French, the word for parasite also means noise). Reciprocity, and the accompanying *hau* (spirit) that anthropology has done much to theorise and describe, are turned into social relations predicated on feeding as opposed to receiving and reciprocating. The production of ethnographic knowledge remains parasitic as hosts are forgotten, remade and returned to, but only for more information – a relationship driven by the hunger to know. In Serres's (2007: 216) words, the host soon discovers that 'his parasites are eating him up', and their noise covers his voice. This realisation troubled me for the better part of fifteen years spent feasting on information my respondents produced, policy documents revealed and media reportage projected. This unending cycle, where hosts and parasites swap places only to temporarily establish the illusion of reciprocity, masks an unabated feeding frenzy.

The masking or unwitting interpolation of 'native' voice with anthropological noise is a difficult aspect of ethnographic ontology. For some time I have sought to explain the eclipsing of voice with noise in the register of a 'native ethnographer' (Fahim 1982; Ohnuki-Tierney 1984; Srinivas 1997). However, given the impossibility of an 'undivided native position' and the inconvenience of simultaneously inhabiting several communities of sentiment (Clifford 1997), I soon became convinced that native advantage notwithstanding, my position remained fraught and that of an excluded 'other'. Perhaps in order to appreciate 'otherness' we have to draw inspiration from the lessons of anthropology of reproduction. Biological reproduction is the quintessence of a parasitic relationship between a host ('mother'/ womb) and parasite ('child'/ foetus). However, the very act of reproduction introduces difference, and, in the case of biological reproduction, difference that is both made of self and in need of being made self. This difference is reproduced as the other on the confluence of structure and cognition. Cultures possess an exceptional ability to cogitate difference as part of structural realms that continually redefine a shared sense of self. In the end, the challenge lies in being able to accept the invitation of a generous host while remaining cognisant of the (ethnographic) inability to reciprocate. It is also worth mentioning that a host seldom expects anything in return. Perhaps the host is almost always aware of her location in the food chain, or, perhaps, contrary to the established consensus around reciprocity, in a parasitic relation, a host is simply socialised into never expecting a reciprocal prestation. I am aware that my methodological location allows me to analyse the parasitic dimension of ethnographic practice. However, I struggle to imagine a situation where ethnographers can meaningfully forge a relationship of reciprocity. The host, or informant, provides much more than mere 'data'. S/he or it offers the material basis for constructing our academic identities, careers and scholarship. I can only speak for myself: this is one debt I can neither repay nor reciprocate in any meaningful sense.

Journey

This books draws on ethnographic contact with the field spanning fifteen years. During this period I returned to India at least once every year to (re)establish contact with some of the IVF clinics, catch up on new developments and renew old ties. The introductory ethnographic phase lasted from 1996 to 1998. The next phase of exploration was from 2003 to 2005, followed by further years of consolidation in 2008, 2010 and 2013. In total, more than 100 couples were either interviewed together or one partner at a time. A further thirty-five medical personnel and officials of the government of India were contacted and interviewed. The fieldwork itself was spread across six Indian cities: Delhi, Jaipur (Rajasthan), Mumbai (Maharashtra), Bangalore (Karnataka), Chennai and Salem (Tamil Nadu). In three clinics in particular – one each in Delhi, Jaipur and Mumbai – I spent time observing the daily 'life worlds' of the clinics and their day-to-day dealings with infertile patients.

Conversations

The research process generated many conversations, mostly semi-structured, open-ended interviews with individuals and couples and lengthy, open-ended interviews with clinicians and other medical personnel. Interviews with the directors of two Mumbai-based adoption agencies were also recorded. With the exception of two interviews with research scientists on the sensitive topic of the politics of conception (explored in Chapter 3), all semi-structured interviews were tape recorded and later transcribed or listened to repeatedly in order to extract pertinent information. The names of the (treatment-seeking) interviewees (where available) and clinicians or scientists have been replaced by pseudonyms to maintain confidentiality. There is, though, one exception: the identities of those covered in media reports are not concealed as these names are already public. Interviews with the treatment seekers were conducted in English and Hindi. Clinicians and scientists were all interviewed in English. I translated and transcribed the interviews from Hindi to English, though some of the grammatical and syntactical structures posed great difficulty (Ercikan 1998). In such cases, I carried out an approximate translation to correspond with the broader meaning.

Experiences

The process of interviewing was, in most cases, less than ideal, as the couples could be approached only in the clinics. As a consequence, the possibility of follow-up interviews was minimised considerably, since many of these couples came to the clinics under difficult personal circumstances (financial hardship, familial pressure, IVF cycle schedules, geographic distance and accessibility, etc.). Limited access forced me to interview cases as and when I could. There was no conscious attempt to interview individuals separately, as couples, husbands or wives (however much this might have been desirable, for example to avoid a bias arising from gender inequity in relationships), yet, due to the sensitive nature of the research and the problems with accessibility, it was not always possible to interview the couples together. On many occasions women came alone to the clinic while their husbands were at work, or only husbands could be interviewed while their wives were undergoing either sonograms or embryo transfers. Additionally, over 60 per cent of the interviewed treatment seekers, especially in phase 1, were living in joint families, which made conducting interviews outside the clinic even more difficult. Though I was occasionally drawn into some couples' struggles with infertility (explored in Chapter 7), the interviewees were on the whole extremely reluctant to yield personal information. This raises the complex issue of what constitutes private as against public in a research project that explores human struggles with potentially stigmatising conditions. It became clear from this experience that, while there is no fixed private sphere, topics and activities regarded as private vary cross-culturally and situationally (Lee 1999). Interviewee responses varied greatly to questions that I viewed as potentially unproblematic. The majority of the interviewees were not prepared to share personal details like names, class background or even employment or income profile. On one level, this was extremely disappointing, especially since the experience of medicalisation in India is best captured and understood in the context of class and gender ideology (Unnithan-Kumar 2001, 2004). However, repeated probing in casual conversations before and sometimes during the interviews failed to elicit this concrete information. The most common form of resistance encountered was either a long silence or an ambiguous reply. This is not an unusual experience for researchers dealing with sensitive topics, especially in situations where respondents feel an element of unease when asked questions about their finances or sexual behaviour (Goyder 1987). Jocelyn Cornwell (1984) argues the case for repeat interviews to get beyond 'public' accounts to discover 'private' ones, but this option was not open to me. Christopher McKevitt (2000), however, argues that while some open-ended interviews can yield narrative accounts, others do not. Drawing on his own research experience amongst elderly stroke patients, McKevitt found that while some respondents in his interview transcripts came across as engaging and produced lengthy narratives, others were reluctant to assume this role, responding to the questions with brief answers and resisting probing questions with smiles and silences.

Silences, or the 'refusal to narrate', and the absence of data such a refusal produces is in itself significant. The individuals who openly shared information on their class and economic circumstances were either well-to-do, or at least middle-class, professionals, working and living in Indian cities or non-resident Indians visiting from the United Kingdom, Kenya, United States and Australia. The remainder of respondents were financially pressed to fund their quests for conception. I could only get fleeting references on financial hardship in some cases, whereas I obtained graphic accounts of financial drain in others, but no systematic data on socioeconomic background could be collected.

This was both intriguing and unexpected, for at the time the query seemed fairly unproblematic compared to some of the painful aspects of stigma and ostracism the respondents were sharing. However, in hindsight this resistance is justified. Although I routinely asserted my disaffiliation with the clinic, interviewees frequently viewed me as connected with the facility. The fact that clinicians often referred patients to me for interviews and that the clinics granted me the freedom to approach patients likely contributed to this (mis)perception. On more than five different occasions, interviewees in Jaipur and in Mumbai showed me medical reports and, despite my persistent attempts to explain my nonmedical background, could not disassociate me from the clinic. As such, some respondents may have withheld information while others may have offered specific details, both on the chance that their replies might result in improved treatment. Specifically, on one hand, many interviewees were eager to describe their financial hardships, perhaps hoping that their comments would reduce treatment costs (Chapters 7 and 8). On the other hand, some interviewees were less willing to discuss this, possibly fearing that the clinic might perceive them as unable to pay for the treatment, and therefore provide lower quality care. Moreover, many interviewees detailed horrific previous medical interventions while overtly praising the clinic in which our interviews were conducted (Chapter 7 and 8). I am not suggesting that interviewees were deliberatively deceptive, rather that they responded strategically. This raises an important methodological question: should interview responses be treated as information about an experience or as constructed narratives (Holstein and Gubrium 1995; Silverman 1993, 2000)? In this case, the responses lie on the cusp of experience and narrative. Even the narratives are intimately shaped by experiences of infertility, social stigma, financial drain and emotional exhaustion.

Given these difficulties, only an overarching range of treatment seekers from different backgrounds could be identified. Individuals and couples interviewed range from the wife of an industrialist in Mumbai to a farmer from a village in Punjab. Taken together these respondents do not compose a social group or class, though they become their own group by virtue of their inability to biologically reproduce. Through the course of these interviews, information on the familial composition (joint or nuclear), marital status and time spent in treatment emerged. The fact that all respondents and clinicians were Hindus surprised me at first. I asked in my diary in 1997, 'Where are the Indian Muslims?' It is now known that several Sharia compliant IVF clinics have emerged in parts of India that attract Muslim ciiental from all around the country. I know of at least one PhD project currently examining (in)fertility and Islam in northern India. While there was no conscious attempt to include only Hindu respondents, the fact that I encountered only Hindu patients and clinicians in more than twenty-three IVF clinics made religion a central theme in my research. I was particularly struck by the bold Hindu religious iconography in the clinics. I subsequently incorporated this link between an individual clinician's faith and the practice of assisted conception into the research. The scope and scale of the research had clearly multiplied and scattered into various locales and domains, and relationships between sites were emerging. Faced with this unanticipated turn of events, I sought solace in Gary Alan Fine's (1993) contention that 'good ethnographers do not know what they are looking for until they have found it', cited in Irvine (1998: 170).

The interview process was congenial once the 'ice was broken', which required long conversations about politics, popular culture and the like. As a male researcher, I recognised my constraints in attempting to interview women on an intimate and painful subject. Women did vocally participate, however, once they decided to be interviewed. With the exception of three women who rejected outright the idea of being interviewed by a man, all the rest engaged in in-depth discussions of their experiences of infertility and medical treatment. The constraints imposed by the 'conjugal setting' of the interview process, on the other hand, are difficult to predict (Hirsch 1999), especially given that the location of these interviews was confined to the clinics. Additionally, some couples were extremely nervous about talking to a stranger about their infertility, an anxiety accentuated by a fear of being identified or discussed in the press. For example, the following entry from phase I – May 1997 – in my field notes is telling:

> I met the wife first in the presence of the doctor. She was concerned whether her name or identity would be disclosed. 'We are still quite young', she said to me [husband 26 and wife 23] 'we don't want this getting published or talked about in the press. Nobody knows except my parents and my husband's parents and we'd like to keep it that way'.

Some other couples were even more reluctant to be interviewed since they were seeking treatment without the knowledge of their families (see Chapter 5). The process however became more engrossing once I began to step out of the confines of interview-based interactions.

Encounters

Many lives are touched in a typical day at a fertility clinic. Both the clinics and treatment seekers inhabit their own life worlds, which interact during visits. To these clinical encounters, treatment seekers bring their own everyday experiences of 'living infertility'.

In three clinics in particular – one each in Delhi, Rajasthan and Mumbai – I was able to observe the daily 'life worlds' of the clinics and their dealings with the infertile. I was aware of the problems associated with positioning myself in the 'classic observer role' as I did not wish to approach the so-called data collection from the perspective of a privileged outsider, a disinterested, disengaged onlooker. Instead I spent time at these clinics quietly absorbing the daily activity, the mundane coming and going of patients and their interactions with the clinical world. This usually entailed 'hanging out' in clinic lobbies, an approach that also raised concerns about indulging in covert as against overt research (Goode 1996; Van Maanen 1988). In only three clinics where the clinicians were aware of my research interests did I have permission to take notes. In other clinics where I was allowed interviews with only the clinicians – often after a very long wait in the clinic lobbies – I took notes, while waiting, on various themes in the waiting areas and on the interaction between patients and clinic bureaucracy. Parts of the clinic were out of bounds. In all three clinics, my access to the laboratory area was severely restricted due to fears of contamination, though I was given a tour of the 'sanctum sanctorum' of the Jaipur clinic. Unlike some other researchers who participated in the daily life of IVF clinics, I was not given an official role or title. Charis Cussins's experience is interesting in this respect:

> On the first day of my fieldwork the director, Dr T., hastily greeted me, and, with no further ado, dispatched his nurse to find a white coat that would fit me. Once enrobed, I was informed that my title was to be 'Dr Cussins, a visiting scientist', and from then on that is how I was introduced to patients. (Cussins 1998b: 69)

It is just as well that I was not given such a formal title and position, as it would have only reinforced the connections that my interviewees were drawing between the clinic and myself. Sitting in on doctor-patient consultations at the clinics with the express permission of the individuals involved – doctors, clinical staff and patients – produced fascinating insights into doctor-patient relations and a unique glimpse into the social unfolding of infertility in a medical setting.

Texts

Approaching 'media as text' allows an interplay between both print and electronic sources. The data is mainly sourced from newspaper dailies, popular magazines, television reports, documentaries, talk shows and serialised-programmes. There is further engagement with government reports, guidelines and proposed regulatory bills as the 'official response' to assisted conception is still under formulation.

The research (Chapter 1 in particular) also draws extensively on English translations of the 'ancient texts' like Mahabharata and *Dhrmashastras*, which significantly includes the *Manu Smriti*, and other codes of law like the *Narada*, *Brihaspati*, *Vishnu* and *Gautama*, *Apastamba*, and *Vasishtha*, etc. that have come to be assimilated under the general rubric of Hinduism. In so doing I am not attempting to assume that there is a Hindu view and that view is made isomorphic with certain texts. After all there is no guarantee that even upper caste followers of Vedic ritualism knew these texts, recognised their importance, read them and implemented every bit contained in them in actual practice. These texts were mostly in the nature of scriptures, formal literary expressions of normative doctrine, and were not intended to be authentic reflections of 'historical' reality.[5] However, in turning to these textual sources I am merely acknowledging the faint echoes of such ideological and normative notions in everyday engagement with questions of fertility and infertility in India. Chapter 1 uses Johann Jakob Meyer's (1971) English translations of Mahabharata and selectively draws on the translated text. This selective approach is important in light of Uma Chakravarti and Kumkum Roy's (1988) critique of the lack of analytical rigour in pre-independence scholarship on ancient texts: 'Thus, while Meyer is aware of the varna bias of his sources ... and its possible implications, he does not even seem to be aware of the existence of an inbuilt gender bias in the same'. Due to this problematic aspect, the book distances itself from Meyer's analysis and focuses on the rich body of translations of the epic.

Similarly the chapter draws on English translations of ancient legal texts from F. Max Müller's (1894) *Sacred Books of the East* series. However, there is an uncomfortable awareness of the possibility that in these 'pre-independence translations' of ancient texts 'from Sanskrit into English, where religious concepts were frequently used, the translation often reflected a Christian undertone' (Thapar 1989: 218). Reference to the *Manu Smriti* also deserves a brief mention. It is essential to note that:

> The East India Company's interest in locating and codifying Hindu law gave a legal form to what was essentially social observance and customary law. The concept of law required that it be defined as a cohesive ideological code. The Manu *Dharmasastra*, for example, which was basically part of Brahmanical *smrti* was taken as the law of the Hindus and presumed to apply universally. (Thapar 1989: 218)

Patricia Uberoi (1993; 1996: 186) similarly argues that legal codes in British India were constructions derived from Sir Henry Maine's reading of classical Roman law in light of *Dharmasastric* texts and nineteenth-century British observations on Indian customary law. Likewise, Lord Warren Hasting's judicial plan of 1772 outlined the 'different traditional laws for Hindus and Muslims' respectively (Conrad 1995: 306). In this sense it is essential to focus on the *Dharmashastras* and 'laws' of Manu in particular because the discourse on personal law that was set into motion by the British still resonates with contemporary socio-legal thinking, spilling into the contentious issue of a common code of law for various Indian communities.

Categories

Another 'textual site' integral to this research is a large body of social scientific literature. At this stage, however, I wish to discuss these only in relation to certain conceptual clarifications, namely a critical reflection on the constructed nature of categories like 'India' and 'Hindu'. This is crucial, especially in the light of growing scholarly debates on the perils of a simplistic reading of these terms. Ronald Inden (1992: 1–2), in his critique of the Indological branch of Orientalist discourse on India, shows how the scholarly writing built a theory of a world ordered in a natural and stable way by constructing essences into its metaphors. In contradiction to this view, Inden (1992: 2) proposes a theory of 'human agency', which constructs agents as 'complex and shifting' and endowed with the ability to 'make and remake' one another through a dialectical process in changing situations. Inden's main contribution lies in problematising the empiricist tendency to discredit Indian agency and, instead, ascribe it to the makers of Orientalist discourses, which, in turn, ostensibly justified the civilising mission of the European 'selves' towards the Indian 'others'.

Inden (1992: 5), however, makes one important oversight. In his over-enthusiasm to ascribe agency to the Indians and to emphasise 'the capacity of Indians to make their world', he defines 'Indian' too narrowly. This is a recurring problem in writings on things 'Indian'. Inden and many others frequently equate 'Indian' with 'Hindu', using the two terms congruously. Often, contemporary writers in a scholarly or journalistic 'retrospective mode' refer to agents from the past as present variants of a category (in this case, Hindu) that, in fact, existed in a completely different form. Thus the two terms – Hindu/Indian – are unwittingly made primordial and timeless in scholarly accounts, a fallacy not entirely unknown to both contemporary political jingoism as well as popular and journalistic discourses on the subject. If Inden deploys the term Indian to mean a nation state in the sense Gellner (1983) ascribes meaning to the term 'nation', then the Indian nation state is not old enough to cover the range of historical and political issues that Inden seeks to problematise as products of Indian human agency. If, on the other hand, Inden employs the term 'Indian' to refer to India as a historical nation but an unexpressed state, historical complexities still point to the emergence of Hindu and Indian as contested entities and not as timeless primordial objects.

Much is written about the relationship between the terms 'Indian' and 'Hindu'. Heinrich von Stietencron's (1991) explanation about the confusion surrounding their interchangeable usage is particularly revealing. Equally insightful is Triloki Nath Madan's (2003) contribution, which outlines historical contingencies underscoring the rise of Hinduism. Richard King (1999) similarly shows how native (Brahamin) informers contributed to Orientalist reformulations of Hinduism as single world religion. Brian K. Pennington (2005) writes that today's understanding of Hinduism evolved from Hindu efforts to portray a homogenous front against colonial British political and religious encroachment. Regardless of these complex historical circumstances, one thing is clear: 'Hindu' and 'Indian' were separate categories that became combined over a period of time.

The terms – Hindu and India – are used in this book in the clear knowledge that they are not timeless or primordial categories against which an alien Western technological 'invasion' can be propped up. Consequently, while referring to classical texts in this book, a conscious attempt is made to resist labelling them as 'ancient Indian texts'. Likewise, the term Hindu is deployed to refer to a body of people in the full knowledge that the term has been transformed in several crucial respects and invested with a range of cultural and political meanings. In its contemporary usage the term Hindu can at best be looked at as encompassing and modifying several disparate strands ranging from *Vedic* philosophy to *Puranic* and *Bhakti* influences (Dalmia and von Stietencron 2010; Sontheimer and Kulke 1991; Thapar 1989). In the context of Das's (1995) argument in the previous section, this amounts to acknowledging a continuous re-animation of tradition and modernity, or rather a continuous way of (re)making and (re)moulding traditional concepts (Hindus) and modern institutions (Indian state), that sustains a continuity with an imagination of traditional self. When I refer to the Hindu cosmology or worldview in this book or to the Indian nation, it is to this modified and transforming face of Hindu/India that I allude.

The Book

This book explores the experience of infertility and assisted conception in India. It tries to 'make sense', like the infertile and the clinicians in this study, of the way in which infertility and biomedical assistance structures and disrupts the pursuit of personal and social fulfilment. In the main, the book seeks to explain how assisted conception, as a means of bypassing infertility, is accommodated, understood and used in contemporary India. In so doing, it attempts is to unravel critically the complexities underpinning these social processes. This principally entails situating the research in a number of diverse locales, such as the political economy of health in India; the biomedical politics within the private sector; the mass media as a field for promoting and contesting assisted conception; ancient norms and ideas and their reverberation in the contemporary Hindu conceptual domain; and the importance of this cultural frame for producing stigma and making sense of assisted conception. Taken together, these locales unravel the complex nature of infertility and assisted conception in India. The book is organised around four interconnected parts that together compose a cultural account of assisted conception.

Part I examines the importance of human fertility in the Hindu worldview and how the lived, stigmatised experience of infertility can be a direct consequence of not fulfilling a cultural expectation of fertility. Chapter 1 slices into what are described as 'cultural conceptions'. The traditional understanding of infertility as it emerges from ancient texts is contextualised in light of emerging anthropological and sociological evidence from India pointing towards reinterpretation of traditional ideas, norms about fertility and infertility and their resonance in contemporary settings. This framework foregrounds Chapter 2, where the lived experience of infertility is examined by focusing on the entrenched stigma associated with an inability to procreate. This chapter exposes the socially debilitating stigma experienced by infertile couples and addresses how they together manage and resist such pressures. In so arguing, the chapter proposes a rethinking of the conventional dualistic understanding of gendered response to social ostracism. In a culture where it is not uncommon for infertile wives to be abandoned by their husbands and their families, the data in this chapter provides evidence to the contrary that necessitates further research.

Part II of the book is devoted to the politics of assisted conception in India. It views the private/commercial character of infertility clinics in relation to the wider public/private sector interaction, aiming to understand the broader biomedical politics of managing infertility clinics as successful private enterprises. Against a backdrop of the political economy of health in India, Chapter 3 examines the politics of conception by tracing the actual controversy surrounding claims and counter claims within the medical domain that appears to have emerged as a corollary of the rapid commercialisation of assisted conception in India, despite its humble beginnings in the public sector. The chapter isolates an incident where scientists/clinicians are embroiled in a contest over the ascription of proper credit on the issue of being the actual brain behind the first test-tube baby in India and documents the struggle to rewrite the history of IVF in India. The playing out of this contentious issue in the media is emphasised to show that the generation of scientific credibility and reward is produced and ascribed both inside and outside the scientific domain. Chapter 4 situates the emergence of assisted conception in the wider interaction of private and public sector health care in India. This chapter views the emergence and spread of assisted conception as reflecting in microcosm the spread of private sector health care more generally. Given that the spread of these technologies is restricted to the private sector, the chapter goes on to argue that this has pressured clinicians into running their clinics at optimal levels as successful biomedical enterprises, especially in the face of what they perceive as the constraints of operating out of India. More crucially, the strain to remain economically viable has fragmented the ranks of reproductive health care practitioners, which has in turn disrupted the crucial referral chain of patients.

Part III takes the book into the domain of those seeking assisted conception and the ways in which both treatment seekers and practitioners make sense of conception technologies. Chapter 5 explores the secret world of 'seeking conception'. It endeavours to understand how within the context of marriage and wider familial location couples pursue assisted conception and what strategies and dissimulations they deploy in managing their fertility treatment and potential births after a long stigmatising wait. The highly invisible and secretive nature of seeking out assisted conception is grounded mainly in the extent of normative conformity to the ideas of relatedness and biological connectedness perceived by these couples. The chapter shows how some individuals manage stigma by withholding information about their infertility and medical treatments from certain loved ones or society as a whole. Chapter 6 provides a conceptual analysis of India's emerging role as the pivot of transnational surrogacy arrangements. The chapter asks what it is to be supplementary and surrogate in India today. In so doing, the chapter interrogates the position of supplementary women and the role of the Indian state in the making of 'the other mother'.

Part IV takes us into the clinical realm. Chapter 7 deals with how treatment seekers make sense of their failed past and present encounters with biomedically assisted conception by examining the emotional and financial costs. The chapter also includes the views of clinicians in order to understand how, from within the profession, charges of medical mismanagement are understood. Chapter 8 speaks from a clinical site. The chapter focuses on the paradoxical nature of clinic/patient interaction that both reinforces high expectations and deepens the ambivalent feelings treatment seekers have about their past and present medical encounters. It seeks to understand issues that the treatment seekers bring with them to the clinic and how the clinicians respond to them. In exploring this, several purportedly antithetical themes such as religion and science, altruism and commercial interests, resistance to clinical practice and an active interest in seeking it out, emerge as actively engaging with each other in making up the 'clinical experience of infertility'.

Conceptions is an exercise in verbalising multiple sites that were hitherto relatively unexamined. In the chapters that follow, I connect the experience and presence of infertility and assisted conception to reveal a fragment of this complex and endlessly mutating picture.

Notes

1. Medical and non-medical discourses have long defined reproductive technologies as 'old' and 'new'. A common assumption is that recent advances in reproductive medicine can conveniently be accommodated as new, with the rest relegated to an old stock. However, to avoid ambiguity, the term 'assisted conception' is used here to mean any biomedical or technological intervention geared towards inducing conception on behalf of an infertile individual or couple. This helps to locate a whole range of biomedical practices of infertility management, from intrauterine insemination (IUI) to in vitro fertilisation (IVF) and intracytoplasmic sperm injection (ICSI) among many other techniques, within an Indian cultural context without recourse to any lengthy explanations about their 'age' or 'newness'. However, the prefix 'new' is crucial in one important respect: medical intervention in the process of procreation draws attention to the cultural 'facts of life' brought into a 'new' context (Strathern 1999). The 'old'/'traditional' (and as the book shows, on occasion, archaic) ideas about relatedness and connectivity give way to 'new'/'modern'/'contemporary' possibilities of forging biological and social relations.

2. The first edition of *The Death of Nature* was published in 1980, making it contemporaneous with MacCormack and Strathern (1980).
3. I am very aware that the Euro-American category is no less problematic than the category of 'the Indian'. I use this term as it has become normalised in anthropological literature and to refer to diverse collectivities and formations in Europe and North America and not as an 'othering' trope. I reflect further on categories such as India, Indian and Hindu in the last segment of this chapter.
4. Dipanker Gupta (2000: 5) writes of the 'mistaken modernity' in India, pointing out that while there have been definite moves away from tradition in contemporary India, what ones sees is 'not yet modern'.
5. I am grateful to Professor Jyotirmaya Sharma for this insight.

PART I

In Hindu India – as in 'other cultures' – cultural norms and ideas are inextricably bound up with how people experience and make sense of disruptions to life processes. The disruption caused by infertility connects the worldly and otherworldly dimensions that together give meaning to everyday existence. Part I provides an insight into cultural conceptions about fertility and infertility. Although these ideas originate in classical texts and oral storytelling traditions, they nevertheless permeate contemporary thinking about human fertility. The social experience of infertility and the experience of stigma associated with such a condition can be located within this wider cultural context. Human fertility is quasi-sacred and inherently gendered with differing male and female inputs underpinning the reproductive process. This worldview ascribes a superior status to men while holding women responsible for bringing pregnancies to fruition. A disruption to this division of reproductive labour heralds a socio-cosmic crisis that stigmatises and ostracizes the inflicted bodies. In attempting to understand the cultural strength of fertility beliefs and the debilitating experience of stigma, one can also better understand why infertile couples readily turn to assisted conception both to fulfill their desire for a family and to salvage their socially fractured personas.

Chapter 1

FERTILE CONCEPTIONS

CULTURE AND INFERTILITY

In India, as in many parts of the world, the centrality assigned to fertility and the ability to translate this fertility into pregnancy and eventually childbirth is one of the most important factors in assigning a woman her personhood. For a man, fatherhood represents the only chance to establish visibly masculine credentials. Taken together, for the married couple, fertility and its outcome are often viewed as a main source of happiness, as worldly and otherworldly merit. However, in India, anxiety surrounding the inability to produce a 'visuality' of womanhood and manhood in the public domain arises also from its perceived cosmic consequences and is thus better understood in the context of Hindu conceptualisations about human fertility. These norms and ideas are firmly rooted in quasi-sacred myths, epics and ancient codes of law, which provide some sense of the urgency with which the Hindu community engages with the subject of infertility and the social complications it engenders.

The importance assigned to human fertility and the quasi-sacredness bestowed upon it by the ancient Vedic and *Puranic* texts has profoundly animated the contemporary Hindu worldview. These textual sources are part of rich oral storytelling and visual iconic traditions in India. As such, they help to structure and reconcile culturally appropriate responses to social and biological issues. This chapter seeks to explore (some of) these fertility themes as they emerge from such ancient sources, aiming to understand how these ideological and normative frames become weaved with a rich tapestry of contemporary cultural thinking and practices in India, a society in which everyday religiosity has particular significance and where the 'sacred' touches almost all aspects of human existence. Reading the past to comment on cultural conceptions in the present is a difficult task. According to Rajeshwari Sunder Rajan (2001), this amounts to reading 'only along the grain of our pressing cultural and personal needs', a process Gillian Beer describes as 'hermeneutic retrenchment'. But if such a reading 'brings sharply into focus a pattern of debate within the work hitherto little understood, or masks discursive elements unfulfilled at the historical moments of the text's production', it may have 'a sound political function ... Such at least would have been my intention' (Sunder Rajan 2001: 332–33). This chapter follows Sunder Rajan's lead in accomplishing productive retrenchment from textual sources that remain relatively ignored while framing contemporary understandings of infertility. It discusses a range of ideas echoing the importance of human fertility and the socio-cosmic crisis left in its absence. In doing this, the chapter attempts to interlace ancient textual sources and contemporary anthropological/sociological studies to introduce social attitudes towards infertility and the cultural approach to managing a failure to conceive.

Fertility: Expectation and Dictation

The cultural importance of women as visible symbols of fertility and continuity, i.e. the actual locus of reproduction and regeneration, was firmly established in the Vedic practices. With themes such as perpetuation of the self, abundance, and life-engendering symbolism associated with the concept of fertility, we find that much of the Vedic period (ca.1750–500 BCE) was firmly organised around an ideological premise where the procreative power of the fields and that of women became central components of social life. In the ancient Vedic literature, and later in the Puranas and the Dharmashastras (law books) alike, woman is often referred to as the *kshétra* (field/soil) and man as the *beja* (seed). The ancient laws of Manu (IX: 36, 33, 333) echo this view most explicitly: 'By the sacred tradition the woman is declared to be the soil, the man is declared to be the seed; the production of all corporeal beings (takes place) through the union of the soil with the seed'.

This metaphoric dualism is literalised in many mythic renditions of divine conception. For instance Sita (literally meaning 'furrow'), the chaste divine goddesses in the epic Ramayana (more on this later), was conceived when her father, King Janaka, spills semen (seed) on the ground (field), which, when ploughed, birthed his divine daughter, imbued with celestial beauty (Doniger 2009). This metaphoric postulation of the field/seed dualism and symbolism occurs also in many contemporary understandings of reproduction. R.S. Khare's (1982) study, for instance, brings together an interesting mix of informant and textual statements to highlight the culture-specific formulations of this analogy. The beja comes to represent the necessary *karma*, and kshétra thus becomes the field where the fate or destiny of the beja becomes known (Khare 1982: 157). Veena Das's (1976a) case study of fifty Punjabi urban households explains the 'Punjabi theory of procreation' in which the woman provides the field and the man provides the seed. Das (1976a: 3) goes on to emphasize that in the Punjabi understanding, 'the quality of the offspring is determined by the quality of the seed. Nevertheless, the field should be able to bear the seed. If the seed is very powerful, it will "burn the field". Hence it is important that the qualities of the genitor and the geneterix are evenly matched'.

Leela Dube (1986) argues that across much of northern, central and parts of eastern India, human reproduction is 'expressed' in terms of seed and earth. Ethnographic evidence ranging from Gond (Dube 1956) and Khasi tribal communities to the Kashmiri Pandits (Madan 1981) and Bengali kinship studies (Fruzzetti and Ostor 1976; Inden and Nicholas 1977), similarly suggests that a specific cultural conception is rooted in a fairly wide geographical region (Böck and Rao 2000).[1]

The field/seed dyad finds further expression in various festivals and rituals where female fertility and sexuality become homologous with agricultural practice. N.N. Bhattacharya (1977) provides an exhaustive compilation of various beliefs centred around female biology and the cult of the mother goddesses. The fertility ritual called *ambuvaci*, which is observed by Bengali women in India from the seventh day of the third month of the Hindu calendar, connects to a belief that for four days Mother Earth menstruates in order to prepare herself for the work of fertilisation. As a result there is complete cessation of ploughing, sowing and other farm work (Bhattacharya 1977).[2] The homology between women and earth/soil is taken further to express what Dube (1986: 41) calls an 'idealised role': 'Like the earth a woman too has to bear pain. The earth is ploughed and furrowed; a woman too is ploughed and pierced. A common metaphorical expression for sexual intercourse is ploughing'. Dube further argues that ploughing is strictly forbidden to women, despite the fact it is not particularly strenuous for them.

The point of similarity between (mother) earth, mother goddesses and women (as mothers) transcends the biosocial fact of reproduction. It inscribes a deep symbolism of nurturance, maternal love and duty, which equates women to goddesses and goddesses to women.[3] The ideology of motherhood therefore becomes one of the many central themes around which the 'two great national Epics of India' – Mahabharata and Ramayana (Meyer 1971: 2) are constructed. Taken together these two epics exert considerable influence on people's lives to this day; the norms and ideas enshrined in these works form an important subtext in the collective conscience. Examples range from the ritualised enactment of the Ramayana every year in most parts of northern India to television adaptations of the Mahabharat and Ramayana in serialised form broadcast on state television from the mid-1980s. It is these, in particular, which illustrate the rootedness of these epics in contemporary Indian life (Sutherland 1991). The state-sponsored television, in the words of Rajeshwari Sunder Rajan, has a

> dual obligation in its representation of women and religion – on the one hand to acknowledging the state's constitutional commitment to equal rights (in [the] case of women) and to secularism (in [the] case of religion), and on the other hand to developing a new idiom of 'nationalism', equated with a valorisation of the traditional (which is preserved, precisely, in and by women and religion) – redefines the two terms [women and religion] flexibly. (Sunder Rajan 1993: 134)

The central female figures appearing in these televised epics and in the popular understanding and interpretation of these works have become not only an ideal of femaleness but also potent symbols of Indianness. Prabha Krishnan (1990), in her critical account of the construction and projection of motherhood in the televised rendition of Mahabharata and Ramayna, raises crucial issues concerning the impact of idealised constructs of Indian womanhood and motherhood. She is especially critical of the stereotypical constructs of ideal and chaste woman in the depiction of Sita – the heroine of Ramayana, who also happens to be a female role model and a prime example of a woman's devotion to her husband in contemporary Hindu thinking. But Krishnan is also critical of the very effective depiction and separation of 'good' and 'bad' mothers in these epics, where the latter are invariably women who are not under direct male supervision. She argues that television in India can in theory reach nearly 75 per cent of the population (the satellite television revolution in the twentieth century, especially networks led by media mogul Rupert Murdoch, has increased this number exponentially). This makes television a powerful propagation medium. Drawing on her personal observation, Krishnan (1990) further asserts that these viewers are not just Hindus; they cut across religious lines and include many Muslims, as well.[4] Thus, the potential of this epic to shape the worldview of a captive audience is 'enormous'.

The subject of motherhood in India has been hotly debated for some time. Academic works range from psychoanalytic analyses of the concept in the Hindu worldview (Kakar 1978; Obeyesekere 1981; O'Flaherty 1980) to the evaluation of the status of women in India (Basu 1992; Dube 1988, 1997; Dutta 1990; Ganesh 1990; Kumar 1994; Lakshmi 1990; Sangari 1993; Sinha 2007) through to the nationalist project of garnering the 'icon of motherhood' to forge the nation as a geopolitical, linguistic and religiously unified entity (Gupta 2001). It is clear that popular culture, at least, reproduces constructs derived from Hindu cosmology, within which a woman is viewed as *Samsarahetu*, the 'source of the world', the cause of the *Sansara*, the world (Meyer 1971). Motherhood is extolled as the highest duty, and women in this sense are viewed as born to be mothers. This passage from laws of Manu (IX: 92, 96, 344) substantiates this view: 'To be mothers were women created, and to be fathers men; religious rites, therefore, are ordained in the Veda to be performed (by the husband) together with the wife'. Manu (IX: 25, 27, 332) goes on to separate woman as a living cause of the very act of everyday life: 'The production of children, the nurture of those born, and the daily life of men, (of these matters) woman is visibly the cause'. A woman thus becomes not only a symbol, but also the source of the visuality of motherhood and fatherhood that has become such an integral part of married existence in India.[5] The reproductive responsibility of women is also closely linked to the proper discharge of worldly and otherworldly duties, which are to be shouldered by a woman alone: 'Offspring, (the due performance of) religious rites, faithful service, highest conjugal happiness and heavenly bliss for the ancestors and oneself, depends on one's own wife alone' (Manu IX: 25, 28, 332). The idealised Hindu normative order conflates the twin concepts of womanhood and motherhood. One is inconceivable without the other; the two must occur in conjunction. Thus, for a woman to realise her full potential and worth, she must become a mother, a transition mediated by marriage.

Marriage for Hindus is the first socially prescribed and proscribed step towards motherhood. It is a sacred duty on two levels. First, the bride giver (father) has a duty to give the daughter away in marriage on time; second, the bride taker (husband) has a duty to beget children from his lawfully acquired wife:[6] 'Reprehensible is the father who gives not (his daughter in marriage) at the proper time; reprehensible is the husband who approaches not (his wife in due season), and reprehensible is the son who does not protect his mother after her husband has died' (Manu IX: 3, 4, 328). The rules for the father – the bride giver – are, however, more strictly encoded in various ancient legal texts. For instance, the laws of Gautama (XVIII: 21, 22, 269) state: 'A girl should be given in marriage before (she reaches the age of) puberty. He who neglects it, commits sin'.

The code of Vasishtha (XVII: 71, 92) goes a step further and states, 'As often as the courses of a maiden, who is filled with desire, and demanded in marriage by men of equal caste, recur, so often her father and her mother are guilty of (the crime of) slaying an embryo; that is a rule of the sacred law'. Kautilya's *Arthashastra* (150 AD) similarly declares it to be the father's duty to marry off his daughter within three years of her reaching puberty. Kautilya (1992: 365) declared that 'A bridegroom shall have the right to have marital relations with the betrothed girl, if seven menstrual periods have passed since the date of the betrothal. The bridegroom shall not then be obliged to pay the dues owed to the father, since the latter loses his rights by wasting his daughter's fertile period'. The discharge of the sacred duty – to procreate after marriage – has clear implications for the couple, but there is more pressure on the husband, the owner of the seed, than on the woman, the receptacle for the seed (Filippi 1996 in Böck and Rao 2000). This is not to say that women are not pressured, but as we shall see in the next section, the timing and the intensity of pressure is bound up with the male and female inputs and their potency. According to the cosmic division of labour, the task of sowing the seed belongs to the husband and the task of fertilising and nourishing it belongs to the wife. The following two sections briefly consider these respective obligations.

The duty of a husband to visit his wife in *ritu* is stressed in most ancient codes of law and in the two epics. Ritu implies menstruation in women, particularly the fourth day onwards, which even to this day in the Hindu view is considered the proper time for conception. However, sexual union with a menstruating woman is forbidden. To be in contact with a menstruating woman (*rajasvala*) and not a woman in *ritu* (*ritugamana*) is a dreadful sin. Interestingly the monthly flow is also construed as a great 'liberator' for women. The cleansing power of menstruation is considerable according to these textual sources. The legal codes of Vasishtha, for example, declare:

> A woman is not defiled by a lover, nor a Brahman by Vedic rites, nor water by urine and ordure, nor fire by consuming (impure substances). A wife, (though) tainted by sin, whether she be quarrelsome, or have left the house, or have suffered criminal force, or have fallen into the hands of thieves, must not be abandoned; to forsake her is not prescribed (by the sacred law). Let him wait for the time of her courses; by her temporary uncleanness she becomes pure. Women (possess) an unequalled means of purification; they never become (entirely) foul. For month by month their temporary uncleanness removes their sins. (Vasishtha XXVII: 17; XXVIII: 9, 1, 2–3, 4, 132–33)

Similar references are found in Manu and Vishnu.

The consequences of approaching and not approaching one's wife in *ritu* are most explicitly laid down in the two epics. Ramayana, for instance, mentions the evil-minded man (*dushtatman*) who does not give his wife her rights after she has bathed for the monthly cleansing (Meyer 1971: 217). The Mahabarata states that whomever does not know his wife carnally during the *ritu* must suffer the pains of hell. The *Garudapurana* accuses the man who fails in this duty of being an embryo-slayer (*brudn hatya*). At the other end of the spectrum, those who do discharge this duty are extolled as virtuous and on the path to heaven.

For the woman, on the other hand, marriage marks a new beginning, the essence of which is lucidly encapsulated in the following verse from the *Rigveda*: 'I loose thee from the shackles of Varuna (the warden of the moral law in the world) by which the kindly Savitar has held thee bound (up to now to thy father's family). Into the womb of the Rita,[7] into the world of good works, I set thee, together with thy husband' (translation in Meyer 1971: 140). The verse mentions a new family life accompanied by duties and obligations. It speaks of liberating the woman from the shackles of Varuna (keeper of virginity) into the rita where family life and activity would essentially entail – as discussed earlier – the fusion of the khétra with the lawful and legitimate beja.

Once the fusion of the khétra and the beja has taken place, the outcome – offspring – facilitates the transition from womanhood to motherhood. The status of a mother is the subject of much glorification in the ancient texts. In Meyer's (1971) translations of Mahabharata, the mother is described thus: 'Of all guru the mother is the highest guru' (I: 196.16); 'There is no higher virtue than the truth, no guru to equal the mother' (XII: 342.18); 'Above ten fathers or even the whole earth in worth (*gaurava*) stands the mother; there is no guru like the mother' (XIII: 105.14); and 'For all curses there are means of averting and destroying (*pratighata, moksha*), but for the mother's, and hers only, there are none' (I: 37.3–5).The importance attached to the mother is understandable since her very essence is hailed as *Samsarahetu*, the 'source of the world'. As the carrier (*dhatri*) and bearer (*janani*) of children, she is also the source of family and happiness, which accompanies the birth of children.

Critiquing Anant Sadashiv Altekar's (1959) assertion that the apotheosis of motherhood has reached a greater height in India than anywhere else, Sukumari Bhattacharji (1990: 51) argues that this apotheosis does not reflect the actuality of women's status in society but rather 'may be compensatory, seeking to recompense society's indifference to the mother'. Drawing extensively on ancient texts, she traces the ritual aspect of conception, gestation, parturition and post-parturition stages in a woman's (mother's) life. She demonstrates how women were continually overshadowed by men and how these rituals were acts of self-sacrifice and ritual observance for the wellbeing of the father and the son. However, some evidence in classical sources shows that the importance ascribed to women in procreation and conception was far greater than that afforded to men (Böck and Rao 2000).

From the patriarchal RigVedic society to contemporary Hindu society, motherhood has stood as a concept to which the wider socioeconomic and religious needs of a patriarchal culture attached themselves. This inherent inequity of ritual and social status between men and women becomes the subject matter of wider cultural thinking where, despite the much exalted status of motherhood, the primacy of male beja over female kshétra always provides a thorny subtext, a reminder of the secondary place of the mother in an ethos dominated by the father.

The epics are also very prescriptive about the nature of reproduction and the primacy of male and female input into the creation of new life. The important task of begetting children is accomplished when both woman and man contribute to the building of the body. According to Mahabharata, bones, sinews and marrow are contributed by father and skin, flesh and blood come from the mother. There are several examples in ethnographic accounts of procreation beliefs that conform to this scheme. Madan's (1981, 1982) study of the Kashmiri Pandits is one such example. Madan found that the Pandits believed that:

> conception occurs when husband and wife reach orgasm simultaneously. Female orgasm is believed to result in the discharge of vital fluids into the womb, which also receives the male seed (bij). Not only were my informants uncertain about the nature of the supposed female discharge, some of them also considered it to be of no consequence. The male seed is believed to contain in it all the requirements for the making of the complete human being: bones, flesh, blood, all internal and external organs, hair, nails, intellect, knowledge, ignorance, health, disease. It has the capacity to provide for the nurture of the fetus and subsequently of the new born child. The mother's menstrual blood provides the soil or bed for the seed to grow in when it ceases to flow out and solidifies into the fleshy sack that envelops and nourishes the fetus. (Madan 1982: 105)

Similarly the Punjabis in Das's (1976a: 3) study believed that the bones of the child are formed by the father's semen and blood is formed by mother's blood. The interesting aspect of this belief is that semen is understood as condensed blood. Leela Dube (1986) observes that the seed is contained in the semen, which is said to have a relationship with blood. The child born, especially the male child, shares his father's blood and can in turn transfer it in due course to subsequent generations. The blood in this scheme, therefore, is made patrilineal. While women, in this worldview, are shown to contribute blood to the maintenance of the foetus, the social definition of the child born is marked by the presence of the father's blood. Sangeeta Dutta (1990: WS84) argues that 'motherhood is far from the liberatory and enriching experience it should be. The concept is very much under male control, motherhood operates strictly within the material framework and is not autonomous. The mother can give birth but cannot give her child a social identity'.

Both the primacy given to the male seed as an agent of producing desired offspring and the importance of the combination of two reproductive fluids (blood and semen) contributed by the married couple can be traced to the laws of Manu: 'On comparing the seed and the receptacle (of the seed), the seed is declared to be more important; for the offspring of all created beings is marked by the characteristics of the seed' (IX: 35, 36, 333); 'Whatever (kind of) seed is sown in a field, prepared in due season, (a plant) of that same kind, marked with the peculiar qualities of the seed, springs up in it' (IX: 36, 36, 333); and 'That one (plant) should be sown and another be produced cannot happen; whatever seed is sown, (a plant of) that kind even comes forth' (IX: 37, 40, 334). An interesting parallel to this ancient position on the metaphorical importance of the seed is found in rural Andhra Pradesh in contemporary South India:

> If the physical appearance of a low caste boy and the quality of his intelligence and capacity for leadership, etc. attract attention as being incongruent with his caste status, people try to explain it by alluding to the history of his mother's illicit sexual relations with some powerful high caste man such as a Reddy or a Kamma landlord. 'After all if you sow seeds of lentils (legumes) you will not get a crop of gram' is the logic that conveys the message. (Dube 1986: 29)

This overriding tendency to assign primacy to the male seed has important implications. It determines that property ownership and inheritance flow through the male line alone. The ancient laws of inheritance are very clear on this issue. Interestingly, the rule that the field must be given to one who has the seed is intimately related to the notion of unobstructed patrilineal descent concentrated in a virilocal residence. The importance of the continuity of the male line can be gauged from certain codes of law like the Narada, which goes as far as to suggest that:

> Women have been created for the sake of propagation, the wife being the field, and the husband the giver of the seed. The field must be given to him who has seed. He who has no seed is unworthy to possess the field. The man must undergo an examination with regards to his virile [*sic*]; when the fact of his virile [*sic*] has been placed beyond doubt, he shall obtain the maiden, (but not otherwise). (Narada XII: 22, 6, 19, 9, 169, 166)

Curiously the distinctively pro-procreative and patriarchal logic underscoring the Narada's injunction is echoed in the contemporary legal domain in India. A recent Madras High Court ruling supports the use of premarital potency tests. Justice N. Kirubakaran described impotence as 'an avoidable human tragedy', pronouncing that 'If premarital clinical examinations by doctors are done, it will prevent not only impotents getting married, but (also) prevent marriages of people suffering from dangerous and incurable diseases. Governments should give first preference to tackling this kind of human problem'. Justice Kirubakaran asked, 'Why should the government not prescribe punishment for people who suppress impotency or frigidity at the time of marriage and cheat their would-be spouses?' (Saravanan 2014).

More importantly, the man, as per the Narada's dictate, is unworthy of possessing the field (woman) in the absence of seed and, therefore, also unworthy of possessing and transmitting property. The woman/field in this sense becomes a primary form of property, as well as the agency of appropriating property of a secondary nature.[8] A further analogy is drawn between the male seed and the actual seed by assigning it the mobility and detachment that the field does not possess. In the story of King Uparicara in Mahabharata, for instance, the seed was sent to his wife for impregnation at a time when he was away in the forest and his wife was in ritu by means of 'pigeon post'. The ability to travel great distances to a woman in ritu to fulfil the sacred duty is the mode the epics use to convey this message. Seed can be detached from its point of origin but a field can only receive and fertilise it, a fact that makes the field dangerous and subject to strict male control and surveillance. A field – like a woman – in this discourse, therefore, does not distinguish between its seed; it simply brings it to its logical conclusion.[9] These two issues are discussed in greater detail in the next section.

The culmination of the union between the man (beja) and the woman (khétra) – the all-important son – in the Hindu normative order marks an important shift in the woman/marriage/mother axis. The cog in this structure, narrowly defined as the son and at its broadest as offspring, connects the physical with the metaphysical. It is the task of making these physical and metaphysical connections that makes the son so necessary, according to the epics. This issue connects to a wider theme in the Hindu normative structure, that of the importance of children, sons in particular, and the ways of begetting them. When dealing with the assigned importance of a son over a daughter, it is not enough to focus on the mother, caught between her own patriarchal indoctrination and the patriarchal expectation from the rest of the family, including the husband. The position of the husband/man himself is crucial. According to most ancient texts – codes of law and the Upanisads alike – the son is the perpetuation of the self. The man, through the agency of his son, recreates himself and in this sense is reborn as and in his son. In this context the *Aitareya Upanisad* speaks of three births of the self:

> In a person, indeed, this one first becomes an embryo. That which is semen is the vigour come together from all the limbs. In the self, indeed, one bears a self. When he sheds this in a woman, he then gives it birth. That is its first birth. It becomes one with the woman, just as

> a limb of her own. Therefore it does not hurt her. She nourishes this self of his that has come into her. She being the nourisher, should be nourished. The woman bears him as an embryo. He nourishes the child before birth and after birth, he thus nourishes his own self, for the continuation of these worlds; for thus are these worlds continued. This is one's second birth. He (the son) who is one self of his (father) is made his substitute for (performing) pious deeds. Then the other self of his (father's) having accomplished his work, having reached his age, departs. So departing hence, he is, indeed, born again. That is his third birth. That has been stated by the seer. (Aitareya Upanisad II: 1.4, 1, 2, 3, 4, 521)

This process, however, is graphically described in the *Yogatattava Upanisad*:

> The breast that was sucked before he presses and finds joy; the vagina from which he was born before – he takes pleasure in that. She who was his mother before is now his wife, and she who is his wife is indeed his mother. He who was his father is now his son, and he who is his son will be again his father. (Yogatattva Upanisad, cited in O'Flaherty 1980)

The obvious erotic and explicit incestuous overtones notwithstanding, we find a theme that makes the life of a man permanent through the agency of his son – an open defiance of death. A man who does not reproduce himself in his son specifically, and in his offspring of any gender more generally, faces the possibility of a genetic death – complete oblivion. Manu (IX: 13, 8, 329) similarly declares, 'The husband, after conception by his wife, becomes an embryo and is born again of her; for that is the wifehood of a wife (*gaya*), that he is born (*gayate*) again by her'. There is also a widespread belief in India that ancestors are born in the form of children.[10] The performance of *shraddhas*, or the sacrifices for the ancestors, in the Hindu faith is one such way of recovering the lost spirits. The son, therefore, becomes an important player in rescuing the dead; it is through him that ancestors win either deliverance (*moksha*) or another opportunity to be regenerated to complete unfinished tasks. Manu (IX: 136, 138, 354) therefore states, 'Because a son delivers (*trayate*) his father from the hell called *Put*, he was therefore called *put-tra* (a deliverer from Put) by the self-existent (*Svayambhu*) himself'. The *Putra*, or the deliverer from the hell called *Put*, comes to symbolise for a man a permanent existence, as his constant regeneration in his son would keep him away from hell. Alternatively, the sacrificial duties performed by the son upon his death would liberate his soul and free him from the unending cycles of birth and death. In this sense, primarily sons, and more generally children of either gender, are very important contributions towards the Hindu notions of self-worth, fruitfulness and salvation. Against this backdrop it is crucial to view the cultural expectation, as expressed in the desire for male children, as a feature of norms of patriarchal unilineal descent. Das Gupta et al. (1998) rightly argue that:

> One dimension of men's pivotal role is that of the sustainer, which emanates from being defined as the appointed breadwinners, regardless of how much contribution women make to the productive process. Another dimension is that of the reproducer. This may sound strange, since it is women who bear children. But simply producing children is biological reproduction. Social reproduction requires that children be given an identity as members of an organised social structure. In a patrilineal society, it is the males who form the framework of the social structure. Thus the reproduction of the family, the household and of the society takes place through the male line: *it is men who reproduce themselves*. This is what underlies the symbolism of the masculine seed and the feminine earth: the woman, like earth, is merely a necessary accessory for the seed to reproduce itself. (Das Gupta et al. 1998: 3; emphasis added)

Such institutionalised gender asymmetry is a 'potent' feature of Indian social organisation and significantly affects both the social and reproductive life processes of women. As the next chapter shows, as a result of this gender inequity, women bear the brunt of stigma and ostracism more directly then men.

A popular dialogue between Bhima and Arjuna, the *Pandava* brothers in the epic Mahabharata, epitomises the importance attached to children. According to Mayer's (1971: 449–50) translation, 'Three are the lights that mankind has: offspring, pious works, and knowledge; and when man is an unclean dead body, forsaken in the wilderness by all, then these three show their profit. For us now the light has been destroyed, by strangers having profanely touched our wife. How indeed could offspring come from a woman that has been touched?' The importance of this dialogue is twofold: First, it makes explicit the notions of female purity and the importance of offspring as having originated from a pure source. Second, the passage highlights the implications of having children and the consequences of not having them. These and related themes are explored in the next section.

Infertility: Infliction and Prescription

The implications of the seed/field dualism and its analogical importance have a profound impact on the lives of Indian women. Whereas fields can be barren, there is no conception of a barren seed in the popular understanding of this dyad. Men are at best viewed as incapable of sowing the seed, but the potency of the seed itself is never in question. In this sense, infertility has never been a male problem in India, a view only now being challenged.[11]

The subject of infertility or barrenness is of central importance to many ancient Indian texts. According to the laws of Manu (IX: 81, 81, 342), a barren wife can be superseded in the eighth year of marriage. In Mahabharata once again we find similar sentiments expressed. Woman, according to this epic, is *ratiputraphala*, i.e. woman with (sexual) pleasure and sons. A barren wife, on the other hand, is worthless; gods and forbears will not accept a sacrificial offering that has been looked at by a childless woman (*aputrika*) because her very glance (shadow) taints the offering. Mahabharata also mentions that gifts offered by a woman without a husband and children rob the receiver of his life-powers (Meyer 1971: 155–56). In the main narrative of Mahabharata itself, we find several central characters who are inflicted with the pain of infertility. The theme of infertility is a source of many rich dialogical exchanges between the central characters of the epic. In Meyer's (1971: 149–50) translation, King Pandu for instance bewails his sorrow to the holy men: 'For him that has no offspring no door to heaven is known or is named; this torments me. I am not free of my debt towards my forbears. When my life is at an end, then it is the end of my fathers'.[12] The concept of *adharmika* or godlessness is exclusively reserved for men who are son/childless; therefore to carry on the blood is the highest duty and virtue, according to the epic. According to certain Puranic sources like the Garudapurana, a man who has died childless becomes an evil ghost (*pretakalpa*). The active role assigned to progeny in ordering the Hindu cosmology (as well as general notions of order) makes the task of overcoming infertility through purely cultural means an important part of the ancient Vedic and post-Vedic society. Legal codes and the scriptures alike deliberate over the thorny problem of infertile couples lawfully begetting children.

Hindu notions of ordering the social universe on the pattern and rhythms of the cosmic universe play a crucial part in determining social ideas of normality and desirability. The cosmic symmetry, order and rhythm, which became the harbinger of the Vedic philosophy and much of the Rigveda, comes to bear severe pressure on notions of 'dharma', or duty. Dharma as a concept is polysemous, encoded with a multiplicity of meanings. Attempts to define the term often stop short of grappling with the word's many facets. Wendy D. O'Flaherty and J. Duncan M. Derrett (1978: 14), therefore, define 'dharma' as a problem, a concept that is vague, indeterminable and impossible to define, 'without broadening it into useless generality or narrowing it to exclude valid instances'. Sudhir Kakar (1998: 37) on the other hand defines dharma as the 'means through which man approaches the desired goal of human life'. The term is commonly translated to suggest 'duty', 'right action' and 'morality'. While each of these translations defines one or more aspect of dharma, the meaning in its entirety remains elusive. Like many similar philosophical concepts that Hinduism has assimilated over the centuries, the true meaning of dharma escapes when we attempt to define it. Dharma can at one level be understood as a social cement holding individual and society together and a 'ground-plan of an ideal life cycle in the sense that it defines the tasks of different stages of life and the way each stage should be lived' (Kakar 1998: 40–42). On another level, human dharma can be understood as being carved out of a perceived dharma of the wider cosmos. This gives us a sense of how the expectation of discharging one's duty as a social being, modelled on the cosmic bodies as scared geography (as opposed to natural), became the basis of *acharan* or conduct. Just as the dharma or duty of *Surya*, or the sun, is to rise in the East and set in the West, so it is ordained on this earth for the worshippers of that cosmic sun God to be unflinching in discharging their worldly duties in the same orderly manner, thus laying the groundwork for an otherworldly existence. Any breach in the cycle of order and structure according to this worldview would be tantamount to the heavenly bodies colliding in the far depths of the universe. Briefly, dharma dictates that the totality of the cosmic order is respected when interpreting it to garner a response (see Biardeau 2003).

Infertility in this sense becomes one of many breaches in the orderly flow of the social and a source of nothingness out of which the creator sculpted the *prithvi*, or earth. Hence, the act of living for most Hindus becomes precariously balanced between the two extremities of social meaning and nothingness. It is therefore not surprising that the contemporary Hindu way of life – as with the category 'Hindu' itself – has been generated from the powerful and contradictory forces of conformity and opposition, an overt flexibility that allows for improvisation in the pursuit of sociocosmic solutions. The implication of this eclectic approach to social life, then, becomes an integral part of a dharma-ordained lifestyle. To cite Kakar (1998: 39) again, '[A] sense of dharma as the spirit rather than the content of activity is, I believe, related to the individual Hindu's notable tolerance of lifestyle other than his own. Hindus tend to accept casually deviance or eccentricity which in the West might be anxiously labelled anti-social or psychopathological, requiring correction and cure'.

An obvious corollary of such flexibility came to be a social engineering of 'codes of action and modes of conduct' that repaired the cultural and cosmic complications produced by infertility. These codes and modes were crystallised in the practice of *niyoga*, or conception by proxy. Niyoga in its strictest sense was the 'appointment of a wife or widow to procreate a son from intercourse with an appointed male' (Kane 1974, in Sutherland 1990: 77). According to the laws of Manu (IX: 59, 59, 337), 'On failure of issue (by husband) a woman has been authorised, may obtain, (in the) proper (manner prescribed), the desired offspring by (cohabitation with) a brother-in-law or (with some other) *Sapinda* (of the Husband)'. It is, however, important to understand that the improvisational approach[13] to creating sociocosmic solutions opens many contradictory pockets in the Vedic normative structure. This section argues that these contradictions offer additional flexibility when synthesised with cultural notions of order.

Wendy Doniger (1995) views the presence of contradiction resulting from the practice of niyoga primarily in terms of a sibling rivalry 'in absentia'. According to her:

> legally and biologically, the person you most want to have sex with your wife, when you are dead, is your brother, because he has your genes. But psychologically, the last person you want to have sex with your wife, even when you are dead, is your brother, because of sibling rivalry (remember Jacob and Esau). For this reason the *niyoga* is the most liminal form of Hindu pseudomarriage, poised on the volatile fault line that distinguishes and connects marriage and adultery: *niyoga* is paradigmatic in myth but stigmatized in *dharmasastra*, secretly longed for but publicly disavowed. (Doniger 1995: 173)

Doniger's somewhat glib argument on the liminal nature of niyoga helps contextualise contradictions that eventually signalled the demise of this practice.

Because the niyoga style of engendering fertility implicitly recognised the existence of a barren or absent seed, it ran counter to the traditional notion of barren field and potent seed. Niyoga was designed to overcome the lack of seed, whatever its cause, rather than solve the issue of the barren field. The male- (phallic-)centric universe had a simple solution to the problem of a barren field – replacement. But the solution to the problem of impotent seed was not so clear; it was impossible to merely replace the male element, given his ownership and entitlement rights.[14] However, this did not compromise the ownership entitlement of a man in whose name a surrogate male is appointed. According to the laws of Manu:

> As with cows, mares, female camels, slave-girls, buffalo-cows, she-goats, and ewes, it is not the begetter (or his owner) who obtains the offspring, even thus (it is) with the wives of others. Thus men who have no marital property in women, but sow their seed in the soil of others, benefit the owner of the woman; but the giver of the seed reaps no advantage. (Manu IX: 48, 48, 51, 336)

Male control and hegemony is central to this discourse. In the presence of a potent seed, primacy is given to the male seed, but in its absence, the field becomes all important. In either case, control remains with the owner of the field. There was, however, a glaring lacuna in the niyoga model: it compromised the much cherished notions of purity and monogamous devotion (*pativrata*) of a wife towards her husband. Niyoga could only be justified on the grounds of *apaddharma*, dharma for times of distress. But in so doing, the problem of sullied purity remained unresolved.

As argued earlier, Manu extolled the mother as the site of fusion of beja and kshétra. We also saw how the concept of motherhood places a mother on a par with goddesses who are in turn addressed as mothers. Therefore any woman not living up to the ideology of motherhood and the purity associated with it stands stigmatised as a barren field. The problem with the niyoga model was that it compromised the purity of the very concept of motherhood. Purity is central to the very being of women according to the ancient textual sources. To understand the demise of the practice of niyoga it is important to understand how the ideas of purity developed in a later Hindu ideology, which locates this purity narrowly in the virginity of a woman but more broadly in her religious devotion to her husband. It is interesting to see primary and secondary distinctions in the case of female virginity as articulated in this ideology. According to niyoga, the cultural permanence of a woman's purity, rooted in virginity, depends on her conduct (*dharma samvat acharan*). That is to say, a pure woman never loses her virginity in the Hindu conceptual and normative order. As a girl or *kanya*, purity is rooted in assumed biological virginity, or primary virginity. In transitioning from kanya to *suhagan* (married woman), the woman also transitions to secondary virginity. According to Khare (1982), virginity, whether physical or biological, is always a formulation of dharma within the Hindu system. That is to say a kanya's virginity is basically understood as a state of dharma rather than as merely a physical condition of continued sexual celibacy. Even though there are legends and mythological heroines in the epic Mahabharta who conceive through means of divine male surrogacy, such as kanyas or suhagins, their actions are considered unblemishing because of their divine or quasi-divine status.[15] As Edmund Leach (1976) claimed, a woman impregnated by God remains a virgin even after giving birth. This immediately clarifies the notion of secondary virginity. As a married woman and even after becoming a mother, the woman remains culturally pure and therefore 'as if a virgin' because impregnation achieved with one's *pati parmeshwar* (god-husband) bestows divine purity or a quality equivalent to that of Immaculate Conception. It is also worth mentioning that in Tamil mythology, for instance, a mere glance is enough to impregnate even a chaste woman if the power of the onlooker is deemed sufficient (Good 2000: 348). The Hindu ideology of *pativrata*, or literally, she who takes a vow (*vrat*) of devotion to her husband (*pati*) (Harlan and Courtright 1995: 8), was instilled in the ancient religious laws of Manu, which still hold considerable sway over Indian women (Dhruvarajan 1989). Manu clearly spelt out the duty of a virtuous wife as one who serves her husband and treats him as her God or pati permeshwar. These conceptions are important because it is around them that cultural ideas about one's personhood and sacredness are created. The practice of *niyoga* went into decline because it came into conflict with these ideals of purity.

There are therefore two contradictory models of fertility – the niyoga model and the Brahminical virgin model. In the previous section, the exchange between Bhima and Arjuna gives a sense of how contentious the issue of compromised purity of a wife can be in relation to the future (unborn) progeny. Female purity assumes even more significance once women are viewed as, in Das's (1976b: 135) words, 'points of entrance, "gateways", to the caste system'. This means that no man of a lower caste could access a woman from a higher caste, as that would endanger the purity of both the woman and the caste group. Similarly Lindsey Harlan and Paul B. Courtright (1995: 6) argue that 'the purity of women is especially crucial to the maintenance of the position of the family within the social hierarchy ... because responsibility for maintaining the blood purity of the husband's line falls heavily upon the wife'. The main threat to the caste group in this sense came from female sexuality; gradually this control extended to include the control of women within the caste and agnatic group. Byron Good (2000: 344) shows how, in Tamil cosmology, divine marriage is explicitly stated to be a prototype of human marriage and the powers of virgin goddesses are 'chained in idealised domestic role of the Hindu wife'. Such entrenched views paved the way for stricter male control and surveillance of women as the notion of guarding one's property gained further momentum. Guarding the woman/property (field) dyad thus became conflated with guarding the purity/virginity/dharma triad. The decline of niyoga is intimately linked to this subtle ideological shift. In the new virgin model, therefore, the pure field belonged only to the owner of the seed and the field. The figure of Sita in the Ramayana in this respect marks a watershed in the Bhraminical valorisation of purity and chastity as primary attributes of a devout wife (Doniger 2009).

The contradictions produced by an improvisational strategy must be grounded in some commonly acceptable notions of dharma, if a sociocosmic crisis is to be averted.

Table 1.1 The Niyoga Model vs The Virgin Model

The Niyoga Model	The Virgin Model
Flexible	Rigid
Impure	Pure
Turns loss [of purity] into gain [offspring]	May scarifice [offspring] for purity
Creates visuality of fertility	May or may not create visuality of fertility

The niyoga model may have created a contradiction by compromising the purity and sacred dimension of marriage, but it was flexible enough to turn this loss into a gain by creating a visuality of fertility. On the other hand, the decline of niyoga and its replacement by the virgin model was a means of resolving a contradiction that could have posed an open challenge to the acceptable principle of dharma in its social and cosmic dimensions. It is sometimes suggested that the practice declined due to a general waning of the human capacity for righteousness, which made it impossible to sustain the rigour of moral intention and the sexual detachment necessary to avoid lapsing into adultery or incest (Sutherland 1990: 80). Little wonder that niyoga was always associated with divine and quasi-divine beings or their embodiment on earth, the Brahmins, as they were thought to have the moral rigour and purity of intent that were absolute requirements for the practice (for a portrait of an ideal Brahmin, see Biardeau 2003, 59-63). Manu remained uncertain about the merits of the practice, and expressed contradictory views on its desirability, which can be attributed to the multiple authorship of the text and to its gradual evolution. However, the issue of waning morality remained central to the justification for discontinuing the practice. Brihaspati's legal code (thought to be from the first century AD) assimilated this presumed lack of morality into the epochal theory:

> The Niyoga (appointment of a widow to raise offspring to her deceased lord) has been declared by Manu, and again prohibited by the same; on account of the world, it must not be practiced by mortals (in the present age) according to law. In the ages Krita, Treta, and Dvapara, men were imbued with devotion and sacred knowledge; in the (present or) Kali age, a decrease of its power has been ordained for the human race. (Brihaspati XXV: i, 12, 13, 369)

Later legal views on the issue completely reject the use of niyoga. The *Vijnanesvara* (between 1121 and 1125) and *Sarasvati-vilasa* codes (sixteenth century) reject the concept of niyoga and assert the woman's right to inherit property, for instance, without a husband or son (Sontheimer 1977: 134, 151).

Citing Sudhir Kakar (1990), Doniger (1995) makes a strong case for the persistence of the idea of niyoga in contemporary India:

> Though the custom gradually fell into disuse, especially with the prohibition of widow remarriage, the psychological core of niyoga, namely the mutual awareness of a married woman and her younger brother-in-law as potential or actual sexual partners, is very much an actuality even today … In clinical practice, I have found that women who are on terms of sexual intimacy with a brother-in-law rarely express any feelings of guilt. Their anxiety is occasioned more by his impending marriage, which the woman perceives as an end to her sensual and emotional life. (Kakar 1990 in Doniger 1995)

The psychological explanation for niyoga undercurrents in a married woman's relationship with her brother-in-law appears inadequate for the purposes of understanding this social phenomenon. Doniger and Kakar overlook the important role played by kinship structures in the articulation of a relationship of 'privileged familiarity': a Radcliffe Brownian (1940, 1949) 'joking relationship' between a woman and her younger brother-in-law. The common term for the younger brother-in-law in most parts of north and central India is *devar*. According to Irawati Karve (1968), the word 'devar' occurs many times in the Vedas. In the marriage hymn, gods are exhorted to make the bride loving to the devar. Elsewhere, the *vidhava* (widow) is mentioned as leading the devar to the bed; the way in which the devar is connected with the vidhava and used in the bridal hymn suggests that he had sexual relations with the bride and that he had either the right or the duty to marry the widow of his elder brother (Karve 1968: 34–35).

However, an important oversight in most accounts on the subject is to ignore the kinship term – devar – itself. In Sanskrit the term devar can be split (*sandhi-vichhéd*) into two distinct words 'dvij' + 'var', which can roughly be translated as the 'second husband'. The perpetuation of a kinship term that inscribes the potential (husband) status of a man onto his social identity, and the social accommodation of a relationship of over-familiarity (especially on festive occasions like *Holi* in some parts of India), reinstates the sexual nature of the relationship that once marked their social interaction. Without adequate research it would be hasty to relegate the entire issue to the deep recesses of the human psyche.

Conclusion

The importance of fertility in the Hindu worldview is deeply rooted. Ancient textual sources amply testify to the quasi-sacred nature of human fertility. Infertility, therefore, disrupts not only the procreation of corporeal being, but also destabilises the meaning giving cosmology.

The gendered nature of the reproductive model, on the other hand, which views male and female contributions to the process of procreation as qualitatively different, reinstates gender inequity by subordinating women. The importance attached to the 'male seed' over the 'female field' makes women more vulnerable to the charge of being barren or incapable of fertilising the seed. Although these themes apparently originate in ancient texts, law codes and myths, they still resonate in contemporary Indian settings. While anthropological and sociological studies show how these ideas are understood in different parts of India, popular culture – especially through the dramatisation of the epics – has succeeded in disseminating these ideas to an unprecedented number of Indians.

What implications do these ancient norms and ideas have for contemporary seekers of infertility treatments? Is it fair to argue that much of this ancient paradigm still holds sway over individuals and structures their response towards their infertility and its treatment options? By alluding to heuristic – niyoga and virgin – models we can at best expose at an esoteric level the ideological and normative traditions that structure the Hindu notions of fertility and its absence. Although there are some emerging indications in this research (specifically located in Chapters 5 and 6) that suggest that the 'tradition of niyoga birth' provides a potential ideological basis for accepting new reproductive technologies, further research is needed before more potent connections can be made.[16] What has emerged with clarity, however, is the fact that there are deeply rooted cultural ideas that make infertility an emotionally debilitating and socially stigmatising condition. How couples experience stigma in the face of eluding pregnancies is the subject of the following chapter.

Notes

1. It may be an interesting research issue to explore whether this spread of a classical metaphorical concept of procreation is indicative of a wider process of 'Sanskritaization' (Srinivas 1989).
2. According to Bhattacharya the belief in the common pattern of fertility between women and Mother Earth accounts for the conception of menstruating goddesses in different parts of India. Bhattacharya offers several examples. In the Punjab, Mother Earth sleeps to the full moon day while she rests and refreshes herself. A similar rite of purification is made, according to Bhattacharya, in the temple of the Goddess Bhagvati in Kerala. In the Malabar region, Mother Earth rests during the hot weather until the rains. In parts of India great importance is attached to the menstruation of Goddess Parvati. Similarly, the menstruation of Goddess Kamakhya in Assam is considered very important.
3. In the Hindu worldview, gods are often created in the image of man. According to Wendy Doniger O'Flaherty (1980: 72), Hindu gods are 'often imagined to be men, to be like men in character … as ludicrous men, men who exhibit all the lowest weaknesses of men … Hindu Gods (even upper case [sic] Gods like Siva and Vishnu) begin, by the medieval period, to become not merely human but banal'. It is therefore not surprising to see women, because of their assigned and ascribed maternal role, equated to goddesses, and goddesses are shown to be like women because they are referred to as mothers.
4. According to Krishnan (1990: 114), 'a Madras [now Chennai] based Muslim entrepreneur is engaged in subtitling the Ramayana in English,

describing this as a labour of love and an act of faith. A Muslim professor of the Jawaharlal Nehru University in Delhi commented that the story of the Ramayana embodied some universal values, and that his family, including his two young sons, were regular viewers. A neighbour travelling to Najibabad in Uttar Pradesh found her train compartment, one Sunday morning, full of Muslim women, regretting that their travel had caused them to miss that week's broadcast of Mahabharata'.

5. As we see in Chapter 2, there is an oppressive cultural expectation that demands fertility as a logical corollary of married existence. Most couples interviewed complained that the social pressure to have children and seek medical help had become a major part of their infertile existence.
6. Many anthropological accounts identify an underlying asymmetry between the status of a bride giver and bride taker, where the latter is superior to the former. While Gray (1980) describes this inequality in hierarchical terms, Östör and Fruzzetti (1995) defend their position by describing the relationship as one of unequal gift giving.
7. According to Meyer's (1971: 140) translation, rita is 'The natural and moral law, governing the whole world, and, according to the Indian belief, having its origins and most important centre of life and activity in the family'.
8. Patricia Uberoi (1996: 185) has shown, in the case of the Hindu Marriage Act in contemporary India, that a judicial ethnosexology justifies the 'legal requirement for consummation to establish the validity of Hindu marriage by recourse to naturalistic explanations of the physical and emotional effects of the act of consummation'. The present-day Hindu Marriage Act fundamentally departs from the Dharmasastric provisions by separating potency and sterility. While potency can be valid grounds for nullity (as also seen above in the recent Madras High Court judgment) – that is, an inability to sustain erection on the part of man and for a woman to be unable to receive it to some degree – male/female sterility is irrelevant to the legal notion of potency. Though as Uberoi (1996: 201) argues, 'judges routinely affirm that the procreation of children is one of the principal aims of marriage; that women have an innate desire for motherhood, which in the proper course should be satisfied'. These tensions are found in a much wider debate surrounding Hindu marriage as sacrament versus contract.
9. An alien seed is like a wild weed growing in a field. Therefore, a woman is construed as needing protection, even surveillance, against weeds (alien beja) finding their way into her womb.
10. Interestingly, according to the *Garbha Upanishad*, the foetus in the womb remembers its past lives and on contact with the wind of the outer (impure) world – upon birth – loses that knowledge. The cries of a newborn infant in many parts of India are therefore interpreted as a

vocal protest and moaning of a loss of sacred knowledge of the self and the cosmic mysteries.

11. The patient interviews bring out this shift in perception about the omnipotent male seed. Men interviewed at the clinics were frank and open to admitting that their sperm counts were low. Even clinicians were unanimous in expressing satisfaction at a significant shift in male attitude towards male infertility. Several doctors interviewed felt that the majority of infertile couples are still inaccessible because of false conceptions about the power of the male seed.
12. Similarly, Pandu sadly speaks to his wife Kunti: 'Offspring, indeed, is the abiding-place in the worlds that concords with the law. I have sacrificed, given alms, practiced asceticism, thoroughly carried out vows of mortification, but all this, it is declared, does not purge the childless man of sin. I, a childless man, shall not reach the pure, fair worlds' (Meyer's translation 1971: 150). Elsewhere in Mahabharata in the story of King Ucinara, Galava speaks to him: 'Thou art childless; beget two sons. In the boat of "son", ferry thy forefather and thee thyself over to the shore. For he that partakes of the fruits of sons is not cast down from heaven, nor does he go to the dreadful hell like the sonless' (Meyer's translation 1971: 150). Elsewhere in Mahabharata: 'For men yearn for sons to this end: Who shall save us from sorrow? For their own good do fathers yearn after sons, who with friendly hearts bring them salvation from out of this world in that beyond' (Meyer's translation 1971: 150). Similarly, numerous references to the importance of sons/children in the epic form a significant part of the core narrative: 'To make offerings to the gods, to give alms, to study the holy writings, and to sacrifice with abundant sacrificial gifts, all this is not worth a sixteenth part so much as offspring. Whatever he brings about with many vows and much fasting, all is fruitless for the childless man ... The sacrifice in fire, the three Vedas, and the propagation of the family are everlasting. All of them (that is, of the other things) are not worth sixteenth part of an offspring. So it is among mankind, and just so among creatures. Thus it is. What is called offspring, that it is which is the threefold *Veda* of the ancients, and of the godheads that which lasteth for ever ... Three are the lights which man has on earth: children, deeds, knowledge ... Let a man wed and beget sons, for in them there is profit greater than any other profit' (Meyer's translation 1971: 150–51).
13. The term 'improvisational approach' does not imply a relaxing of control and rules. On the contrary, the process of improvisation is resorted to so that rules can be sculpted and made more effective in the face of a dharma crisis.
14. There is a prevalent saying in India: if a son dies, that is the end of the line; but if the daughter-in-law dies there will be a marriage in the house (Dhruvarajan 1989).

15. All mythological heroines remained virgins because of their own pure qualities and devotion towards their husbands. Draupadi in the epic Mahabharata regains her virginity five times so that she could be 'pure' for each of her five husbands. Likewise Kunti remains chaste because, like a dutiful wife, she begat sons from the gods upon being implored to do so by her husband. It can therefore be argued that these women remain pure more because of their religious devotion to their husbands and by conforming to their every wish, even to requests for begetting through the practice of niyoga, than because of their quasi-divine status. Mrinal Pande, drawing on Sanskrit scholar Vishwanath Kashinath Rajwade's unfinished treatise on marriage in ancient India, argues that unlike in common parlance today the word kanya means a young virgin, in the Mahabharata, as the sun god visiting young princess Kunti explains to her, the root of the word kanya is kam or to desire. Pande extrapolates from this to show that in the text 'a kanya is a young woman who has the right to claim whosoever is the subject of her desire' (Pande 2016). While an undoubtedly empowering (re)interpretation, there is enough contradictory evidence in the text that renders this interpretation at best one possible explanation. In large part this contention is utterly unsupported by the patriarchal attitudes towards women in the Mahabharata.
16. As observed in the introduction, reading a recent entity called Hinduism back into a randomly chosen past tends to conflate, in the words of Gregory Schopen, carefully contrived ideal paradigms with historical reality, giving rise to a perspective where textuality overrides actuality. In other words it is assumed that if a text proposed an ideal, it must either continue to be in practice up to the present day or at least must have been so in the historical past. In most cases, there is little evidence of a canonical text and its ideals being either fully or partially implemented in the lives of people, including those practising a religion with fervour (I am grateful to Professor Jyotirmaya Sharma for this personal communication). It is precisely because of this reason I point out in the introduction that my intention is not to see textual sources as historical reality or experience but rather as a source to better comprehend how ideological dogmas, philosophical thought processes and normative as well as practical injunctions capture fleeting shards of canonical notions and recapitulate fragments of 'ancient' thought or 'traditions' and continually borrow and stretch ideas to give birth to new expressions, experiences and theodicies.

Chapter 2

GENDERED CONCEPTIONS

STIGMA, BLAME AND INFERTILITY

Mark Tully (1996), in his collection of short stories, *The Heart of India*, paints a vivid sketch of gendered experience of infertility in India:

> When the first song was over, Ram Lakhan Yadav, a man of about thirty who had been sitting at the back, taking no part in the *faag*, rose and picked his way through the singers towards the gap between the two groups where the percussionists were sitting. He was carrying a pair of cymbals.
>
> Chote Lal Yadav said, '*Arre bhai*, sit down, we don't need any more cymbals. Two are quite enough. If you too come in now, we won't be able to make ourselves heard above all the banging and clashing.'
>
> A young man, Hoshiar Singh, sneered, 'Get out of here, Ram Lakhan. Holi's the season for cutting the crop – and where's your crop? Don't you know how to plough? Something wrong with the seed? Didn't you irrigate the field? What's the problem? People like you bring us bad luck. We'll have poor crops this year if you play Holi with us. Wait until your house produces some children before trying to play those cymbals'.
>
> Ram Lakhan pulled the young man to his feet and punched him in the face. Before a full-scale fight could develop the singers were on their feet, pinning back the arms of the two men. Ram Lakhan was frog-marched off the veranda and given a parting kick to see him on his way.
>
> In the small inner courtyard of the house next to Ram Lakhan's his wife was standing against the wall watching women pressing the pastry for *gujias* into moulds and frying *papadums* and *kachoris*. A child

> darted to the pile of freshly cooked gujias and stuffed one into his mouth. His young mother caught him up in her arms, hugged him and said, 'What will we do if you go on like that? The men will be very angry if there are not enough gujias for everyone who comes to the house today. They will smack you if I tell them what the problem is'.
>
> There was a tussle going on in another corner between one of the brothers of the house and his younger sister-in-law. She was trying to stop him pouring a pot of coloured water over her, but let go of the pot for one moment to prevent the border of her sari from slipping off her head and found herself drenched with yellow dye.
>
> Ram Lakhan's wife thought, 'I have no brother-in-law to play Holi with, no children to hug. I look like all these women here. I've got the same gold nosepin, the same bangles, the same silver anklets. I wear the red *sindoor* of a married woman in my hair. But really I'm nothing like them because I have no children, and there's no family in our house'.
>
> Rani and Sima, two of the younger wives of the family, came over to her. Rani asked, 'Why don't you have any colour on your face or your sari? Doesn't anyone play Holi with you?'
>
> Sima giggled and said, 'Nobody plays Holi with a barren woman. It brings bad luck'.
>
> Ram Lakhan's wife stared silently at the ground.
>
> Sima poked her in the ribs and asked, 'Have you been sitting under our mango trees? They should be flowering now, but they aren't, and people say that if a barren woman sits in a mango grove, the trees won't flower'.
>
> Both giggled like schoolchildren they really were, and Rani said, 'Come on, we are wasting our time. Her mouth is closed as tight as her womb'.
>
> Ram Lakhan's wife walked around the edge of the courtyard, her head turned towards the wall, until she reached the front door. No one noticed her going. It was as if she had never come to play Holi with her neighbours.

This passage expertly captures the gendered normalisation of the stigma of infertility in rural India in small towns and large urban centres across the country. As a social scientific concern, infertility in India remains conspicuous by its absence (Unnithan-Kumar 2010). There are only fleeting references to the issue of infertility in studies on family, gender, reproductive and fertility issues (Das 1976a; Jeffery et al. 1989; Madan 1965, 1976, 1982; Patel 1994). With the notable exception of Deborah L. Neff's (1994) study of the matrilineal Nayars in South India, Sayeed Unisa (1999) on the psychosocial consequences of childlessness, Veena Mulgaonkar (2000) on treatment-seeking behaviour amongst the urban slum populations in Mumbai, and Catherine Kohler Riessman (2000) on the experience of infertility amongst women in Kerala, there appear to be few social or anthropological studies of infertility and its status in a pronatalist culture. This is an important gap, given the severely disabling consequences of infertility in the developing world (Inhorn and Bharadwaj 2007) and in the context of in-depth understanding of reproductive and fertility behaviour in India (Unnithan-Kumar 2001, 2004).

This chapter attempts to look at infertile bodies and revisits common understandings of gender and stigma in relation to infertility. It locates the issue of childlessness in a wider cultural context that ostracises infertile bodies. In so doing, it endeavours to show the complex reality of living with infertility and the stigma that accompanies it. Moreover, I argue, this necessitates further research and critical reflection on the finer processes of stigma ascription.

Stigma and Infertility

'Stigma', according to Erving Goffman (1963), results from either physical deformity, individual character deformity or deviation from group identity. Charlene E. Miall (1985) suggests that infertility is more closely associated with Goffman's physical deformity classification, whereas Whiteford and Gonzalez (1995) associate this stigma with breaking from a group norm. They argue that this is particularly true of a pronatalist, medicalised society 'where the only external expression of infertility is the absence of children' (Whiteford and Gonzalez 1995: 29). Robert Scott (1978) on the other hand argues that the 'stigma (of infertility), carries with it a series of moral imputations about character and personality ... the fact that ... stigma leads [non-affected people] to regard [the affected] as their moral inferiors' (Scott 1978: 385 in Whiteford and Gonzalez 1995: 30). These readings of infertility-based stigma are all accommodated by Goffman's broad, lithe theoretical interpretation.

Some aspects of Goffman's approach, however, are now questioned in non-Western settings. Riessman (2000) critiques Goffman's Eurocentric assumption that individuals who find themselves in potentially stigmatising conditions strategically manage information about themselves. She argues instead that the 'theory (a product of Western thought) assumes a self-determining, autonomous individual with choices and a mass society that allows for privacy – in Asian contexts, these are problematic assumptions' (Riessman 2000: 113). For infertile South Indian women, selective disclosure of an 'invisible' attribute (infertility) was not an option, as they were repeatedly questioned about their family status in a variety of public and private contexts (Riessman 2000: 118). Data from the present study similarly suggests that the luxury of selective disclosure is seldom available to infertile men and women in the Indian context.

Unlike in Euro-American settings, infertility ceases to be a 'secret stigma' (Greil 1991) since in a patriarchal pronatalist context the absence of children in a marriage becomes more visible than their presence. To further explore this issue, it is important to distinguish between 'stigma' and 'blame'. While women may be blamed for being barren or men (more rarely) for being sterile, stigma can attach itself to a married body. In other words, whereas blame is specific and remains the primary site of female (and sometimes male) oppression, the stigma of infertility can expand to include both the man and woman in an 'infertile union'. Stigma in this sense becomes what Arthur Kleinman calls 'sociosomatic', resulting in the 'delegitimation' of the stigmatised rather than rendering their social identities spoilt (Kleinman et al. 1995). That is to say that, though stigma – like in the Euro-American context – remains a moral category, the process of delegitimation affects the person, the family and all aspects of social intercourse. Thus, the absence of children can be remedied by social intervention (which could, for example, be medical) or the creation of social distance between the affected and the rest of the familial unit, lest the 'moral blame' extend to implicate the conjugal unit or family. As discussed below, the latter recourse is predominantly evoked in the patriarchal familial context in India, where a woman's inability to contribute living members to the family and to the society at large is punished – regardless of the cause of infertility – by the real threat of abandonment. Marriages that resist such 'normative prescriptions' find that the process of delegitimation affects all aspects of their social interactions.

In what follows, the gendered experience of infertility and its associated stigma is examined further. Subsequent chapters 'privilege the suffering' wrought by its social unfolding, which risks obfuscation if it is somatised as mere disease (Kleinman 1995). In doing this, the chapter examines suffering caused by the stigma associated with infertility, as represented both in social-anthropological accounts and in the narratives of the couples most severely affected. It emerges that, rather than remaining passive victims in the face of stigma, couples resist and 'disavow dominant perspectives' (Riessman 2000) about the right course of socially responsible action in the face of failed conception.

What is the Gender of Infertility?

In India infertility is often construed as a female problem. What little has been written on the subject reflects this. Tulsi Patel (1994: 78), in her study of fertility behaviour in a Rajasthan village, argues that barrenness is considered a 'dreaded condition', 'a curse', and cause for 'emotional and social doom' for a woman. According to Patel:

> In a male dominated society a barren woman's status gets further lowered as it is always her fecundity that is doubted. Rarely is male fertility questioned. Men are rarely expected to undergo fecundity tests while a few women [*in her study*] have been made to do so when they did not bear any children for several years after marriage. (Patel 1994: 78)

Jeffery et al.'s (1989: 87) study of women and childbearing in North India similarly found that 'to fail to conceive or to have no living children' was usually 'calamitous' for a woman:

> In bearing children, especially sons, the bahu [*daughter-in-law*] continues her husband's line and provides the chaulha [*hearth*], future generation of workers. Failure is just cause for a man to return his wife to her parents and several women in Dharmnagri and Jakri (who ultimately bore children) recall worrying times when their husbands were pestered to replace them. (Jeffery et al. 1989: 87)

Madan (1976) discusses 'Hindu women at home' who fear not only rejection but the threat of divorce on being considered childless:

> Having been married, a wife is next expected to prove her worth by bringing forth children, if not sons, at least daughters. A barren wife is no good. We have an incident reported from the life of a West Punjab Hindu doctor, educated in England, who was married in 1925. The biographer, the doctor's own son, describes how his mother was still not pregnant after two months of marriage. Her parents persuaded the doctor-husband to have her examined by a gynaecologist who

> pronounced her incapable of conception. When they returned from the doctor's office, Mamaji clasped her hands and said 'do with me what you like, but don't send me back to my parents'.
>
> 'What are you taking about?' [asked Daddyji]
>
> She said she knew that a woman was like a pair of shoes – when she wasn't useful a man threw her away and got another…
>
> 'Please take a second wife', she begged. 'I will stay in the house and be a sister to her, and look after your children'.
>
> 'That may be the practice among city people, but not among us country people', he said.
>
> 'But we Hindu women are like breeding cows, she said, between her sobs. 'Our value is in our sons'.
>
> Luckily for this lady, she bore her husband several children, including the renowned author of the biography I have quoted from, namely, Ved Mehta. (Madan 1976: 76–77)

The incident reported above dates back to the first half of the twentieth century, but it is not far from contemporary Indian reality in the twenty-first century. This episode ties in with the gendered understanding of fertility and infertility as explored earlier; however, emerging evidence suggests that the lived experience of infertility is more complicated. There appears to be a subtlety in how gender is understood by the infertile and how the idea of gender is drawn upon to make sense of their predicament. For instance, there was no firm basis for seeing infertility in terms of a stark gender contrast. Whether the cause of infertility was male or female, the couple was 'in it together'.

Fieldwork in one of the North Indian IVF clinics provided access to confidential patient correspondence files. Many painful letters detailed the suffering couples endured on account of the stigma surrounding their condition. One letter in particular stood out as significant in its reference to the issue of societal pressure to remarry. Its author was a junior railway clerk residing in a small town in the economically backward North Indian state of Bihar. Though the letter was written in Hindi, a small excerpt is translated below:

> Doctor *sahib*, please help us. God will bless you with a long life and good fortune. We are fed up of this existence. Everybody tells me to get married again, but I love my wife dearly and I don't want to leave her. Doctor *sahib*, please give the gift of one child, just one, we ask no more of life.

The letter is a straightforward plea for treatment, so it is possible that the grief is manufactured. What stands out from this letter, however, is its explicit reference to remarriage, a recurrent theme in interviews. For example, consider the following excerpt from an interview with a couple (Arvind and Parul), interviewed in a Rajasthan clinic:

> AB: What was the problem?
>
> Arvind: Nothing happened, and then you have to listen to things because of society.
>
> AB: What you mean by 'because of society'?
>
> Arvind: You know, a woman's position is as good as nothing. Like other women interfere, like you don't have a child, you are barren [*banj*].
>
> AB: Who are these women who talk like this?
>
> Parul: In the family [*Ghar ghrihasti mai*], relatives, near ones, even neighbours.
>
> AB: What do they say?
>
> Parul: They say, 'He will leave you. You don't have children, why aren't you having any?'

Arvind and Parul persisted with treatment to ward off social pressure from women within the family who insinuated that Parul should be abandoned. Arvind's assertion, that 'a woman's position is as good as nothing', reflects his deep understanding of his wife's difficult circumstances. Their conjugal bond had faced social ostracism for nearly eleven years (they were married in 1986). While many studies highlight the particular consequences of infertility on women, others expose more complex dimensions of infertility, its stigma and its gendered associations. Biological causality notwithstanding, does infertility have social consequences for women alone? The question remains unanswered: what is the gender of infertility?

Drawing on more than ten years of interviews with couples from a range of socio-economic backgrounds, I argue that the gendered experience of infertility is an oppressive contradiction, in which social indifference and social concern, stigma and pity, social isolation and social interference converge to create an expressively undesirable condition in need of cultural management. The centrality of stigma to the experience of infertility is a consistent theme in the lives of all the interviewees. The narratives that follow give an insight into how infertility cuts across social markers as both an infliction and a lived experience.

How Infertility Affects Women

Stigma, on one level, has a unique ability to remain subtle and even masquerade as pressure (and therefore escape detection for a considerable period of time) by individuals who experience well-meaning but often thoughtless concern at home. A couple – Ravi and Geeta – from Lucknow in Uttar Pradesh in North India, interviewed in a clinic in Rajasthan, summed up this complex aspect of stigma:

> Ravi: ... I'll tell you that society puts it across. Anyone who comes asks, 'How many do you have?' So probably a lady gets pinched very badly.
>
> AB: So is it because of a collective pressure or a personal desire that you feel the need to have a child of your own?
>
> Geeta: I don't care about what people say. Let them talk; a lot of people talk. He goes out on trips, then I am lonely [pause]. What should I do?
>
> Ravi: I would put it across as it might be the loneliness. Something of her own is not there, like, well she says, 'You are not there in my absence', probably her way of putting it, 'I don't have anything of my own'. I feel after my four years [of marriage] my relatives ask, 'What's up?', 'What's the matter?' They might not ask her, but they might ask my mother, 'What's the problem', like, 'What is the problem and what are you doing?' So the first question is put across through her ... the collective pressure in the family is put across to her in terms of 'What's the matter?' Then speaking about her own thing that, 'I want a child', everybody desires a child, that's probably the second factor. But it's the first factor in the initial stages that plays the part ... probably that society puts it across very thoroughly and then after a point you forget the society and your own feelings come across.
>
> Geeta: Now it feels, quickly I should have a child. I just want one that's all, we don't even want two, just one ... nobody says anything, like my husband's relations and other relatives-in-law [*sasural walé*] they will not say anything to their son. They will only blame the daughter-in-law, 'Why aren't you conceiving? What's the matter?'

The distinction between personal need and social expectation appears confused in this extract. The concerns expressed by Geeta become significant in light of the comment that her in-laws would 'blame' only her, the daughter-in-law, and not their son. Stigma and its accompanying shame make the desire for 'something of my own' not only part of the solution to the problem but also a part of her survival strategy in the family.

The experience of Maya, a [*Maharashtrian*] Hindu woman interviewed in a Mumbai clinic, reveals another dimension. Maya and her husband are professional architects, and on the day of the interview she was visiting the clinic alone as the couple took turns looking after their firm. Maya's social experience of infertility was one of exclusion:

> Maya: When you are educated you think of life on a larger scale. These are all petty matters, the social attitude, they don't socialise with you because of this matter [infertility], they don't call you for functions – that makes no difference, that's petty.
>
> AB: Have you ever experienced such...
>
> Maya: Yah! Yah! I have experienced [it]. We have Hindu religion. We have some ceremonies and all to be done, so what happens is that there is a particular ceremony on the seventh month of pregnancy [and] there is a function arranged, to that [function] all women are invited. Certain families, they don't invite women who don't have children, so that's when they miss you from their list of guests ... so okay [it] doesn't matter anymore because it doesn't [pause] it's a petty thing because they are petty minded, it's a very petty thing ... It doesn't hurt because we've got over it, it doesn't matter. Initially it hurt, it doesn't matter, it shows how petty they are, they are not growing up. They are not looking at the world on the larger scale...

Maya consistently claims that it does not matter what people think or do, and yet her assertions barely veil her sadness and anger. The stigma and exclusion is in line with the low status accorded to barren women in Indian society.

According to Patel (1994: 78), a barren woman is 'considered an ill omen both for the household and the larger society. It is inauspicious to run into her early in the morning or on auspicious occasions, such as rituals of childbirth, wedding and marriage, or while setting out of the house to the fields for sowing, or another village or city'. Unisa's (1999) quantitative study indicates that infertile women try to avoid ceremonies. Out of 315 women questioned, 164 [52.1 per cent] refused to attend any ceremonies. Bhatti et al.'s (1999) research also supports this. For Maya, her social and occupational status as an architect is rendered less significant than her lower status as infertile.

Similarly, Neelanjana, who worked as a nutrition consultant for a non-governmental organisation, recounted how village women assumed that she would be cast out of her marital home and ultimately be in need of her own father's protection:

> I meet people in the villages, like, in fact I take this problem of not having a child very philosophically and can laugh about it, discuss it ... even at the grassroots level ... I was talking to village women and one of them was a traditional birth attendant. She asked me, 'Are you married?' I said, yes. 'How long?' I said, five years. She said, 'Do you have any children?' No! The second question she asks me – she didn't ask me about my husband or something – she says, 'Do you have your father alive?' Yes, my father is very much there ... It wasn't judgmental; she wasn't looking down on me, but she was empathizing with my situation. She said, 'Where will this girl go?' So I laughed it off...

The traditional birth attendant described in this story was voicing an all-too-familiar fear that permeates the lives of infertile Indian women. The force of community disapproval can, in fact, irretrievably disable the lives of infertile couples, whose only desire is to be left alone. A highly educated doctor named Rajkumar, interviewed in a Mumbai infertility clinic, spoke of the torment he and his wife were enduring at the time. While his wife – a doctor herself – was resting after an embryo transfer, he spoke of their experience of infertility:

> It is a *majboori* [compulsion, to seek treatment] – what can you do! I am a doctor, my wife is a doctor. We don't have any problem, but society always interferes in your life. The need to ask, 'You don't have children, why?' is always there. Even the patients said, 'Oh! the *doctrni* [lady doctor] is barren!' So you do feel. The patients who come say, 'This doctor is barren, what treatment can she possibly offer us? I don't want to be delivered by her' ... I [as a result] don't stay for more than two years in a place. I ask for a transfer; before someone says anything it is better to go to a new place, so that nobody should say that the doctor doesn't have any children. In the past, whenever my wife went for deliveries, she was told that, 'Don't let this woman touch you, she is a *banjh*' [barren woman]. She feels it. So we had to get a transfer because people found out that this *doctrni* is unable to produce children, that she is barren.

The stigma of infertility and the force of social ostracism can penetrate and even subvert otherwise fixed social hierarchies in India. Social markers of class and caste, as well as elite professional boundaries, do not safeguard against social stigma and disablement, as seen in the case of Rajkumar and his infertile physician wife. The oppressive cultural expectations of fertility, therefore, make ideas such as reproductive rights, agency, privacy and choice deeply problematic in contemporary India, even among the upper class. In a cultural context where the continuing absence of children in a marriage becomes sufficient grounds for social interference, selective disclosure of one's infertility in an attempt to manage one's 'spoiled identity' is simply untenable. Clearly, the stigma attached to infertility and its particular effects on women is severe. Whether it is the family, as in the case of Geeta and Ravi, or relations and friends like those of Maya, or simply 'society at large', as Rajkumar describes above, the symbolic violence that women face appears to be both socially and emotionally crippling.

How Infertility Affects Men

Men – contrary to popular belief – are no less affected by the stigma of infertility. Ajay and Shanti, a couple from a small town in Rajasthan, had this to say:

> Ajay: People in the family talk a lot. On our side people talk all the time...
>
> Shanti: They ask, 'What happened about your treatment? You've shown yourself in such a big hospital, what happened?' What answer should we give them?
>
> Ajay: There are thousands of things these people say...
>
> AB: Who are these people? Relatives or...
>
> Ajay: Relatives, brothers and friends. You see, when a person is lacking something in his life or a person who has a shortcoming in his life, everybody talks things about such a person ... *A condition such as mine puts a question mark on you, in every way.* People start saying, 'He's like this, he's like that'. If a person is lacking in any way, like in his life, or family a thousand and one shortcomings and troubles are associated with him... [emphasis added]
>
> Shanti: They say very derogatory things.

> Ajay: The main problem is the social pressure. You see, in the society I have my brothers, etc. Now *I stand apart from everyone, cut off from the social mainstream.* In the family if there is a marriage or anything, you see if you have a child it has so much display value. A person who is behind a person who is off the track, there is a family and the person who is a little different from the rest he has to listen to a lot of things. Nowadays the way the world is people don't think about your wellbeing, but they are the first ones to contribute to your misery [emphasis added].

Throughout the interview, Ajay poured out his pent-up frustrations on being infertile. The cause of infertility in their case was (genital) tuberculosis that had affected Shanti's fallopian tubes. To describe his wife's infertility in terms of 'a condition such as mine puts a question mark on you' tells us something important about how Ajay perceives his wife's condition as his. The contagion of stigma appears to have spread and inflicted the 'married body' rather than Shanti (wife/woman) alone. His wife's inability to conceive also implicates his manhood, a topic on which he is silent. Given the couple's fourteen-year childless marriage, together with the popular understanding of the gender-specific nature of infertility, Shanti should have been abandoned by now in favour of a fertile bride. As they are from a patriarchal joint family in a small Rajasthan town, Ajay's sentiment and his wife's courage in dealing with the highly antagonistic and hostile domestic climate suggests there is more complexity to gender oppression and equally to resistance to patriarchal norms, particularly since this is not an isolated case.

A Punjabi couple from the city of Faridabad in Haryana – Jeet and Sonia – were more forthcoming in sharing their fears and mutual support, once again making it difficult to view infertility as exclusively a woman's problem without support from the man:

> Sonia: People do talk like, 'You should have had, you should have [a baby]'...
>
> Jeet: They speak in a taunting way.
>
> AB: How are you coping with this pressure?
>
> Sonia: Sometimes we take it as a joke and laugh it off, sometimes we keep quiet and say nothing, sometimes we say the treatment is on, sometimes we simply say it is in God's hands. We have to deal with it somehow.

Jeet: People keep on talking, and we have to deal with it but at the level of immediate family we are facing no such problem ... We have no problem adopting but publicly it is difficult. People would say, you have adopted because you couldn't manage to produce one yourself, you both must be incapable or lacking in some way...

Sonia: It is also emotional...

Jeet: You are impotent, they can say anything. To escape all this it is better to have a child of your own.

AB: Are you tense about the treatment?

Jeet: Yes, a little bit.

Sonia: No, not a little bit; it's quite a bit! I feel because of me he is suffering. He never says anything to me and he never ever said anything to me like, 'You don't have a child,' or [pause] I feel bad, because it is my weakness, all his reports are okay. I feel because of me he is suffering and that he is worried.

Jeet: Psychologically, she is under pressure. She feels that because of her we don't have a child. It becomes a one-sided thing with her.

Jeet and Sonia are under intense social pressure to explain why they do not have a child. For Jeet, the fear of being labeled impotent adds to his anxiety and hence his need for a child to establish his masculinity and his wife's fecundity. Sonia's guilt magnifies her emotional crisis though Jeet's continual support in viewing the situation as theirs, rather than as a 'one sided-thing', as he puts it, does not support the assumption that men remain unaffected by deepening stigma. This further problematises the issue of gender-specific blame for infertility among marriages in India.

Faced with culturally entrenched stigma and socially debilitating community ostracism, it is not uncommon for Indian couples to withdraw into a world of their own. Unable to bear the endless torment of social disparagement, a couple from Gujarat, Ram and Sujata, had stopped going to social functions, a highly unusual state of affairs for an Indian couple:

Ram: Sometimes it makes us very sad. People ask things like, 'When will you have a baby?' We get very depressed but still we have got a hope. That's why we are here and we are taking every care, rest is up to Almighty...

AB: What has your experience been like [to Ram's wife, Sujata]?

Ram: We avoid people.

AB: Has it effected your social life?

Ram: It has. We ... will not mix in social functions.

Sujata: Unnecessary talk all the time.

Ram: Sometimes all people are not equal, some may talk in polished language, some might talk in a rough way. People will not understand that this is also a kind of disease, but this particular disease they will take it some other way. People are having cancers, people are having TB, people are having kidney problems, people are having brain hemorrhage, so many things, but this particular they will take the other way.

AB: Why do you feel that is the case?

Ram: That we felt sometimes. That is why we generally will not go to social functions. We have cordial relations with everyone otherwise. Not that we are not friendly relations, I am also very social man. We will not go to meet people often.

Ram and Sujata see the medicalisation of their infertility as the only tenable option in the face of growing social opposition to their childlessness. Society's inability to see infertility as a disease, disability or handicap – comparable to the common and socially acceptable conditions of cancer, tuberculosis, kidney problems or strokes in India – is particularly disconcerting for Ram. He obliquely hints at how (in) fertility and sexual dysfunction are often conflated, when he states, 'This [infertility], they [society] will take the other way.' In Ram's case, he had undergone corrective surgery for impotency, which apparently cured his sexual dysfunction. But throughout the interview, he remained tight-lipped about his own experience of social ridicule. Even though the truth of his impotency was not common knowledge in his family or community, his sensitivity towards his own past sexual disability compounded the anxiety of social disapproval, as his wife's inability to achieve pregnancy had implicated his manhood yet again.

Veena Das in her study of Punjabi kinship notes that:

sexual virility as a value of the backstage is highly prized among Punjabis. So much so, that even a statement to the effect that a particular man seems to be somewhat weak, can be used to make insinuations that he is sexually inadequate. In cases of childlessness,

> these insinuations are not rare, for while the childless woman may be accused of sterility by her immediate conjugal family, her own natal family or other members of the *biradari* may blame her husband, by saying that he was always a weakling. (Das 1976a: 8)

This is also in line with the ancient legal code of *Narada* and the recent Madras High Court ruling as described in Chapter 1. The fear of being considered impotent is central to the anxiety that some men experience in the face of an infertile marriage (Ramasubban and Rishyasringa 1998). The pressure to acquire a new wife/field and prove their adequacy is partly in line with this anxiety. However, there are interesting exceptions to this gender stereotype. Some men openly oppose the idea of a second marriage through the course of these interviews, while others like Arvind, above, quietly support their wives while ignoring such social pressure. The most interesting case was of a farmer – Harjeet – from Punjab, who had sold part of his agricultural land to fund IVF cycles:

> Harjeet: I thought a lot about this [treatment]. You see, my wife, she has a different 'plan'. She says our younger sister-in-law is picking fights, abuses her and generally troubles her, on this issue [infertility]; she [i.e. the sister-in-law] says take medicine. Sometimes they [sisters-in-law – three married brothers including Harjeet live together with their mother] say get married again, but what's the point when there are no sperm in my semen.
>
> AB: Did you tell your sister-in-law that...
>
> Harjeet: Yes! I tell her but she doesn't listen. I have said no to a second marriage. I have told them [sisters-in-law] in so many words that if it has to happen [i.e. a baby] it will happen with my wife or nothing at all.
>
> AB: Do you feel your wife is going ahead with the treatment because of the pressure at home or she is herself very keen on a child?
>
> Harjeet: She is doing it because of the sister-in-law is giving her a hard time at home.
>
> AB: Have you ever considered adoption?
>
> Harjeet: I am prepared.
>
> AB: Your family members are not supportive of the idea?

> Harjeet: No! Even the family members agree. My mother, my sisters, my brothers-in-law they all say, 'Try and convince your wife to consider adoption'. They say, 'Why spend two lakh rupees? The adopted child will also be yours'. But my wife doesn't agree. Then I have to listen to her.

This narrative assumes greater significance in the light of Patel's (1994: 78) assertion on the position of an infertile woman: 'In quarrels and squabbles she is insulted for her failure in fertility performance. The dart of barrenness is thrown at her to whittle down her strength and to latently glorify fertility. She is under constant pressure from household members, relatives and neighbours to produce children'. Little wonder that Harjeet's wife is putting up such stiff resistance to the 'dart of barrenness' thrown at her by her younger sister-in-law even in the face of overt family support to not seek treatment and to accept her own infertility (she is unable to ovulate) by adopting. Harjeet's support ('Then I have to listen to her') and that of his mother, sisters and brothers-in-law brings out the complex and paradoxical nature of stigma. Living in a joint household, therefore, and in an atmosphere of 'fertility competition' with an abusive and younger sister-in-law makes infertility unbearable for Harjeet's wife. It is also significant that Harjeet owns up to his infertility, rather than follow the more conventional route of making the 'barren field' the cause of infertility. As is clear from Chapter 1, while there is a cultural conception of a barren field in the Hindu worldview, there is no corresponding concept of a barren seed. A man can at best be viewed as incapable of sowing the seed; the potency of the seed is rarely in doubt.

A migrant – Hariram – from a village in Uttar Pradesh, North India, seeking treatment together with his wife in Mumbai, said, 'Fifteen years ago we faced a lot of problems. People used to say get married again, my mother, she died, she too used to say, "Have a child"... so one or the other problem one has to face when the family is involved ... but one has to understand whatever god wills happens'. Hariram had been married for twenty years and had not resorted to remarrying as a solution to his wife's 'barrenness'. This is significant, given that Hariram and Harjeet both have rural backgrounds where abandoning barren wives is not an infrequent practice, as Jeffery et al. (1989) and Patel (1994) amply demonstrate.

These narratives highlight the difficulty in reducing infertility to a simple opposition between a dispensable/substitutable infertile woman and socially undamaged (in)fertile man. While women remain substitutable on account of their infertility in India, the data above provides some evidence to the contrary. Jeffery et al. (1989) and Patel (1994: 79) acknowledge that childless men suffer 'humiliation' but that their position is not as 'stigmatised' as that of barren women. Equally, there are important exceptions in situations where divorce or the fear of abandonment does not follow a barren woman (Jeffery et al. 1989: 88).

However, this data suggests something different. Here, there is a clear sense of sharing the stigma, though it must be acknowledged that the experience of its intensity is connected to gender. While the attitude of men like Rajkumar, Ajay and Jeet towards their wives's infertility makes it difficult to assert that sigma is experienced more by the female body than the male, given the institutionalised gender asymmetry permeating Indian society (Chapter 1), nonetheless the consequences for women in general are more severe. Even though there are men like Ajay, who sees his wife's condition as his, Rajkumar, who goes to the extent of opting for professional transfers so as to shield himself and his wife from stigma and ostracism, and Jeet, who views his wife's condition as inherently 'theirs' while reacting to his wife's guilt pangs as a 'one-sided thing for her', the fact remains that men are socially enjoined to abandon barren wives, thus perpetuating the inferior position of women. This makes it difficult to answer the question: what is the gender of infertility, when a man can choose to walk out of a 'barren marriage' with his dignity intact, an option unavailable to a great majority of women?

Conclusion

The stigma of infertility in the lives of couples who turn to assisted conception attaches itself to much more than mere reproductive disruption; it becomes the source of symbolic violence that frays the fabric of the mundane everyday. Even though the overriding tendency in India is to blame the woman for failed conception, the stigma of infertility penetrates to a point where the social identity of wives is rendered barren and that of husbands sterile. In the present, as in the past, this presents men with an opportunity to abandon a barren wife and de-stigmatise themselves. In the case of an infertile man, this amounts to a public accommodation of masculine pride. A public assertion of virility and a public denial of infertility are made easier by an entrenched patriarchal normative order, a process where male infertility is grafted onto the female body, thus rendering it socially barren.

The evidence presented in this chapter complicates this reality. It points to a gender equation where the conjugal bond is not browbeaten by the fear of censure or patriarchal intolerance. This subversion of a commonly understood 'rule of patrilineal marriage' (thou shall abandon a barren wife) parallels evidence from Egypt and the Middle East, where infertile couples are also able to resist, reject and undermine patriarchal interference. Marcia C. Inhorn (1996a, 2012) in her study of infertility and patriarchy in Egypt argues:

> The success of so many infertile marriages bespeaks the strengthening of conjugal connectivity in Egypt at the expense of patriarchy, which is being undermined. Although patriarchal religious, legal, and cultural norms allow men to replace their infertile wives, many men refuse this option out of feelings of love, loyalty and commitment. (Inhorn 1996a: 149–50)

Married couples who either resist a pronatalist normative structure or turn to medically assisted conception appear unwavering in their commitment to each other. Assisted reproductive technologies, and IVF more particularly, become a sieve through which only the strongest conjugal partnerships can pass. I base this assertion on my earliest encounters with treatment-seeking couples [N 43] from 1997 through to 1999. This data set reveals that the average duration of marriage in the sample is ten years [mean: - 9.9487] with a range distribution of twenty-one years separating the maximum [23] and minimum [2] limits. This becomes significant if we examine the number of years these couples had been in treatment. The average duration of years in treatment is more than seven years [mean: - 7.1053] with a range of nineteen years of treatment seeking. This means that, out of an average married duration of ten years, the interviewees had spent on average seven years in treatment. In this respect IVF can be imagined as a delicate filter that allows only the strongest conjugal relations to persist on the cusp of infertility and stigma. It is because of this unique interface that couples are able to face up to both well-meaning but thoughtlessly expressed concern and callous social attitudes. Not surprisingly, therefore, delegitimation of their social identities becomes an almost predictable outcome of nonconformity to the 'rule of patrilineal marriage'. As a consequence, these marriages endure the worst kind of social exclusion and humiliation. Stigma becomes 'contagious' (Das 2001) and engulfs the conjugal unit. However, rather than be subservient pawns in the hands of a delegitimating society, these couples – as we shall see in Chapter 5 – actively persist in seeking treatment within the confines of their infertile union by forging tactical alliances both within their marriage and with preferred members of the wider family. This is a crucial part of a larger process of treatment seeking that remains a thorny subtext for the greater part of their infertile lives.

Part II

The 'global' technologies of assisted conception are always transferred into 'local' cultural contexts. In the Indian context this has meant that these technologies have been received and promoted in the wider sociopolitical environment. Part II locates assisted conception in relation to the private and public sector interface in India as one way of understanding the spread of fertility techniques in a densely populated, developing country. In other words, the chapters in this segment pay particular attention to three crucial aspects: first, to the controversy surrounding the birth of the first 'test-tube' baby in India and the contest over proper credit ascription and the rewriting of IVF history in India played out in the mass media channels; second, to the spread of assisted conception within the private sector reflecting the wider biomedical politics of public/private sectors; and third, to the pressures and politicking internal to the functioning of infertility clinics within the private sector. In doing this, it is suggested that the need to promote these technologies of conception and the contesting claims to scientific credibility through media channels can be viewed as born out of an urgency to run clinics at an optimal and financially viable level.

Chapter 3

CONTESTED CONCEPTION

THE MEDICAL POLITICS OF TEST-TUBE BABIES

The history of in vitro fertilisation (IVF) in India is arguably as old as the history of IVF itself. Its origin was controversial and its subsequent development no less so. In vitro fertilisation laid the foundation of assisted conception in India and created the battleground on which wars for the legitimate ownership of the first 'test-tube baby miracle' were fought. Early feminists like Michelle Stanworth (1987a) rightly argued that the use of the 'curious term test-tube babies' conjures an odd image of a foetus growing independently of the body of a woman – a miracle of science rather than nature. Her contemporary, Deborah Lynn Steinberg (1990: 78), similarly argued that the term 'test-tube baby' misnames the site of fertilisation, which does not occur in a test tube, and communicates an extra-corporeal image of the process of conception and pregnancy that contributes to the erasure of women from the entire process. And yet, as explored in the Preface, the term has become normalised in both scientific and non-scientific (media) discourses on infertility in India. One important implication of the term 'test-tube baby' is that it makes ownership of the expert primary and that of the woman/couple secondary. The political struggle over the ownership of the first test-tube baby charted in this chapter amply demonstrates how these babies are viewed as scientific trophies rather than as mere scientific solutions to infertility.

Assisted conception in India became a contested terrain in part because of the reckless pursuit for credit (reward) and credibility (ability to do science) by its practitioners (Latour and Woolgar

1979).[1] This pursuit has been accentuated by an entrenched multimedia rhetoric on assisted conceptive techniques as a long-awaited solution to the biosocial problem of human infertility. This chapter represents my attempt to chart the trajectory of assisted conception in India by stringing together various key moments in its growth. It attempts to unveil the politics of conception by focusing on the contested nature of the claims of various medical practitioners responsible for producing the first test-tube baby in India. The story of the first IVF baby in India reveals a scientific rejection of claims unsubstantiated by peer review (see also Bharadwaj 2013a, 2013b, 2013c). I reinforce the ideas that the pursuit of peer-endorsed credibility is not always a pivotal motivation for scientists and scientific work and that the generation and ascription of scientific credibility is inherently multicentred. In so asserting the importance of politics and power relations in the practice of science, I ultimately emphasise the ways in which scientific 'facts' are constructed and contested. This chapter also shows how the ability to do science and the pursuit of reward can extend beyond the scientific terrain, especially when faced – as seen in the previous chapter – by the demands of making IVF practice economically viable and commercially sound. As explored in Chapter 4, the development of assisted conception in India is largely contingent on several interrelated factors. First, the 'experts' successfully left the state sector in order to function with an otherwise unattainable degree of autonomy and freedom. Second, once out, they used the media not only to carve a niche in the infertility market but also to set in motion a contest for respect, status and credit hitherto unknown to them. Indeed, many media accounts of assisted conception appear as no more than attempts to promote the reach and penetration of various practitioners in the infertility market, creating a media/medicine nexus (Bharadwaj 2000). Third, since 1991, India, in line with its policy of economic liberalisation, has incentivised the technological management of infertility. Fourth, the stigma attached to infertility and an almost oppressive cultural expectation to contribute living children to society (Bharadwaj 2002) has increased existing demand for treatment in the face of new technological breakthroughs. Thus, to summarise, the collapse of the state-sponsored IVF programme, coupled with the experts leaving the public sector, accompanied by success in the private sector primarily as a result of liberal state policies and lack of regulatory mechanisms, soon fueled a contest for proper credit allocation and recognition, the roots of which go as far back as 1978.

Rewriting the Past

With the birth of the first 'scientifically documented' test-tube baby, Harsha, on 6 August 1986, India officially entered the new world of assisted conception. The use of the term 'scientifically documented' is deliberate as it was repeated ad nauseam in scientific circles to negate the parallel claims of a similar breakthrough made by a doctor in 1978, months after the birth of the world's very first test-tube baby, Louise Brown, in Britain.

On 3 October 1978, the birth of the world's second test-tube baby was announced by Dr Subhas Mukerji in Calcutta. The news was widely reported in the media in India and to some extent abroad. Mukerji's claim, however, was contested because he did not publish the bulk of his research in standard peer-reviewed journals. Ironically, nineteen years later, the story of Mukerji's test-tube baby was retold by Dr T.C. Anand Kumar, the man most closely associated with India's first 'scientifically documented' IVF baby. It was Anand Kumar and his collaborators in Mumbai who produced a baby girl, Harsha, as India's 'first' test-tube baby. By Anand Kumar's (1997: 526) own admission, 'Harsha was described as India's first "scientifically documented" test-tube baby because the details of Mukerji's work were not then available'. Delivering the Subhas Mukerji Memorial Oration at the third National Congress on Assisted Reproductive Technology and Advances in Infertility Management, held in Calcutta on 8 February 1997, Anand Kumar appealed to the scientific establishment to credit Mukerji posthumously for creating India's first test-tube baby. Two months later, Anand Kumar (1997) followed this appeal with the publication of an article in the journal *Current Science*, titled 'Architect of India's first test tube baby: Dr Subhas Mukerji (16 January 1931 to 19 July 1981)'. The story of Mukerji's long-forgotten past was resurrected with the publication of this article. Anand Kumar argued forcefully that Mukerji did produce India's first test-tube baby in 1978, a claim Anand Kumar had personally come to believe.

Mukerji was a medical graduate of Calcutta University, where he also obtained a DPhil. He was awarded the Colombo Plan scholarship to work in the MRC Clinical Endocrinology Research Unit in Edinburgh under Professor John A. Loraine, a reproductive physiologist. In his paper, Anand Kumar (1997) offers exhaustive documentation of Mukerji's presentations at various scientific and public fora, along with a detailed description of his research interests and analysis of the IVF technique that he deployed to produce a baby girl, who was given the pseudonym Durga. Anand Kumar undertook this systematic exercise to demonstrate that, even in the absence of published scientific papers in leading journals, Mukerji's work was truly monumental and pathbreaking. According to Anand Kumar (1997: 529), Mukerji was 'far ahead of his time in successfully using an ovarian stimulation protocol before anyone else in the world had thought of doing so'. He continues:

> It may be noted that Subhas Mukerji reported the successful cryopreservation of a 8-cell embryo, storing it for 53 days, thawing and replacing it into the mother's womb, resulting in a successful and live birth as early as 1978 – a full 5 years before anyone else had done so. This small publication of Mukerji in 1978 clearly shows that Mukerji was on the right line of thinking much before anyone else had demonstrated the successful outcome of a pregnancy following the transfer of a 8-cell frozen-thawed embryo into human subjects transferring 8-cell cryopreserved embryos. (Anand Kumar 1997: 530)

After this breakthrough, Mukerji's happiness was short-lived. The government of West Bengal appointed an 'expert committee' under auspices of the Indian Medical Association and Bengal Obstetrics and Gynecology Association to investigate the veracity of Mukerji's claims. The inquiry committee met on 18 November 1978, to review critically Mukerji's report to the Director of Health Services (DHS), West Bengal Government, and rejected Mukerji's claim. Anand Kumar questions this as the committee was headed by a professor of radiophysics and composed of a gynaecologist, a physiologist and a neurophysiologist. None of these committee members, he argues, 'could have had any background or insight into modern Reproductive Technologies, a subject upon which they were to hold an inquiry' (Anand Kumar 1997: 528).

Mukerji tried to explain his position and, in a letter to the DHS dated 1 December 1978, stated that he needed adequate time to prepare the report on his work. However, since Mukerji was forced to assemble the report in about two weeks of the committee's judgement, he felt that he had inadequate time to plead his case in detail. Anand Kumar however claims:

> With very sound reasoning, Mukerji did not reveal all his data because he wanted to 'publish these in recognized scientific journals after the reproducibility of the work is reasonably assured'. [Mukerji] went on to state: 'The final concentration of DMSO used before freezing as well as the exact indigenous method of cooling were deliberately omitted from the report, like (also) the steps for removal of

> DMSO before thawing. Certain essential intermediate steps, during the whole procedures also involving the use of undisclosed and enriched media were completely omitted. I had to be careful to guard our unpublished data, because by that time I became aware of the penetrating efficiency of the tentacles of the mass media'. (Anand Kumar 1997: 528)

Mukerji paid dearly for withholding this crucial information. Not only was his claim rejected by the committee, but the DHS imposed strict restrictions, preventing him from attending any conferences without prior permission. Anand Kumar provides a detailed account of events leading up to Mukerji's mental and emotional degradation:

> Mukerji was invited by the Primate Research Center of the Kyoto University, Japan, on 25 January 1979 to attend a closed meeting at their expense to discuss details of Mukerji's work. Mukerji applied to the DHS for permission, which was promptly denied via their letter of 16 February 1979. The letter directed Mukerji not to leave the country without prior clearance from the Government. Subhas Mukerji shortly afterwards suffered a heart attack. His request for special leave was declined but his request for transfer was promptly accepted and, at 'pleasure of the Governor of West Bengal' he was transferred to the Regional Institute of Ophthalmology as Professor of electrophysiology on 5 June 1981. The Government, preventing him from presenting his work at scientific meetings, denying him leave to write up his results, and humiliation he was subjected to by his colleagues in Calcutta were some of the things that the sensitive Subhas Mukerji could not bear. His transfer to a department in which he had no expertise was the last straw on the proverbial camel's back for Mukerji. This transfer order was dated 5 June 1981. Mukerji gave up fighting the system and ended his life on 19 July 1981, 44 days after the transfer order was issued. Much of Mukerji's work remained unpublished not because he did not have data but because he was not given a chance to do so by his administrative Ministry in the Government. (Anand Kumar 1997: 530–31)[2]

The impact of Anand Kumar's appeal extended beyond the medical community. Sixteen years after Mukerji's suicide, a Calcutta English daily, *The Telegraph*, reported:

> India's medical establishment is under pressure to recognize the doctor's work [sixteen] years after he committed suicide, following a leading scientist's assertion on this count. Dr T. C. Anand Kumar, an authority on human infertility management and assisted reproductive technology, has rekindled the debate on India's first test tube

> baby by crediting Dr Mukherjee [as spelt in the report] with engineering it. (Mukherjee 1997)

The same article reported that Dr Mukerji's wife was living in 'a twilight of physical pain and bitter-sweet memories and believed that all the moves to recognise her husband's work posthumously would not "bring him back"'. She, on the contrary, hoped for the establishment to encourage a more supportive scientific environment that the one that drove her husband to his death.

This sentiment notwithstanding, Anand Kumar's assertions at the Calcutta conference made it to the major national dailies and the regional press – assertions such as, 'Let me tell you that Subhash Mukerji must be given credit for producing the first test tube baby', and 'All other achievements dwarf in comparison to what he achieved'. The focus simultaneously shifted to Mukerji's miracle Durga, whose identity and that of her parents had been hidden for eighteen years. Headlines such as 'Test Tube Baby's Parents Reveal All, Resurrect Scorned Scientist' in Calcutta's *Telegraph* (Mukherjee 1997) and 'Test Tube Baby, Now 18, is Ready to Talk' in New Delhi's *Hindustan Times* (19 February 1997) added to the drama. Some media accounts unanimously identified Mukerji's biggest shortcoming as his inability to produce the baby as evidence to consolidate his claim. He either did not understand then, as we now do, or resisted, the notion that babies legitimate the use of new conceptive technologies in very powerful ways (Stanworth 1987a: 27a). Moreover, the parents of the Calcutta baby, Durga, fearing social ostracism, had not allowed Mukerji to go public with the details back in 1978. Anand Kumar himself spoke of the Indian 'psyche' that considers barrenness to be a curse. His remarks were widely covered in the media. The *Hindustan Times* article cited above wrote:

> After hearing the lecture, Durga's parents met him [Anand Kumar] to explain why they did not want Durga's identity revealed at that time when IVF was a novel procedure and how they felt differently now. According to Anand Kumar, Durga who is [a] 'delightful young lady of 18, well educated and articulate', did not have objection to revealing facts of her birth 'if it helped advancement of knowledge'. But she did not want the Press to intrude on her or her parents' privacy'.

There were four elements working against Mukerji. First, he did not have a physical baby to show to the world because of patient confidentiality. Second, he did not have enough academic publications to support his claims. Third, important peer reviews were absent because of his lack of publications. Finally, bureaucratic hostility prevented Mukerji from presenting his work to the world at large.

Twenty years later, Mukerji is news as a result of Anand Kumar's efforts. Even more interesting is the evangelical zeal with which Anand Kumar campaigned to clear Mukerji's name. The situation is further complicated by the fact that, by raising the Durga issue, Anand Kumar stands to lose his claim of association with the first scientifically-documented test-tube baby, Harsha. Recognising Mukerji as the scientific father – of the very first Indian and only the second ever test-tube baby in the world – requires a degree of peer recognition and scientific validation from the Indian scientific community that would mark a fundamental shift in the definition of the first 'scientifically documented test-tube baby in India'. That is to say, the present claim to the first test-tube baby would have to be abandoned in favour of the earlier claim of Mukerji, and Harsha would have to be replaced by Durga. This construction of the first scientific baby produced from a test tube is at the heart of the contested terrain of assisted conception in India. These battles are fought to salvage and restructure scientific reputations under the thinly disguised rhetoric of scientific and peer documentation. I attempt to problematise these strategies and clashes of ambition in the following section.

Birth of a Contest

As has been seen above, there is an ongoing campaign to credit Mukerji for engineering India's first, and the world's second, test-tube baby. The genesis of ascription of 'proper credit' may be traced back to the birth of India's first 'scientifically documented' test-tube baby, Harsha, when the actual credit allocation, following the media aftermath of the breakthrough, completely disrupted the credibility cycle of the scientific team responsible for the feat. What emerged was a fundamental distinction between the multi-sited nature of both credibility production and credibility allocation. There was a divergence between credit and credibility as it emerged from peers versus the media.

Baby Harsha was the product of a collaboration between an institute controlled by the Indian Council for Medical Research (ICMR) and a Mumbai public hospital. The scientific team is popularly believed (for reasons that will become clear below) to be headed by the collaborating pair of Dr Anand Kumar, the medical director of the Institute for Research in Reproduction, Mumbai (IRR), and Dr Indira Hinduja, a gynaecologist from the King Edward Memorial Hospital, Mumbai (KEM). The rest of the team comprised both senior and junior scientists. With the publication of the IVF project results in 1985–1986, India's first test-tube baby became a peer-reviewed reality. Even though the information first appeared in the ICMR Annual Report and did not offer the exact scientific details, it opened the way for scientific engagement and peer review. The publication cited the contributing team members before more detailed data on the technique and other accomplishments were revealed:

Figure 3.1 Indian Council for Medical Research Annual Report

Title of Project	11.8. In vitro Fertilization & Embryo Transfer: A collaborative project between the KEM Hospital and the Institute for Research in Reproduction.
Project Leader	Dr T.C. Anand Kumar
Project Staff	Dr J.V. Iyer, Dr G.M. Ranga
Project Collaborators	Dr I. Hinduja, K.E.M. Hospital Dr C.P. Puri, I.R.R. Dr T.D. Nandedkar, I.R.R. Dr K. Gopalkrishnan, I.R.R. Dr R. Asok Kumar, I.R.R.
Time of starting	August 1985
Approximate duration	Five Years
Provisional date of completion	1990

The article goes on to state that the 'In Vitro Fertilization and Embryo transfer technique has been perfected and performed as a collaborative project between the KEM Hospital and the IRR. This has resulted in the birth of the country's first ever, scientifically documented, test tube baby' (ICMR 1986: 74).

The project leader and project collaborators are clearly identified in the article. Dr Hinduja is but one amongst five collaborators working under the project leader, Dr Anand Kumar. The inclusion of the KEM Hospital as a collaborating partner recognises Hinduja's links with the hospital. Together IRR and KEM created India's first scientifically documented test-tube baby.

India learnt of this breakthrough on *Doordarshan*, national television's evening news, on the evening of 6 August 1986:

> The first test-tube baby in India was born to Mrs Mani Chawda, a twenty-four year old housewife at KEM hospital Mumbai. Our Mumbai correspondent reports:
>
> 'A pretty and healthy baby girl weighing 2.8 kgs has become India's first scientifically documented test-tube baby. She was born to Mani Shanti Chawda at KEM hospital this afternoon at the hands of Dr Indira Hinduja. The baby was delivered by cesarean section. This tiny bundle is India's first successful case of conception using the in vitro fertilization technique where the sperm and ovum are fertilized outside the mother's womb and foetus transferred inside her for development. Dr Hinduja successfully used the technique in close co-operation with Dr Anand Kumar and his institute for Research in Reproduction in Mumbai. We spoke to Dr Hinduja and the child's father Shanti Kumar'.

The very first media account shifted the balance in favour of Dr Indira Hinduja. Throughout the news report, Dr Hinduja was shown with the baby and the hospital staff and, even as she was interviewed on camera, project leader Dr Anand Kumar could only be seen standing quietly next to her. In subsequent coverage, the reporter found it more newsworthy to interview the father of the baby than the project leader, whose name was mentioned only in passing as a close collaborator. Thus, in the evening news, Dr Hinduja practically walked away as the project leader who, in close cooperation with Dr Anand Kumar, had produced India's first scientifically documented test-tube baby. In a matter of hours, from being one of five project collaborators she became the person who delivered India's first test-tube baby, and Dr Anand Kumar fell from the position of project leader to that of a close collaborator.

The media frenzy subsequent to these developments further developed the account in *Doordarshan*'s evening bulletin.[3] All the leading dailies were splashed with pictures of and news items on Hinduja, the newborn wonder and her parents. Anand Kumar and the rest of the collaborating scientific team were lost to the public gaze in this media melee. Nor did media interest abate with time. With the dawn of the 1990s, the field of assisted conception was fully embraced by the popular media. Media coverage of infertility and scientific advancements in its management had become louder and shriller. The uproar and interest generated in the media by assisted conception was further accentuated by the entrance of newer players in the field. Hinduja had become a cult figure as far as IVF and other related reporting was concerned. No media account could begin without paying tribute to the groundbreaking achievement of the lady 'who did it first'. Some common examples are:

> Dr Indira Hinduja of Mumbai is the only doctor in India doing micro-fertilisation. She has a number of other medical firsts to her credit: the first test tube baby in India, the first GIFT baby, the first IVF baby from donor sperm. (*The Week*, 13 December 1992: 30–35)

> [T]he woman who headed the team responsible for the birth of Harsha Chawda, India's first officially recognized test tube baby. (*Sunday Times of India*, 6 February 1994)

> Dr Indira Hinduja who was responsible for the birth of Harsha Chawda, India's first test tube baby in 1986. (*Sunday Times of India Review*, 7 January 1996)

Hinduja's superstardom was not confined to the print media. She has continued to make appearances since 1986 on television chat shows and interviews. A serialised programme which ran to a few hundred episodes dedicated to the theme of parenting even features her in episodes concerning infertility. In one such episode the Chadwa couple was interviewed:

> Anchor: The Chawda couple has a special place for Dr Hinduja in their heart: Mani Chadwa (Mother): I was never … I was not meant to have a child … but madam did the test tube and gave me a baby. We consider Indira Hinduja God. She is our God. Madam made it possible, everything she did, I feel she (Harsha) is her daughter…

In another episode, Hinduja was extolled: 'After all what is a test-tube baby? Let us meet the person responsible for the sensational news; the world's second and India's first test-tube baby's creator, Dr Indira Hinduja!' With this dramatic, high-pitched voiceover, the 'goddess' of artificial conception was unveiled to the audience. This brief introduction gives an excellent insight into the role played by media hyperbolae and uncritical glorification. Yet this misrepresentation of 'documented' facts is curiously in consonance with Mukerji's claim of producing the world's second test-tube baby and India's first. In one of her earlier television appearances in the 1980s, Hinduja was asked directly at the start of an interview about Mukerji's claim:

> Q: Is this India's first test-tube baby or have there been such cases in the past?
>
> Hinduja: First of all I would like to say that this procedure was a product of collaboration between [the] Institute for Research in Reproduction, which is ICMR's branch, and the other one KEM, Mumbai. These two institutes together researched and established this. Your second question was whether this is the first baby. I would like to say that [on] 6th August 1986 the child that was born was scientifically documented, [the] first IVF baby in India.
>
> Q: It was heard that in Calcutta a similar baby was born. That was not documented ... it was not scientifically documented?
>
> Hinduja: Yes, I would only say this: that this procedure was not repeated and no other child was born because of this procedure.

Hinduja took the path of least resistance in answering these questions. The fact that the 1986 baby was a product of collaboration between two institutes clearly provided the credibility that Mukerji lacked. Besides, the viability of any IVF project could only be measured by the success of the subsequent applications. Once again, on that count, Mukerji was silent, while Hinduja could boast a number of ongoing pregnancies and live births. What is interesting, however, is that this line of questioning and answering disappeared in subsequent media accounts. The term 'collaboration between two institutes' is absent from most accounts that emerged in the print and electronic media. Hinduja became virtually synchronous with India's first test-tube baby. Mukerji on the other hand remained completely invisible until the beginning of 1997, when for the first time since 1978 the media reported the details of his past, details made available to them by Anand Kumar.

Contesting Claims

On 4 November 1990, in an English-language magazine *The Week*, an article appeared entitled 'An ill conceived move: research rivalry leads to winding up of test tube baby project'. The article blamed the ICMR for concluding the test-tube baby project at the IRR, Mumbai. The article began by rather dramatically asserting that the IRR is barely a 'test tube's throw away' from the King Edward Memorial Hospital of Mumbai and yet a 'yawning gulf' has suddenly emerged between the two, whose joint effort saw the birth of India's first test-tube baby (Rao 1990). The article went on to quote the director of ICMR:

> Dr A. S. Paintal, director of the Indian Council of Medical Research (ICMR) under whose wings IRR has been hiding cosily all these years, had this belated explanation: 'The major reason for winding up the IVF (in vitro fertilization) unit is that Dr Indira Hinduja's (she was the brain behind India's first test tube baby) project has already proved its success. And we thought she could continue her studies outside whereas the IRR's funds could be utilised for other important projects'. (Rao 1990)

There are two very interesting points to make here. First, as early as 1990 it appears to have been firmly established even in the official (ICMR) circles that the test-tube baby was Hinduja's project. It is surprising that the director above describes the project, funded by a government council (ICMR) and executed by an institute (IRR), supported in collaboration with a public hospital (KEM), as 'Dr Hinduja's project'. It tells us something significant about the inroads made by the media and popular representations of India's first scientifically documented test-tube baby into the official vocabulary. It can alternatively be referred to as the synonymous effect, a product of media reporting that made Hinduja synonymous with the first test-tube baby project. Second, it exposes the enunciatory function of the media. The all important bracket, inserted into the objective quote of the interviewee, is made available for the less informed reader who, in case they have missed the crucial detail about the central role played by Hinduja, should be made aware of 'the brain' behind the project. The article goes on to show how slashing ICMR's Rs. 340 million budget by 20 per cent is used to justify the project's termination and further asserts that the figure of Rs. 10 million 'gobbled up by IVF is inflated perhaps to justify its killing' (Rao 1990). Citing modest expenses on the project (from the IRR annual report), the article goes on to argue that the test-tube baby research was never a 'white elephant' for the IRR. The root of the problem is attributed to a conflict of interest within IRR:

> Another vital aspect is professional jealousy: the impression that Hinduja, who is on the rolls of the KEM Hospital, has been hogging the limelight and depriving the IRR scientists, who have been handling the lab side of the IVF project, [of] their share of the glory. Ironically, there was perfect harmony within the IVF unit, but the so-called experts within the IRR who have nothing to do with the IVF project have been fomenting trouble. This led to increasing non-cooperation, raising of hurdles, deprival of facilities and at times open antagonism, which steeply brought down the tally of IVF babies. (Rao 1990)]

This article makes a firm case for perfect harmony within the IVF team. However, when I contacted some of the team members, they gave very different accounts on the condition of strict anonymity. One team member, for instance, when first contacted on 13 April 1998, spoke of the 'arrogant' and 'uncompromising' attitude of the gynaecologists that led to the collapse of the project. 'The publicity-hungry individuals associated with the project', the informant went on to say, 'created an atmosphere of dejection and frustration' amongst the real scientific 'think tank' behind the project. Those involved were reported as pulling in different directions. Whereas some were more interested in 'promoting themselves', others were too 'disgruntled' because their 'behind-the-scenes hard work was not being appreciated' and they were being 'systematically sidetracked', even as the bulk of the limelight remained on a chosen few. I contacted this respondent again on 21 April 1998 and requested an expansion on the earlier interview. S/he now talked of moves to 'stifle people who wanted to be heard', citing a research officer (ARO) who wanted to be included but was transferred without reason and replaced by someone who would not question the authority of the top project management. The respondent added that 'no data' came 'from the top'; all the hard work was done in the lab, and the data as it came through was simply being 'passed on' to the principals. S/he continued:

> Nobody was trained, neither there was any second in line to take up from where the top people involved in the project left off. Repeated pleas were ignored, and people did not even have access to biological material to research with. They decided who got what and when the whole thing got over, the entire IVF lab was dismantled and

> equipment was distributed within the institute to different departments on a piecemeal basis.

The above two interviews with the respondent in question were not tape recorded as the person was extremely anxious about talking on record. However, my notes record a deep sense of disappointment and anger in someone associated with a scientific team purportedly 'in perfect harmony'.

There was some success in interviewing another individual, who also asked to remain anonymous but gave a brief recorded interview, which revealed considerable grudges and resentment about the project:

> You see, if at that time we had also trained up some people to take over, like when a person goes away that would have been much better ... that couldn't happen ... But that was very sad the way she was given publicity, which is wrong. Why [did] the council and the government ... not [question] our director? Why should she get so much publicity? All the facilities, everything at the cost of the other research, all the money was diverted to this IVF programme and then, my God! The credit should have been given equally to the institute. That is why our current director more or less goes on emphasizing that ... He goes on projecting our institute at the Ministry that it was our institute, our funds, our this, our effort and that has brought about [the IVF baby].
>
> Q: Who was the director when this was happening?
>
> A: Anand Kumar ... He was there, I don't know, he got carried away by the lady. We have a scientific advisory committee who usually assess[es] our projects and gives advice, healthy criticism. There it was also questioned that you have ... developed a technology, you are enforcing it, you are doing it but the technology is ... not going for further research. Who are the next in line or would you conduct a workshop so that other people are trained, so that if one person goes, the technology carries forward? But he just gave some vague reason.

The tendency to eclipse the 'other' emerges as the basis of this contest for credibility. On the one hand, the scientific team claims that it was kept at arm's length from credit (reward) and that their credibility (ability to do science) could not attain its potential because they were marginalised. On the other hand, the principals, Anand Kumar and Hinduja, appear to pursue an approach of mutual obfuscation. There are few documented media accounts where one openly refers to the other as a collaborating partner. The earliest accounts, like the *Doordarshan* evening news of 6 August 1986 and other similar stray reports, refer in passing to both as collaborators. But the closest the protagonists come to acknowledging the other in interviews and in other accounts on the issue of the first test-tube baby is to name the collaborating institutes. The two institutes have been bestowed with a metonymic quality as they almost step in to represent the two collaborators. Anand Kumar for instance made the following assertion in his article on Mukerji:

> The organisers of the recent Calcutta meeting believed that I was pre-eminently qualified and experienced to delve into whatever material was available regarding Mukerji's past work and throw light on it. The reason for this assumption perhaps lay in my having played a key role in the birth of another test tube baby, Harsha, on 6 August 1986. This birth was announced by myself, when I was the director of the ICMR's Institute for Research in Reproduction, and Dr. G.B. Parulekar, Dean of our collaborating institution, King Edward Memorial (KEM) Hospital, Mumbai ... I published our technical report and procedural details in the ICMR Bulletin. The work leading to Harsha's birth was executed by a team of scientists from the IRR and clinicians from the KEM Hospital working under my direct guidance and supervision. (Kumar 1997: 526)

The argument is bluntly clear on three counts. First, the name 'Hinduja', which had become synonymous in the media with the birth of the first test-tube baby, is absent. Her 'claims' are openly resisted by reminding the readers of the contents of the report published in the ICMR Bulletin (cited earlier in this chapter). The primacy of peer-reviewed documentation over popular media accounts is openly asserted. It is also noteworthy that Hinduja is conspicuously absent, even while the KEM hospital and the name of the dean of the collaborating institute is included. Second, the distinction between IRR and KEM is constructed on a clear-cut scientific hierarchy of scientists over clinicians. A sense of 'our' (IRR) scientists and 'their' (KEM) clinicians is asserted to reclaim the 'reality' that was glossed over by media representations, such as Hinduja as 'the brain' behind the project. Third, and most significantly, is the emphasis on phrases such as 'key role' and 'my direct guidance and supervision', which completely underplay the importance and even the extent of the contribution of the collaborating hospital and its now famous collaborating partner, Dr Indira Hinduja.

Hinduja, on the other hand, pursued a similar but more subtle line to assert the primacy of her contribution in the breakthrough that led to Harsha's birth. In a television interview, for instance, she was asked:

> Q: This technique is not taught in India. Where did you learn it from?
>
> A: I did not go abroad to learn the technique. I learnt from my own experience. First I started with animal experiments, in humans, people who used to come for sterilization. We tried to study their eggs, tried to study fertilization, and when it was found that something is happening then we started enrolling infertile couples. (*Doordarshan* documentary, 1986)

Clearly Hinduja is not 'a mere clinician' as Anand Kumar implies, and this is further supported by the fact that she has a successful practice of her own. However, these accounts consistently fail to acknowledge anyone beyond herself. Dr Indira Hinduja 'did it on her own'; Dr Anand Kumar 'got it done under his direct guidance and supervision'; and the disgruntled team of scientists 'couldn't do anything' as they felt completely side-tracked. There is a complete breakdown of credit ascription to the 'other'.[4]

Conclusion

Thus, credibility production is multi-sited. The credibility generated by media accounts can obfuscate peer-reviewed scientific endorsement. The peer-documented credit that Hinduja and Anand Kumar shared is different from the credit generated by media accounts, which focus on Hinduja alone.

Credibility, or a scientist's ability to do science is only a point of departure. Its continual upkeep and regeneration, through a quest for credible reward and recognition, are the mainstays of scientific enterprise when it acquires a commercial face. This helps us understand how scientists respond to demands made outside the scientific terrain. There, the market (infertility patients) judges the credibility of an expert not on what his or her peers have to say – though that is centrally important to the scientists' survival in the field – but more on media representations of the experts.

By raising Mukerji's claim, Anand Kumar stood to lose his own association with the birth of India's first test-tube baby. However, it can be hypothesised that Anand Kumar lost nothing at all, as his credibility – which is well documented in peer citations – remains intact. The professional credit of being associated with the first scientifically documented test-tube baby is more or less secure. What he lacked, however, was credit of a different kind, that no amount of peer citations can generate. This credit or reward is what his scientific partner, Hinduja, walked away with. Hinduja basked in the spotlight of the media (and is also recognised as an able scientist by her peers).

When I first wrote this account in 2002, I concluded that it is difficult to speculate whether official recognition of Mukerji would deny Hinduja what was denied to the rest of the collaborating team all along. And should this happen, the media's attention might shift to the man (Anand Kumar) who dismantled one claim (Hinduja's) and replaced it with another more substantial claim (Mukerji's). In 2002 I was not entirely certain 'whether this hypothesis [would] stand the test of time' (Bharadwaj 2002: 331). However, in 2015 the controversy seems to have been settled. On 26 January 2010, Anand Kumar passed away, ending his illustrious career. A glowing obituary in the *Indian Journal of Medical Research* (2010) observes:

> A man who stood for truth had the greatness to give away his fame and glory of being the pioneer of India's first test tube baby when he discovered all the hand-written notes of Dr Subhas Mukerjee. Dr Mukerjee from Kolkata had claimed to have created a test tube baby in 1979 (the second in the world) but his claims were neither substantiated nor recognized by scientists or the authorities leading to the man ending his life prematurely. Dr Anand Kumar had the courage to research his predecessors' findings and scientifically present it to the world giving Dr Mukerjee his due place in medical history. Such generosity and honesty are very rare and precious attributes of Dr Anand Kumar. (Mehta 2010: 466–67)

Anand Kumar succeeded in crediting Mukerji as the pioneer of Indian IVF. In 2002, the ICMR acknowledged Mukerji's contributions in the National Guidelines for Accreditation, Supervision and Regulation of ART Clinics in India. In 2004, the ICMR director delivered a Memorial Oration named after Mukerji. In 2005, as a rather belated sign of recognition, the West Bengal Health and Family Welfare Department erected a plaque in Mukerji's memory. In 2007, Mukerji's life story and work was published in the *Dictionary of Medical Biography* by the London-based Wellcome Trust Centre for the History of Medicine. These accolades further cemented the claim that Mukerji was responsible for the second test-tube baby in the world within two months of Steptoe and Edwards's breakthrough. In the same year, 2007, his work was recognised by the Brazilian

Medical Society in Sao Paulo. Predictably, a controversy that was born and bred in the mass media had a very public culmination under media spotlight. In April 2011, India's 'first test-tube baby' broke her silence and appeared in the cover story, 'The Doc Who Gave Me Life and Killed Himself', in a popular Indian weekly magazine, *The Week* (3 April 2011). The magazine editorial reads:

> Angst lay buried in their bosom for 30 years, heaving with muted melancholy every now and then. They allowed hope to bloom instead. Now, two women who are part of one of India's biggest achievements have decided to bare their heart ... in this week's cover story, both reveal the beauty and the beast behind what is now accepted as India's first test tube baby. One woman is the test tube baby; the other is the wife of the man who was hounded and called a fraud, making him end the misery by taking his life ... It may be a story straight out of the Roald Dahl stable – dark, depressing and sad – but it is also about hope. It has many heroes: a crusading Sunit Mukherjee, who continued to believe that his friend Subhas the pioneer was a genius; the wife who stood by her husband who chose his research over her; Kanupriya's ['the first test tube baby'] parents who decided to take a gamble; T.C. Anand Kumar, who chose to give up his claim to history to hand it over to a man who had been discredited; and finally Kanupriya, who was brave enough to come out and lend her voice to this cause. 'Dr Anand told me Subhas Mukherji did this because he had to, for the greater cause of humanity. It wasn't just for me' she says. 'I can't let him go down in history as a wannabe', Kanupriya adds. 'Neither should India'. (Matthew 2011: 3)

It is safe to say that this attempt to reconstruct credibility was successful. In the end, scientific credibility and peer recognition were available in abundance to the main protagonists of this story. What was lacking, however, was credibility of a different kind – the kind that only the loving eye of the camera and the affectionate outpouring of the journalist's pen could bestow.

Notes

1. The terms 'credit' and 'credibility' are used here as developed by Bruno Latour and Steve Woolgar (1986) in their seminal text, *Laboratory Life: The Social Construction of Scientific Facts*. Latour and Woolgar make a fundamental distinction, at least analytically, between credit as reward and credit as credibility. They reserve credit as reward for those instances in which there is a sharing of rewards and awards that is also symbolic of

peer recognition of a previous scientific achievement. Credit as credibility, they argue, means scientists' actual ability to do science. Interestingly, they give primacy to the notion of credibility as encompassing scientists' ability to do science, investment strategies, the scientific reward system, scientific education and so on. At the same time, they assert that both credit (reward) and credibility originate essentially from peers' comments about other scientists.

2. Anand Kumar was not the first to report on the events leading up to Mukerji's suicide. Gena Corea (1985b) described in great detail how Patrick Steptoe and Robert Edward's success led to a scramble among gynaecologists and physiologists across the world. Drawing on Mukerji's interview given to CBS reporter Jay McMullen and on *Sydney Morning Herald* reporter Rajan Gupta's report on Mukerji's suicide, Corea (1985b: 139) gives an account of Mukerji's claim and eventual suicide. Similarly, the 1990 award-winning film, *Ek Doctor Ki Mau* (A Doctor's death), was loosely based on the life of Mukerji. The film's director, Tapan Sinha, saw Mukerji's work as an indigenous effort in pioneering IVF technology at the same time as Edwards in the United Kingdom. In the film, the protagonist pioneers a vaccine against leprosy and faces ostracism at home. The last-straw scenario is depicted in the form of two American scientists receiving credit for discovering the same vaccine.
3. Television news bulletins and other programmes mentioned in this chapter for the purpose of elaborating the argument could not be cited, as either the exact date of telecast or the channel on which they were broadcast could not be ascertained. The accounts were obtained during fieldwork from the informant doctors, who had copies of the various television programmes telecast since 1986 – on the subject of infertility and test-tube babies in India – on a personal videotape.
4. Frances Price (1993) contends that in the context of IVF there is a fundamental departure from conventional assumptions about a doctor's role since the so-called doctor or IVF specialist/clinician is 'partnered' with a scientist, and as a consequence there is a division of labour between them (see also Chapter 8). The contest for credibility between Anand Kumar and Hinduja can be viewed as the breakdown of such a partnership.

Chapter 4

Politics of Conception

The State and Biomedicine

The presence of clinically managed infertility in India surprises some. With more than one billion people, India is considered 'overpopulated' and is pursuing an aggressive state-sponsored policy of population control. India is also plagued by poverty and by growth pains typically associated with transitional economies. Thus, infertility and its high-tech management does not resonate with the global perception of the country.

The precise magnitude of infertility and the presence of assisted conception in developing countries is ambiguous. The Indian case is particularly unclear due to a near total absence of research in the area. The reason for this neglect lies partly in the nature of social science debates that have crystallised around the constructed polarities of North and South (Bharadwaj and Glasner 2009). In some of these debates, the West and the developed North is positioned against its binary opposite, the East and the developing South, where the latter is viewed as preoccupied with fertility concerns and the former with the problems of infertility (Lingham 1998; Raymond 1993). Thus the manipulation of fertility is often explained in the context of:

> population policies in the North and South ... [where] women as procreators are central to pro-natalist and anti-natalist population policies ... [Therefore] it is not surprising that developed countries practice pro-natalist policies domestically and anti-natalist policies [are practiced] in the developing countries ... pro-natalist technologies (like IVF) are developed for the white middle-class women of

> the North to achieve 'motherhood', and anti-natalist technologies (injectables, implants, vaccines) are developed to control the fertility of poorer women from the South. (Lingam 1998: 206)

Arguments such as this help to explain the monolithic, Eurocentric, neo-Malthusian discourse of Western population policymakers interested in the 'hyperfertility' of non-Western populations and who view Third World women as unworthy of high-tech Western infertility interventions (Inhorn and Van Balen 2002).[1] However, this position also conceals some of the on-the-ground realities in the countries of both the North and South. Inhorn, for example argues that:

> infertility is inherently political in that it threatens the perpetuation of the body politic. Thus, even when the State attempts to 'control' fertility among a reluctant populace, infertility is rarely viewed as a tenable option, as apparent in the recent proliferation of 'high-tech' infertility clinics in purportedly 'overpopulated', developing countries. (Inhorn 1994b: 459)

Infertility and its medical management may not appear to be in line with the commonly perceived official state policy in India, but it is nonetheless being accommodated under the Reproductive and Child Health (RCH) programme of the Indian Government. A number of complex socioeconomic and political factors underlie this gradual acceptance of infertility as a legitimate reproductive health concern alongside an otherwise antinatalist population policy.

This chapter argues that, to understand the presence of assisted conception in contemporary India, it is important to comprehend the nature of biomedicine in India. It begins with a focus on the role of public sector health care, and locates the emergence of assisted conception in the public/private dialectic that has come to characterise the health care system. In doing this, the chapter relates the evident growth of a high-tech fertility industry in an ostensibly overpopulated country to a number of state policies and, in turn, the private sector's response. The chapter then examines some features of assisted conception in the private sector through a discussion of the strategies that clinicians deploy to establish their work not merely as a branch of biomedicine but also as a successful enterprise. In brief, the chapter argues that the expansion of private sector medical care is closely related to the existing pattern of public/private sector interaction and that the emergence of assisted conception in India is a feature of this dynamic. While much new and cutting edge research has problematised the rise of biotech and pharmaceuticals and corporate hospital care in India, few accounts dwell in any meaningful detail on the political economy of health care and delivery in India. A few, now dated but nevertheless pioneering, accounts on political economy of health in India provide a useful foundation for grappling with the kinds of concerns that drive the argument in this chapter. This book does not regurgitate official health care provision policy; rather it addresses the structural fault lines that run across the health care and biomedical landscape in contemporary India. The figures and statistics are bound to shift and change, but the fault lines remain deeply entrenched in health care policy reforms and initiatives.

The Politics of Biomedical Development in India

Health care provision is acknowledged as the responsibility of the Indian government. Health care, however, is incorporated under the 'State' list of legislation and jurisdiction, different from the 'Union' and 'Concurrent' lists, thus enabling various state governments to assume control and responsibility of health provision for their populations (Venkatratnam 1987). The Indian government in this sense is responsible only for the health of people residing in the Union Territories and for 'Concurrent and Central Subjects', as detailed in India's constitution. However, excessive centralisation means that, although health is a state matter, the states are at best sleeping partners in the process of centralised health care planning and policy implementation. Central guidelines are taken as directives and uncritically applied to the state populations. The genealogy of health planning in postcolonial India can best be summed up as a series of 'Expert Committees' set up by the central government to review the services and delivery systems in the country. For more than five decades these committee reports and recommendations have structured and nurtured health care services and their planning. This process was set in motion by the Bhore Committee in 1946, whose recommendations provided the blueprint for health care policy. This framework has been modified from time to time by subsequent committees once the Planning Commission of India was in place by 1950.[2] Nevertheless, until 1983 there was no formal health policy in India, and only after the signing of the Alma Ata declaration on Health for All by 2000 did the government embark upon the establishment of a formal health care policy.[3]

For the most part, health planning in India has stressed preventive and public health programmes with a rural bias (Jeffery 1988). Indian governments have emphasised rural health care in successive five-year plans. Especially since 1980 rural health needs have received special attention in the shape of massive infrastructural investment and programmes for 'providing primary health care facilities to achieve specific targets'. These targets are: 'a primary health centre (PHC) for every 30,000 people and one sub-centre (SC) per 5,000 people in the plains, and one PHC for 20,000 people and one SC for 3,000 people in tribal and hilly areas' (ICHI 1997: 38). These targets are thought to have 'been more or less achieved in most Indian States' (ICHI 1997: 38). However, due to apathy and neglect, the infrastructure cover has made little difference, and rural PHC health provision remains underutilised due to poor facilities, inadequate supplies, poor management, lack of monitoring, and the promotion of personal interests of the PHC staff coupled with indifference (Banerji 1974; Boerma 1987; Nichter and Nichter 1996; Qadeer 2011; Stark 1985). In addition, as Duggal and Anita (1993) indicate, the PHCs do not serve the health care needs perceived by the people. The PHCs and subcentres essentially provide and promote preventive health programmes. This means that 'curative services are not a priority in this delivery structure, even when they constitute the main need of the people ... The staff of the PHCs and sub-centres spend a major portion of their time in family planning and immunisation work and the least on curative services' (Duggal and Anita 1993: 58).[4]

While the Indian government's commitment to primary rural health care in terms of its willingness to allocate resources cannot be questioned, its failure to realise health benefits for the rural majority from such an investment is more problematic (Baru 2010). A good example is the maternal health programme. The Indian government is trying to tackle conditions of childbearing through better maternal and child health services. The medicalisation of childbirth in India has entailed the establishment of (100 per cent state-sponsored) subcentres, primary health centres, community health centres, staffed by full-time/part-time professionals or para-professionals, along with a universal immunisation programme and the training of traditional birth attendants. In relation to childbearing, the ultimate goal is full antenatal screening by doctors and nurses, with most babies delivered under medical supervision in medical institutions. This ambitious plan is part of the Indian government's commitment to rural public health, yet a staggering 100,000 Indian women die each year in pregnancy and childbirth (NFHS 1992–1993: 226). World Health Organisation (2014) estimates show however that India currently contributes 17 per cent to the maternal mortality rate (MMR), that is, 50,000 deaths per annum. These figures are notoriously difficult to verify; often maternal deaths in rural areas remain undocumented, leading commentators to estimate the actual MMR rate as double of what official figures show. This helps clarify why critics of government health policy focus on elitist and urban-oriented curative hospital based services. Such criticism highlights rural/urban differentials in health sector expenditure. This discrimination goes back a long way. For example, Rao et al. (1993: 107), drawing on ORG data for 1982–1983, argue that 'at the national level, as much as 44 per cent of total health sector expenditure was incurred purely in urban areas, as against 15 per cent in rural areas'. Similarly Duggal and Anita (1993) show that from the first five-year plan to 1986, the number of hospitals increased from 2,694 (117,000 beds) to 7,764 (594,747 beds). In terms of availability to the actual population, the improvement is relatively modest, since in 1951 one hospital served 134,001 persons (3,085 persons per bed) and in 1986, 99,176 persons (1,295 persons per bed). Over time, they argue, the rural-urban differential has only increased. In 1956 the proportion of hospitals in rural areas was '39 percent (and 24 percent of beds) but in 1986 only 21 percent of the hospitals (and 18 percent of beds) were located in rural areas, one rural hospital serving 351,500 rural persons and one rural bed serving 5,478 rural persons' (Duggal and Anita 1993: 56). In contrast, they show that in the same year (1986) one urban hospital served 29,115 urban persons and one urban bed served 392 persons in the urban areas (Duggal and Anita 1993: 56).

Historically, in terms of expenditure, allocations to rural primary health care have been almost 50 per cent of the health budget (Berman 1991; Chatterjee 1987; Jeffery 1988). This complicates the picture, as rural/urban inequity in health care cannot be attributed simply to paltry economic allocations to the former in relation to the latter. In the absence of any credible empirical research in this area, one can only propose a hypothesis for future research; that is, if there is a bias then it may be at the level of health planning and policy, which discriminates and distinguishes between the rural and urban health care needs in terms of preventive and curative needs, rather than in terms of resource allocations. More importantly we need deep ethnographic understanding of the role of the private sector embedded in the 'intricate web of power relations' that are blocking equity in access to health care in India (Baru 2012: 64). Generally speaking, however, the unfulfilled curative needs of the Indian population are being met by growing private sector health care in both rural and urban areas, resulting in a scenario where private sector health care is 'burgeoning but at the cost of public health care' (Sengupta and Nundy 2005). National health accounts for India corroborate this trend and show that health care is provided predominantly by the private sector and to a lesser extent from external sources. The report finds that 'expenditure in the private sector contributes to 78.05 percent of total health expenditure, public sector accounts for 19.67 percent and external flows 2.28 percent. In totality, health expenditure formed 4.25 percent of Gross Domestic Product (GDP)' (Government of India 2009). While the nature of health policy skewed in favour of preventive health care may explain the reliance on the private sector for curative needs in rural India, the situation in urban areas is more complex. Sunil Nandraj (1994) argues that the poor quality of public sector-based curative services, in addition to the public sector's inability to keep pace with the growing demand for health services, is resulting in the spread of private sector health care in urban areas. This, however, does not mean that the 'private hospitals are better equipped, more efficient and manned by better qualified and more humane staff [but rather] public hospitals [have] simply failed to keep pace with the demand' (Nandraj 1994: 1680). In fact, Baru et al. (2000: 2,509) persuasively shows the 'questionable management practices with regard to workers as well as patient care' in private hospitals in Delhi. Duggal and Anita (1993: 56) also argue that the 'the private health sector has grown from strength to strength because there is a vast unmet demand. The government has failed to meet this demand but the private sector has served it, whatever the manner and quality'. As such, the private sector is responding to the unmet health needs of population groups and delivering care that remains largely uneven and inconsistent (Shah and Mohanty 2010).

One unmet or poorly met need is infertility management, which evades the majority of the treatment seekers in rural and urban areas. The government's priority and commitment towards family planning and family welfare means that precious resources could not be spent on any curative aspect of health care that ran contrary to this remit. However, the story of the private sector's entrance as a chief contributor to infertility management cannot be understood as a simple response to an unmet health need. The development of biomedical management of infertility in India follows a more complicated route, one that is part of the rapid expansion of private sector health care itself.

State Policies and the Spread of the Private Sector

Despite its avowed commitment to providing health care and planning, the state in independent India did not curtail private interest in health provision. On the contrary, under the shelter of a mixed economy model, the private and the public health care sectors have established a protracted symbiotic coexistence (Baru 1998, 2008). The closing decades of the twentieth century, however, saw rapid growth in private sector health care (Baru 1998; Bhat 1993; ICHI 1997; Nadkarni 2010; Nandraj 1994; Nandraj et al. 2001).[5] According to some early estimates, the private health sector accounts for nearly 70 per cent of all primary medical care and over 40 per cent of all hospital care (ICHI 1997). In the early 1990s, the share of the private health sector was estimated to lie between 4 and 5 per cent of the gross domestic product (Nandraj 1994). More recently, India's health care sector was estimated to be worth US$75 billion (in 2012–2013) and projected to grow to US$300 billion by 2020 (RNCOS Business Consulting Services 2013).

The rise in the number of private hospitals in India gives an idea of the steady growth of this sector. In 1973 the number of beds in public hospitals stood at 230,161; this figure rose to 365,696 beds in 1993. Compared to this, the number of beds in the private sector increased from 66,926 beds in 1973 to 210,987 in 1993. The difference in growth between the private and public sectors in particular is noteworthy (Baru 1998). An emerging body of evidence, mainly micro-level data focusing on private sector growth in regions of India, such as Ahmednagar district in Maharashtra (Foundation for Research in Community Health 1993) and Hyderabad in Andhra Pradesh (Baru 1998), is providing a closer look at the finer processes of private sector expansion. More recent developments in the 'in-patient care market' suggest that corporate hospitals account for 10 per cent of the private hospital markets (Kanjilal and Mazumdar 2013). Top players, including Apollo Hospitals, Fortis, Max, Escorts, Wockhardt, Reliance and Aditya Birla Group, have accelerated their ambitious expansion plans (Drummer and Cook 2008; Kanjilal and Mazumdar 2013; Lefebvre 2010).

There is, however, a continuing paucity of India-wide data indicating growth trends in private sector health care. This is significant, especially given that scholars researching various facets of health care sectors in India agree on the rapid spread of such private services. The evidence, it appears, for such macro-level generalisations is based as much on the existential experience of Indian researchers as on empirically grounded research in the area. Another important factor is the general lack of regulating mechanisms controlling the application and spread of the private sector health care (Baru 2012; Kanjilal and Mazumdar 2013). Traditionally bodies, such as the medical council of India (MCI) and the state medical councils responsible for maintaining and updating the medical register, have failed to maintain a register of qualified medical practitioners, leading to partial and inconclusive documentation of the spread of private practice in India (Pandya 1995). There is also longstanding and unresolved speculation that the number of hospitals in the private sector is higher than the available data suggests, mainly on account of underreporting (Nandraj 1994). Despite this, the private sector continues to respond to the health care needs of the population in India. Particularly in rural areas, the absence of curative services means that people turn to either government hospitals or poorly qualified or unqualified private practitioners. Numerous studies indicate the high level of dependency on the private sector, dispelling the illusion that the public sector is the primary health provider in the country (Baru 2010, 2012; Duggal and Amin 1989; George et al. 1993; Thankappan et al. 1987; Vishwanathan and Rohde 1990; Yesudian 1990).

The privatisation of health care in India also feeds off specific state policies (Shah and Mohanty 2010). In the most recent decade the government offered several incentives in line with its policy of economic liberalisation. Reduction in import duties on high-technology medical equipment has significantly altered the face of private sector health care. In 1996, for example, the *Economic Times* (5 September 1996) reported medical equipment imports as amounting to 4 per cent of GNP. The report observed that medical care in India has become 'so high-tech ... that almost all medical products are imported. That is, 85 per cent of equipment, 90 per cent of consumables and 98 per cent of medical devices'. Similarly, in 1998 the *Indian Express* (January 1998) reported a healthy growth in the medical equipment sector. Estimating the industry to be in the region of 600 crore rupees, the report spoke of a projected annual growth rate exceeding 20 per cent, 'attracting big-time multinationals to tap this market'. By 2013 more realistic estimates collated by the Federation of Indian Chambers of Commerce and Industry and Ernst and Young showed that 75 per cent of medical devices in the country are imported (Biospectrum 2013).

The private health sector was further promoted by state recognition of medical care as an industry (Baru 1998). The Union Budget of 2003–2004 conferred industry status on hospitals and incentivised financial institutions to provide long-term capital for hospital projects (Shah and Mohanty 2010). It is now possible for individual doctors and private nursing homes to take loans from banks and other financial institutions to upgrade and expand their services. Moreover, industries were allowed to diversify into the health sector and invest in multinational collaborations. The emergence of corporate hospitals has been termed by some as the 'medical industrial complex' (Relman 1987). Apollo Industries in India, for instance, has earmarked 1,250 crore rupees to build over 100 hospitals, of which fifty will be in metropolitan cities, approximately thirty-two will be specialist hospitals in other large cities, with the rest in small towns, according to the *Indian Express* (January 1998). The state has also consented to foreign collaborations in the health sector. According to an article entitled 'Government Gives its Assent for 55 Foreign Tie-Ups' in the *Times of India* (September 1995), as early as in 1995 the government had assented to fifty-five foreign partnerships, of which six were in the health sector. Significant amongst these were the proposals of Ranbaxy Laboratories for a joint venture with an overseas firm to manufacture anti-cancer drugs and of Indraprashtha Medical Corporation Ltd and Sir Edward Dunlop Hospitals (India) Ltd. to run a chain of fifty-six state-of-the-art hospitals, polyclinics and diagnostic centres throughout the country. Also according to this article, a 100-bed cardiac care hospital near Delhi is estimated to cost US$25 million and stated to be financed, owned and operated by a consortium of overseas companies and Indian medical personnel. Since 2000, foreign direct investment (FDI) has been permitted up to 100 per cent under the automatic route for the hospitals sector in India (Sunitha and Ajil Babu 2013). According to Sunitha and Ajil Babu (2013: 38), 'The health care sector received Rs.5022.15 crores in FDI inflows from April 2000 to December 2011 and this increased to Rs.5417.92 crores "by accounting 0.75 [per cent] in total FDI inflows"'.

Since independence, the Indian state has not only invested in infrastructure but has also contributed significantly towards the training of medical and paramedical personnel, which in turn has provided a base (albeit indirect) for the rapid growth of the private sector (Baru 1998). It has been argued that the government policy of training medical personnel with taxpayers' money has effectively subsidised the growth of the private sector (Duggal 1989 in Duggal and Anita 1993).

Medical careers in India's public health sector are far from smooth. Writing in 1977, Roger Jeffery commented that:

> Allopathic doctors do occupy a very privileged position in India and they are striving to achieve a status more closely akin to that of their British and American counterparts. However, they show no signs of being able to improve on their current position, and may well be forced to retreat. The main causes of this situation are the dominant position of the State in India, and the internal disarticulation brought about by Imperial rule in Indian society. (Jeffery 1977: 561)

Jeffrey was alluding primarily to the status of doctors employed in the state sector; his assertion largely, to this day, explains the level of disenchantment within the public sector health workforce. The move away from the state sector and into private practice in contemporary India reflects this sense of disenchantment. Even when in state employment, doctors often continue to practice privately (Venkatratnam 1973, 1987; Baru 1998). The government over the years – as a result of this practice – has tried with little success to eliminate public sector doctors working privately (Chawla 1996). In Andhra Pradesh, for instance, two attempts were made, in 1968 and 1984, to ban private practice of public sector doctors, but on both occasions vehement opposition from the doctors led to a revocation (Baru 1998). Similarly, Rama V. Baru (1998) provides evidence from Utter Pradesh, where since 1975 three successive attempts by the government have failed in the face of opposition from 'top specialists'. Similarly, governments of New Delhi and Madhya Pradesh tried banning private practice by public sector doctors, which 'resulted in an exodus of doctors from the public to the private sector' (Baru 1998: 50). With better pecuniary returns, minimal state interference and control over one's working conditions, the private sector continues to lure a significant number of doctors. This tussle however began to bear fruit as the Supreme Court in 2011 ruled that private practice by a government doctor was neither 'criminal' nor 'corrupt' (Venkatesan 2011).

Against this backdrop, a peculiar feature of Indian health services must be confronted. Roger Jeffery writes that:

> health services are not central to class interests in India, either as benefits to be fought over or as important elements in the reproduction

> of a class-based social structure. The main protagonists are the various kinds of medical practitioners who fight over shares of the cake, rather than the broader ideological issues. (Jeffery 1988: 167)

This observation is made about internal conflicts in the public sector, but, as we shall see in Chapter 4, it is equally true for the burgeoning private sector in the case of assisted conception.

In light of this public and private interaction, the arrival of assisted conception in India can be better understood, especially since high-tech infertility management in India originated in the state sector. This may appear surprising given the Indian state's longstanding commitment to population control. The first scientifically recognised breakthrough – in producing an IVF baby – resulted from a collaboration between the Institute of Research in Reproduction (IRR) controlled by the Indian Council for Medical Research (ICMR) and a Mumbai public hospital. ICMR's annual report of 1986–1987 justified the practice of IVF in a state-controlled research institute by positioning the diagnosis and treatment of infertility as 'complementary to an effective Family Welfare Program' (ICMR 1986: 47). Many argued that this research would lead to a better understanding of the nature of human infertility so that more effective contraception could be developed. The rationale behind this approach was that knowledge of the causes of infertility would provide new insights into the control of human fertility through clinical and non-clinical interventions. In a 1987 interview, IRR director Dr Anand Kumar states:

> The IVF-ER technique has now provided a major and justifiable reason to investigate infertile couples thoroughly and thus has offered many opportunities to identify and study factors contributing to infertility. And, *an understanding of these factors may provide clues as to how to induce infertility in fertile couples as a means of family planning*. There are [a] number of lessons to be learnt from Nature's Workshop which has created the infertile couple. (Lingam 1990; emphasis added)

The IVF project (and its support by the state) was justifiable as long as its development was couched in a vocabulary in tune with the official line of developing effective anti-fertility interventions. The promise of using a pronatalist technology to perfect and deliver antinatalist technologies, however, remained a mere promise throughout the project and was never actualised. Infighting amongst those associated with the project contributed to the final demise of the public sector's fleeting but significant tryst with assisted conception, and this illustrated simultaneously the links between infertility developments and the pursuit of personal status (See Chapter 4). By the end of the 1980s assisted conception was almost entirely overtaken by the private sector. The main protagonists responsible for India's first 'official' IVF baby moved fairly rapidly out of state employment and established thriving private practices of their own, while capitalising on their achievements undertaken in the public sector. Newer players who followed these pioneers benefited from the reduction in import duties on high-tech medical equipment to upgrade their practices, along with loans from banks and other financial institutions to help pay for their expansion plans and move into more super-specialty areas like assisted conception.

Private Practice: Making it Work

A transition from the public to private sector in any sphere accentuates demands for survival, sustainability and profitability. The issue, however, is not simply that the availability of newer medical technology makes the market in medical care an attractive form of investment, as seen by some early commentaries on the topic (Phadke 1993 in Nandraj 1994). When I first began researching IVF in the mid- to late 1990s many physicians in private practices in the West, for instance, were arguing that in entering private practices they were essentially opening small businesses, which brings with it the responsibilities of being an employer, a business person and a physician, and yet, their medical training woefully equip them with these skills (Berrien 1987: 334). In the case of assisted conception in India, this means that individual clinicians not only developed strategies to take advantage of the favourable climate created by the state policies but, having done so, then tried to stay afloat and survive. To do this a clinic needed to replenish itself continuously on two fronts: first, by ensuring an optimal clinical infrastructure, and second, by ensuring a steady inflow of patients for economic viability. In the early years (especially phase I and II) I found that it was not always possible to guarantee the smooth running of the clinic. In the early part of the 1990s infrastructure was a huge problem and, in certain respects, remains a source of worry for smaller players. In the past, clinics faced numerous problems, such as delays in procuring disposables, culture media and spares for the equipment, due to an over-reliance on imported products. Dr Chandra, director of an IVF unit in Delhi, described how infrastructure-related problems routinely faced by the clinic had improved slightly, though she still found the timely procurement of even basic items for embryo manipulation very difficult:

> Procurement of stuff like 'culture media', which has to come from abroad and has to be at a certain temperature, that is still a problem because when you bring in the media you don't know whether the customs has cleared it in time because they leave the boxes (at the airport) and inform you in a day or so. By then everything is ruined. But now agents are coming in, and we hope that they will be able to get the stuff cleared in time and store it at the right temperature because if that doesn't happen then you are not going to get anywhere. If the media is all wrong, you can't get your results.

Likewise Dr Suman, interviewed in her Delhi clinic, commented on the problem of importing 'raw materials', like media, especially since it is routinely held in customs warehouses for long periods of time – her estimate was eight to nine days – thereby yielding inferior results due to poor quality refrigeration.

Dr Sukumari, an IVF practitioner in Bangalore, was more broadly disappointed with the government's attitude towards infertility management. Despite the government policy vis-à-vis liberalising imports of medical products and lowering of import duties, the ART sector did not benefit, in her view, from such moves. In addition, she felt that an over-reliance on imports added to the stress of running a state-of-the-art infertility facility:

> Why there are not that many clinics even though the population has so much infertility? The major factor is government apathy to the whole programme, so where they could cut down customs duty and make it sort of life-giving category, we still pay hefty customs duties for the ingredients. For example on plastic we have to pay 40 percent, or if you've got to get some equipment it costs almost 80 percent on customs. How can we import so much? It takes minimum six weeks so we really got to plan six months ahead before we decide that we need something. So anything you need in an emergency there is nowhere you can go and get it straight off the shelf. Actual aspiration needles, disposables for example, we may have a sudden rush of patients sometime and we don't have, or you have the media prepared and kept and you have a short shelf life of media so obviously the hospital pays for it. Then you have to get new media and then new media again if you have not used it, and then there is a sudden rush of patients, you are short of media and then you can't get it! In 1991 when I started the clinic, including the water I had to import. Media is fine, the water in which the media is to be mixed – that also I went

> and got from abroad. So there was a situation when I got ten cases of only water as I came from the UK, so you can imagine the extent we have to go to and you become the domestic, you become the helper, you become the office boy, you become the boss, you become the medical director, you become the administrator, you become the tax consultant – you have to do many things...

However, Dr Sukumari was not alone in her frustration in running an ART programme in the 1990s. It was evident from my visits that delays in supplies frequently frayed the tempers of consultants and made routine practice highly stressful. An excerpt from field notes at a Delhi IVF unit run by Dr Neeta explains how altercations between the suppliers and the doctors can cause disruptions. On 5 June 1998, Dr Neeta, on calling her medium supplier, learnt that it was out of stock, which precipitated a ten-minute shouting match over the phone. Slamming the phone down, the doctor, visibly upset, bemoaned:

> I am fed up, tired, and I don't know what to do with these people. He committed that third of every month the medium would reach me, now he is saying he can't do it. These people lie to you! They are basically dishonest and don't speak truthfully. I have been trying to get through to these people that I need the medium. My patients are scheduled. What answer should I give them? Now he is saying [to] use B2 medium. These people are dishonest, they are compulsive liars; on purpose they mislead. I told him the very first day, 'Give me one date, should I keep eighth for the patients?' 'Yes!' Liar! Now there is no medium! He did not even bother to call and inform me – at least he should have done that. Now he is saying, 'Why are you shouting at me? Everybody in Delhi uses a different medium as and when it is available,' but I am not everybody. I want the medium I have ordered. I feel so sorry for the patients the amount they suffer [because of such delays]. He is saying [that I should] use the washing medium for the egg culture. How dare he suggest that! What will happen if the eggs don't hatch? What answer do I have then? Shameful! This morning when my assistant called them they told her that we could use other medium, as the one he promised is not in stock. All my energy is spent chasing this kind of stuff. The representatives feel that I am making so much fuss, because all the other clinics adjust to other brands, but I refuse to be like the rest. This is highly unprofessional.

Dr Sukumari and Dr Neeta established their clinics in a newly economically liberalised India in 1991. They faced many obstacles, most unexpected. Their gripe seems quaint if we fastforward twenty years to 2010–2011, where 'not only is it cheaper now to set up an IVF lab – about Rupees 40 lakh or less ($66-67,000 approx.) – it's also far easier' (Pratap 2011). For example, duty on imported equipment that was once as high as 115 per cent has fallen to 25 per cent even though exchange fluctuations and vagaries of international market keeps the impact of these changes largely mixed (Pratap 2011). Several established and new infrastructure players in the field are delivering ART setup on a 'turnkey' basis. From representing leading international brands to procuring and setting up clinics, these 'one-stop shop' solutions have made it easier for newer IVF specialists to enter the field. However, the decrease in setup costs notwithstanding, it is simplistic to assume that somehow IVF clinics are now inexpensive to create. The constant need to fund expansion keeps costs high in the face of patient recruitment. In other words, the added demands of running the clinic at an optimal level has remained unchanged for the more than fifteen years I have been observing IVF practices in India. Dr Sachin, a consultant heading three IVF units in Southwest and a fourth in North India, routinely divides his time between various clinics. In doing this he follows pre-programmed cycles. For example, twelve days before he is due to arrive at one of his clinics, a batch of twenty patients are put on Metrodin followed by an HCG (Human Chorionic Gonadotropin) shot on the tenth night. On his arrival, the doctor goes straight into egg retrieval, followed by culture, and by the fourteenth day the embryos are transferred. This is a high-risk strategy of managing four clinics simultaneously and requires a high level of investment to keep the programme running smoothly:

> We have to keep stand-by equipment everywhere, because it is a batch – it's a big risk! See, if there is one patient and the incubator fails, okay, I can explain to the patient that there was a laboratory problem. But if there are thirty patients and you have only one incubator and the incubator goes knocks (*sic*) you can't explain to each one of them how each one lost 35,000 rupees on drugs. So everywhere we have stand-bys, two to three incubators, UPS (uninterrupted power supply), stand-by generators, three ultrasound machines, everything in duplicate and triplicate, foolproof, you know, so nothing can go wrong.

Backing up operations is a common practice in IVF clinics across India. Given the highly unreliable nature of power supply, clinics with embryo freezing programmes take extra care to have UPS systems to prevent mishaps. Dr Sushila, an IVF practitioner in Bangalore, found the vagaries of electricity supply the most stressful aspect of doing IVF in India. Fluctuating voltage and routine power cuts necessitated efficient backup management: Dr Sushila said, 'We have three UPS machines, two generators, one is 25 kva and the other is 40 kva, and then for everything you have to have a backup and for a backup another backup! If we did not have these problems we would have done so much more'. The key to success, however, is to recruit enough new patients to fill an expensive ART programme put in place often at a great financial cost to the clinician. This is the hardest part of setting up a new centre. Dr Sachin summed up the pressures of setting up a private practice:

> Any person who starts an ART centre has very, very high stress level. The reason is that there is a pressure for results if you succumb to that pressure and start doing, you know, that kind of thing – mixing gametes and whatever which can happen in some centres – then you are lost in the long run. Patients find out, everyone finds out, and you have [a] bad reputation. But if you bear the pressure because there is a learning curve, a growth phase for any ART centre is minimum 2.5 to 3 years, 1000 days, come out of that then there is no problem. [The] first three years are very testing. Patients come and they take half a cycle and then drop out, walk into another centre – they'll talk there (that there are no results here) or you can get only very elderly patients, they are the ones who wait for results to come. This is not only here. I am running four centres and everywhere we started the first year has been bad – all 39, 40, 41 years old. The younger ones say let some results come, let some IVF pregnancies occur then we'll come for treatment. Unless you get young ones you can't have a good ongoing pregnancy rate so it becomes a vicious cycle. It breaks someday, but you have to really withstand the pressure. It's too much!

The implications of these uncertainties faced by clinicians running ART facilities helps to clarify a number of ongoing developments in this sector. In the 1990s and early 2000s a great deal of money was invested by clinicians entering the field, either from personal resources or borrowed from financial institutions, to fund expansion plans and to ensure the smooth day-to-day operations. This compounded the problem of costs incurred in inducing conception, especially since they were passed on to patients, which in turn deterred many patients from pursuing treatment. To this day, filling an IVF programme with patients means using innovative clinical methodology capable of inducing conception and sourcing patients from untapped reserves, along with implementing other cost-cutting measures to hold on to infertile recruits (see Chapter 8). This trend in the private sector is gradually resulting in a string of transnational collaborations with ART clinics in the West, which in turn are looking at India as a new potential growth area in the twenty-first century for expanding both clinical practice and research. For example, recently Morpheus ART, a German-Indian medical company, has set up centres in India and currently offers a 'second cycle at "no extra procedural cost" if the first cycle did not result in pregnancy' (Pratap 2011). Similarly the Bourn Hall Clinic – credited with creating the world's first IVF baby, Louise Brown, in 1978 – is making large investments in India and is expected to set up over fifteen centres across the country. Some clinicians view partnerships with clinics in the West as inevitable, especially given the stringent controls on research and development in Euro-American countries. Dr Chandra, for instance, spoke of how some experts in the West are 'very keen to come in because things that are not allowed because of government policy there they can try out here. So you do find people trying to find out if they can do a particular thing and have an association here to do it because the government policy is not stringent'. Though she did not specify what 'thing[s]' these people wished to do in India, the rapid technology transfer from the West to India appears to occur without any governmental control. Dr Lalit, head of his own IVF unit in Mumbai, also alluded to these benefits:

> There is a report in England that they are not allowing testicular spermatid [stem cell spermatozoa] injections, so one unit has affiliated with some unit in India – I don't know which one in India. You know Simon Fisher started injecting and so they have put a ban on that, so to bypass that they have come to India. I think there is some controversy in England saying if you don't allow we are going to go to some country that does ... So its better you allow it and regulate it and use it for good purpose because technology cannot be suppressed ... There are scientists for whom there is only one frontier, that of science, there is no frontier of country if he is obsessed with the work and if his country were to prevent him he'll go somewhere else ... So the British team is coming here and doing it. You cannot suppress scientific quest for knowledge.

While the use of immature germ cells, spermatid, in intracytoplasmic sperm injection (ICSI) procedures yields results, and reportedly a number of healthy offspring, ethical concerns led the United Kingdom to ban the use of spermatids for ICSI altogether (Vloeberghs et al. 2013). However, the benevolent march of noble scientific curiosity into the developing world in the face of bureaucratic resistance requires a separate research inquiry. The production of medical knowledge and its consumption requires the direct involvement of citizens and subjects (Das 2000). Western IVF research could well follow the experience of anti-fertility vaccine clinical trials in several parts of the world, including India, where the bodies of poor women become the points of application of a developing knowledge under test (Viswanath and Kirbat 1998). While the spread of transnational surrogacy is now a well-established concern (see Chapter 6), serious risks associated with 'routine' fertility procedures such as oocyte retrieval are also receiving critical attention globally (Nahman 2013) and in India (Chatterjee and Janwalkar 2014). In addition to ethical concerns surrounding the outcomes of long-term research collaboration, and the eventual rewards that such efforts would bring to the interested parties, a more immediate commercial dimension of this North-South collaboration has begun to emerge in India. Inaugurating its first India centre, Bourn Hall Clinic Chief Executive Mike Macnamee was reported as describing India as 'the most under-served market in IVF' (Pratap 2011). Private equity investors are also seeking to invest in the infertility market in tandem with big corporate hospitals across Indian cities. Individual expansion plans of celebrity doctors who feature prominently across Indian mass media can only materialise through equity investments or, as the recent trend suggests, through strategic connections with big corporate hospitals where these clinicians run their practice on a rotational basis. However, these developments notwithstanding and big corporate and equity interest in ARTs aside, there is much more to running an IVF practice as a successful, viable business than financial investment. Dr Sachin's estimated 1000-day cycle of an IVF clinic remains the rule of thumb. For example, Reliance Life Sciences IVF practice, an initiative of Indian multinational giant Reliance Industries, underperformed and closed due to lack of adequate oversight in 2010 (Pratap 2011). Despite these pressures in an uneven IVF landscape, doctors continue to forge collaborations and press ahead with expansion programmes, contributing to the globalised birth market (Sarojini et al. 2011). Dr Manker, a clinician from Ahemdabad, Gujarat, has gone on to set up a private limited company with a percentage share-holding in collaboration with a famous Australian ART centre. The unique selling proposition of this unit is to provide reasonable and affordable IVF to as many parts of the country as possible. Identifying the cost of IVF as the biggest hurdle in recruiting new patients, Dr Manker and his team used the collaboration to bring in a whole range of treatments that spread the initial investment across the group of four partners. The size of the group means they could draw in more patients; the higher the patient intake, the more easily the infrastructure costs could be distributed amongst the incoming patients, thus considerably reducing the cost per patient. The crux of this programme, however, was to bring down the cost of drugs, the single most expensive input in an ART intervention. Favouring clomiphene citrate over the expensive GnRH (gonadotrophin releasing hormone) analogues for inducing ovulation worked out to be a much cheaper stimulation protocol mechanism, making the treatment extremely competitive. The Australian collaborators had spent a great deal of time researching the use of clomiphene citrate in inducing ovulation, and this expertise, according to Dr Manker, worked in their favour. This effectively meant that by inducing many cycles with the help of clomiphene citrate they could bring down the drug cost by 50 per cent. In addition, a good freezing programme imported from Australia further helped in reducing cost, as embryos could be stored for future use. However, using clomiphene citrate instead of GnRH analogues has its own problems and shortcomings, according to other clinicians. When asked if such an approach could double up as a sound practice for lowering drug/treatment costs, clinicians produced differing responses. Dr Suman for instance opined:

> It is a good idea, but clomiphene citrate is not the drug of choice for every patient. Again you have to be selective; it may not help you to go through seven cycles of clomiphene citrate and you may achieve nothing and one Hmg may do the trick, so depends on the patient selection. You cannot standardise it.

Dr Sachin, on the other hand, had more practical concerns about clomiphene citrate vs GnRH:

> Yah! But then if the cost of bringing down [affects] the success rates, I would not be in favour of changing it. Success has to be maintained. If we can simply maintain the 32 percent pregnancy rate [using clomiphene citrate], all for it. There are lot of other critical parameters with CC alone or Hmg alone. In a busy ART centre we would not like to experiment like that. There is too much competition right now. I must be the youngest probably in Mumbai doing IVF so the pressure is really very high. In this area alone you can go walking from here to six of the best IVF centres in the country, so you can imagine the pressure. And in that kind of pressure what ultimately counts is success rates, everything else is immaterial. If I start experimenting trying

> to bring down costs and do something here and there, which I think might bring down the cost, but if my success rate goes down I am finished! So I can't take that risk!

Indian pharmaceutical players such as Sun Pharma, Alkem Pharma and VHB Life Sciences have established a presence in the IVF hormones sector, and this helps to lower costs (Pratap 2011). However, the bulk of the medicine and equipment used in Indian IVF is imported. Like Dr Sachin, many clinicians feel that using domestic products is too risky as a result of brand perception and a preference for established imported products (For a more detailed discussion on this, see the Afterword.) In the context of the foregoing, the emergence of low-cost IVF (LCIVF), a decade-long struggle to make IVF affordable and accessible, is an important step in the right direction (see Inhorn and Patrizio 2015). However, as the foregoing also shows, it will be an uphill task to persuade practitioners like Dr Sachin to embrace the low-cost variants as lowering costs can also precipitate the fear of lowering success rates.

The pressure to keep up with ongoing pregnancies, therefore, becomes a vicious circle, to which Dr Sachin referred, as pregnant patients become central to recruiting new hopefuls and any cost-cutting measure could easily sound the death-knell for a clinic. Clinicians like Dr Sushila also feel pressured to keep the pregnancies going in order to ensure the commercial viability of the clinic:

> They [patients] are spending a lot of money. If they weren't spending their money there wouldn't be so much pressure on us ... They will say [if there are no results], 'You've cheated us'. Then they come ask you, 'What is the percentage [of success]?' The thing is if you don't get enough people you don't get enough pregnancy. In the sense, if you do get 20 people you may get five pregnancies. What if we did not keep up a certain figure all the time? They must see some kind of advertisement, say for example, somebody they are coming for the first time and somebody will say [presumably at the clinic], 'Oh! IVF patient pregnant or IUI patient pregnant!' – that kind of thing. It is not as though it's a put-on show or a drama or anything because it happens in the hospital. It is a small hospital, and everybody knows everybody and they know what is happening and they know IUI patients. Four of them became pregnant and none of the IVF patients became pregnant. If this kind of thing goes on next time I can't get any patients for IVF, so I have to keep the fire burning all the time!

The predominantly commercial nature of clinical interventions and patient/consumer expectations means that new kinds of 'risks' are created for clinicians. For instance, on 28 July 2011, a New Delhi fertility expert was asked to pay rupees 15 lakhs ($24,500 approximately) in damages for a failed IVF procedure. The Delhi State Consumer Disputes Redressal Commission ruled in favour of the thirty-five-year-old plaintiff who claimed that the expert in question proceeded with the embryo transfer despite her insisting on deferring the process until she had recouped from an infection (Chowdhury 2011).

The commercialisation of babymaking entails being able to deliver the promised goods. This in turn creates pressures to acquire new infertile bodies. For clinicians like Dr Manker, this means tapping unexplored markets. To do this, he and his partners set up a chain of local collaborations with doctors in smaller cities and towns to source untapped infertility patients. According to Dr Manker:

> We have recently started with four satellite centres, which are not big cities but comparatively smaller, basically town level cities which do not have facilities for IVF. But they have a gynaecologist who has an infertility practice, who does trans-vaginal sonography and that doctor tends to the adjoining rural areas, so what we have done is to call them to our clinic and taught them the art of monitoring itself, not the actual IVF procedure but monitoring the patient response like how she is responding to the drugs. So what they do is once the patient comes to him and he may feel that the patient needs IVF they would send the patient to us just for an initial screening and adjustment, and we decide a protocol for that particular patient and we pass the patient over to the local doctor. That doctor then stimulates and monitors so that the patient need not come to our place during the entire cycle. Only when the patient is ready for [egg] pick-up, the patient then comes to us, stays at our clinic only for three days and goes back. So access is easier because the local doctor drains [exhausts or empties] a large local area. We ultimately plan to go even into smaller towns provided we get doctors who have the capacity to monitor patients. That forms the crux, unless the monitoring is good we cannot really help them.

'Draining' a local area with alliances therefore replicates in microcosm the approach adopted by the Australian partner of draining the Indian market with local collaborators. For the Australian clinic, India was one of several business interests in Asia. Dr Manker explained that his overseas partner had similar commercial interests in China and Malaysia. Whether it is a local clinician or a global player, the search for new markets and patients and a consistently high success rate is central to effective and profitable functioning.

The situation is further problematised on account of a weak infrastructure in the country and its subsequent effects on the costs of investment in equipment and other essential backup. Given these constraints, what can possibly explain the growing trend amongst gynaecologists in India to upgrade their practice to include high-tech infertility management?

Naomi Pfeffer (1987), commenting on what infertility experts in the West stood to gain from the introduction of in vitro fertilisation, argued that, since investigating and treating infertility had long been afforded low status in the medical hierarchy, the new techniques provided gynaecologists with an 'exciting high-status area of research as well as a technically complex practice which only they could use'. She argued that, prior to the introduction of these techniques, a gynaecologist hoping to specialise in reproductive medicine had little to boast of, but pressures towards specialisation within gynaecology brought with it not only official recognition, but higher specialist status – and also greater financial compensation – by demarcating the skills of the reproductive medical specialist from those of the general practitioner and the general obstetrician-gynaecologist (Pfeffer 1987: 87). In the Indian case, the rapid movement of gynaecologists into a new super-specialty can similarly be viewed as aligned with a potentially elevated status and greater financial reward. This trend has resulted in greater demarcation and guarding of professional boundaries between niche expertise and routine gynaecological work, with a corresponding polarisation in the field of reproductive medicine. It ties in with Jeffery's (1988: 167) contention, above, on how 'various kinds of medical practitioners fight over shares of the cake, rather than the broader ideological issues'.

A tug of war over professional territories and expertise has, as a consequence, turned patient clients into a commodity around which both sides – gynaecologists and infertility practitioners – feel they must tighten their grip in order to secure survival in the field. Acquiring new patients and holding on to existing ones is therefore central to this professional struggle. Moreover, gynaecologists doing routine work are viewed as incapable of handling infertility cases. According to Dr Suman:

> Most of the people are not even aware of what is assisted conception. You would be surprised at the type of questions that we are asked from our [gynaecologist] colleagues. They have no idea about IVF and other assisted reproductive techniques, simpler ones even. That is why they cannot manage the patient themselves, but at the same

> time they have this feeling that if the patient goes to so-and-so the patient is not going to come back to them, and I think it is maybe an ego problem, as they would say, or feeling of competition with others, but for the patient it is very sad. They end up coming to us very late once they have passed their prime reproductive age. That is why we say we don't have very many patients coming to us.

While Dr Suman draws a boundary between routine gynaecological understanding and super-specialty insights into infertility, underpinned by a fear of losing out to the competition, other clinicians viewed it as an issue of professional jealousy. Dr Kamraj, an IVF specialist based in Madras, articulated this most forcefully:

> There is something called, well something that you are not able to eradicate, you can say jealousy or whatever. I am sorry to say but doctors try to push you out. So to be honest, I have not had even one reference from Madras itself – none! All these years, my first baby is now six or seven years old. Now of late, maybe just recently one or two references from Madras but from doctors whom I don't know at all. But my own doctor, a doctor who is helping me in my caesarean when I am not in station, until today has not referred even one case [from her practice] to me, not even one case! And she is practicing ObGyn like me. You mean to say she never gets tubal blocks? She's never had an ectopic pregnancy? She's never had pelvic inflammatory disease? She will take them to my rival institutes!

Gynaecologists who fail to refer their patients to fertility specialists generally do so out of plain fear of losing patients for good. The crux of the problem is that both routine-care gynaecologists and gynaecologists who specialise in reproductive morbidity and infertility continue to practice routine gynaecological and infertility-related work. Dr Lalit clarifies:

> [Currently] four to five thousand IVF cycles [some estimate that this figure in 2010 stood at 90,000 cycles] are being done in this country where the potential is for 200,000 cycles which people can actually afford ... [This is] because of lack of communication, lack of awareness, lack on the part of the gynaecologists to refer ... It is not a weak referral system; it is a system where doctors feel if they referred their patients they would lose the general part of infertility patients. Also it is a natural response; I won't blame them ... The general gynaecologist does cater to 80 percent of the population of the infertile couples which can be treated by AID [Artifical Insemination Donor]. Also suppose the patient comes to my outpatient and says, 'I am infertile'. I would treat him. I won't say, 'Okay you don't come to me. I am only

> doing IVF, or I am doing only micro'. Probably if I start doing that, [gynaecologists] will refer more cases. That's the point to be noted, maybe if I tell [patients], 'Look, I am not doing routine treatment', I will get referrals ... We have to be financially viable. At the present stage we have to do routine treatment as well to make it financially viable because the referrals are not good. It is a Catch-22 situation.

Panic among gynaecologists who either do not aspire to set up IVF centres of their own or who do not possess the resources for such an expensive upgrade in their practice is therefore understandable. Not every infertile individual needs high-tech medical intervention, and yet in keeping with the line of holding on to their clients, cases that do need to be referred to specialists end up languishing with general practice gynaecologists precisely because of a fear of losing business.[6]

Some clinicians have tried to find a workable compromise with gynaecologists and have in the process worked out a division of labour that allows them to share infertile patients and profit from them at the same time. Dr Sukumari, for example, has benefited from this experience:

> Most of the self-styled infertility specialists also do obstetrics practice, and there is an innate fear within the person who refers the case that the case is lost forever. This kind of feeling makes them so insecure that, even if they know that a person is doing only routine infertility work, but because that person is attached to a nursing home and that person has access to gynaecological and obstetric work, they just don't bother and play an active part in restraining the patient. But here the system has changed because here eight out of ten patients are referred patients to the clinic. It is because I insist that they have a doctor before they come and see me so that I can liaise with the doctor with reference to the treatment and then get back to the doctor for further antenatal management. I send them back to their doctors. I don't want to run a maternity clinic here.

Dr Manker, similarly, is among a group of clinicians who have successfully adapted to the psychology behind weak referrals. He has tailored his practice to overcome the fears of local gynaecologists by making them partners in the game of drafting new infertile recruits by 'draining local areas' so as to keep an expensive ART project running at its optimum level. In addition, large wealthy clinics in major Indian cities are now routinely holding workshops, scientific symposia and academic conferences to publicise their facilities. In so doing, they not only invite active media participation, they also court a sizeable chunk of invited members of the 'gynaecological community' to work out a mutually beneficial mechanism referrals for infertile patients in the private practice of these gynaecologists (Bharadwaj 2000).[7]

Conclusion

Over the years, the Indian state's support for private interest in (bio) medicine has significantly altered the face of investment in modern high-tech medical facilities. The recent decade has seen more rapid growth in predominantly curative private practice than among preventive public health initiatives. This in turn has not only established a trend where individuals and industries alike are making investments in the private medical sector, but has also encouraged those seeking curative medical support to evade the public sector. This development cannot be dismissed as a difference of interests between private and public health sector priorities; rather, it is the product of a long sustained interaction between the two.

The journey of assisted conception from its humble public sector beginnings to a virtual private sector monopoly is located in this broader context. A technology initially developed at the government's expense and behind the smoke screen of a search for effective contraception soon broke new ground by passing into the hands of enterprising gynaecologists, who saw an unprecedented opportunity to enhance their professional, financial and social standings.

The normalisation of infertility and its high-tech medical management in the private sector has had a knock-on effect on the Indian state. Emerging information indicates that the government is reconsidering its role in assisting conception. With the Ministry of Health and Family Welfare and its nodal units struggling to look after the health needs of one billion citizens, the Indian state must finally contend with the idea that aspects of health, such as reproductive health, that have potential family welfare consequences for individuals – such as those due to infertility – deserve attention, even if they sit uncomfortably with its stated policy interests of population control. The first direct reflection of this policy shift can be seen in the recommendations of the National Committee on Research in Human Reproduction, instituted by the government. In its 1997 Reproductive Health Research Needs Assessment report, the committee lists as a priority the management of infertility in the national programme. The report justifies this inclusion on the grounds that:

> A significant proportion of couples of reproductive age suffer primary or secondary infertility in our country. This problem can be overcome to a great extent by developing graded facilities for investigation and management of infertile couples at different levels of primary health care infrastructure with proper referral support facilities including those requiring Assisted Reproductive Technology (ART) procedures. (Government of India 1997)

This signals a significant departure from the posture previously adopted by the state on prioritising population control as its sole reproductive health concern for the greater part of its post-independence existence. In 2004 the president of the Federation of Obstetric and Gynecological Society of India similarly observed how official policy was still obsessed with family planning in the face of the 'growing problem of infertility' (Panicker 2004). More recently the National Institute for Research in Reproductive Health (NIRRH), part of the Indian Council for Medical Research, observed that infertility is a problem not only in urban, but also rural, India. The NIRRH claimed that the the government wants to ensure that people in both rural and urban areas 'get access to economical infertility treatment at state-run health centers' (Iyer 2013). Judging by the success of its population control programme and safe motherhood initiatives it remains to be seen whether the state will once again traverse the familiar road of spending precious resources on its stated objectives without succeeding in securing substantial health benefits. In the meantime, the private sector continues to strengthen as more private capital is invested to sustain and expand it. The presence of assisted conception within a supportive climate of private health sector expansion necessitates a closer examination of the conditions that have assisted the emergence of technological management of infertility in India. It is to this issue that we now turn.

Notes

1. Germaine Greer (1984: 52) observes in *Sex and Destiny* that 'one of the more unthinking expressions of Caucasian contempt for other peoples is the assumption that they are all hyper-fertile and "breed like rabbits"'. This 'mindset' was challenged head on by the landmark Cairo declaration and International Conference on Population and Development

(ICPD) Programme for Action in 1994. While most countries post Cairo abandoned the notion of 'population policies', there is some evidence to suggest that the mindset that dreamed up these polices remains intact. For example, while the notion of pro-natalism became somewhat problematic in the post Cairo global order, some Western countries have adopted proactive 'demographic security polices.' Similarly, while India abandoned targeted and target based anti-natalist population polices in the late 1990s, these do reappear to this day in the guise of 'expected levels of achievement.'

2. Some of the committees since the Bhore committee of 1946 include: Mudaliar Committee 1961, Chadah Committee 1963, Mukerjee Committee 1965, Jungalwala Committee 1967, Jain Committee 1968, Kartar Singh Committee 1973 and Shrivastava Committee 1975.
3. Prior to this, the directions on health issues were provided by the Constitution of India, the National Development Council (NDC), the Planning Commission, the Central Council of Health and Family Welfare, and the Consultative Committees attached to the Ministry of Health and Family Welfare (ICHI 1997).
4. See also Bajpai (2014) and Qadeer (2011).
5. This is partly attributed – as discussed – to the rural/urban differentials in and overall response to public (curative) health coverage.
6. See Chapter 7 for further discussion on this and how this affects patients who feel mistreated by gynaecologists.
7. My earlier research highlights the beginning of this trend.

Part III

Multiple conceptions animate the life-giving and life-altering domain of the assisted search for conception. This assistance appears and disappears in many guises, but most notably as biomedical technologies, tactical alliances within and without families, and problematic intimacy with 'surrogate strangers' who may be adopted or made supplemental. Part III examines how, despite culturally entrenched normative ideas about relatedness and connectedness, complexities underscoring assisted conception are tacitly understood and reconciled within the conjugal unit and the wider family. In doing this, those who struggle with infertility actively persist in seeking treatment, thereby making sense of repeated disappointment within the wider contexts of social hostility and logistical urgency. The chapters that follow examine the conceptual underpinnings of IVF, donor gametes, adoption and surrogacy arrangements and how they assimilate into intersections of family and kinship, state and citizenship, market and clinic, morality and ethics, and the public and private.

Chapter 5

CHANGING CONCEPTIONS?

'ADOPTION' OF ASSISTED CONCEPTION

On 28 June 1997, a leading fertility expert from Mumbai, appearing on a daytime talk show, argued that it was unfair to put the burden of adoption on the shoulders of the infertile. Not only does Indian society look down upon the practice, but adoption accentuates the stigma of infertility. The only way to destigmatise adoption and make it an acceptable family founding alternative, she asserted, was to encourage fertile couples to openly adopt children alongside conceiving children of their own. The infertility expert in question had touched a raw nerve, a contentious issue lying at the heart of the lived experience of infertility in India – that is, is child adoption an acceptable alternative to infertility and is it a culturally desirable solution?

Child adoption receives varying degrees of social scientific attention across cultures. While adoption remains one of the least researched and poorly understood aspects of contemporary Indian reality, a steady trickle of literature emanates from diverse cross-cultural locales. Judith Modell's (1994, 2002) anthropological account of adoption and interpretation of kinship in American culture views the 'fictive' kinship bonds created by adoption in the context of what she calls the 'as-if principle in American adoption': namely, the adoptive family is viewed 'just like' a biological family, the child 'as-if-begotten' and the parents 'as-if-genealogical'. Thus, open adoptions in America increasingly undermine the 'structures and ideologies that have sustained a fictive kinship in American culture' (Modell 1994: 225–36). More recently, Modell has examined the politics of child fostering in Hawaii. There, fostering is seen as protecting the child in the eyes of the state, but it is viewed less positively by the Hawaiian people in her research, as fostering simply 'disappears' the child forever (Modell 1998).

Marcia Inhorn's (1996a, 1996b) work in Egypt sheds light on the complexities of permanent quasi-adoptive child fostering in a region where the adoption of children is both prohibited under Islamic law and culturally unacceptable. Skramstad's (2000) research in the Muslim West African country of Gambia similarly observes that fostering, while a well-established practice, remains, as in the case of the Egyptian urban poor in Inhorn's study, an inadequate substitute for biological motherhood. Similar studies are situated in a wide range of geographic locales, like issues surrounding adoption and identity in Britain (Haimes and Timms 1985) and informal fostering arrangements in Sierra Leone (Bledsoe 1990).

In India, on the other hand, social science research has woefully neglected the issue of child adoption, and much remains to be done to better understand how child adoption is perceived in the context of intractable infertility. Shalini Bharat's (1993) study of sixteen adoption agencies located in five cities/towns of Maharashtra State is perhaps one of few accounts to delve into the quantitative aspects of adoption trends in India today.[1] Bharat's (1993) research quantitatively details 4,526 cases and broadly suggests that the majority of Indian child placements are in foreign homes (67 per cent) as opposed to Indian homes (33 per cent).[2] The research also reveals that the majority of children up for adoption are homeless, destitute and unwanted. She identifies a worrying gender inequity in placements especially in relation to children adopted under the Hindu Adoption Act (details to follow) where two-thirds of the adopted children were found to be male. Given the limits resulting from this lack of research, Bharat's study emerges as an invaluable empirical contribution to the understanding of adoption practices and trends in contemporary India.

The infertile, who, prior to the advent of high-tech conception possibilities, turned to adoption as the only means of forming a family, are now either delaying adoption as the last resort if 'all else fails' (namely, routine gynaecological and other medical interventions like IVF and ICSI) or turning reluctantly to adoption on account of financial hardship, since assisted conception is available only to the more middle-class and affluent urban elite. In either case, adoption is grudgingly accepted, and it is not entirely clear why this is the case. The societal stigma attached to adoption is yet another dimension that remains largely unexamined. There is only hearsay evidence available on the severity of societal disapproval of the practice and how it stigmatises infertile individuals further, given that they already face social ostracism on account of their inability to reproduce.

This chapter seeks to understand how individuals grapple with the option of adoption in the context of reproduction gone awry and examines the cultural roots of this complex issue in contemporary India. It explores the stigma associated with infertility treatments that involve donated gametes to adoption – the inclusion of a 'third party' that fractures culturally conceptualised boundaries of family. This chapter shows how individuals deal with infertility and its medical management by focusing on the workings of private/invisible and public/visible demarcations, often established with the tacit compliance of the family and the wider community. In doing this, the chapter argues that the separations between the private and the public or the invisible and the visible are not spatially removed so as to constitute opposing categories; rather the private/invisible realms are maintained by the interested parties in order to construct a credible public and visible persona. Adoption, it is argued, is often feared as fracturing efforts to build the visuality of credible and normatively compliant fertility.

Practical Conception: Making the Visible Invisible

In India, infertility – like fertility – is publicly visible and hence an object of social control and management. Fertility not only makes conception and reproduction visual entities, but also makes human sexuality publicly visible. The absence of offspring in a marriage therefore becomes more visible then their presence. This means that any measures to restore the 'visuality' of fertility must traverse socially defined and approved routes well within the bounds of marriage. As in many cultures across the world, Hindu cosmology views an intimate connection between the body and the progeny. This corporeal connection between married body and its offspring is at once biological and social (Chapter 1). A 'double conceptual bind,' such as this, coalesces the biological and the social in a way that results in a consequent symbiosis between the visible and invisible. It allows for a cogitation of the visible social triad of mother/father/child as underscored by an invisible, immutable biological triangle of womb, semen and foetus.

Infertility becomes a stigmatised condition (Chapter 2) when these superimposed triads are destabilised by a married partnership. Married couples who turn to assisted conception do so to restore the (visible) 'social triad' and to create an illusion of culturally 'unproblematic visuality' of fertility. It is, therefore, not uncommon for individuals to seek medical help to induce conception if cohabitation does not produce a pregnancy within few months of marriage (for details see below). Once the decision to seek treatment is undertaken, the focus shifts to coalescing the management strategy with normative values, while justifying the treatment firstly to the self and secondly to the community at large. Both the resort to assisted conception and its presentation are attempts to manage infertility and the stigma attached to it in a manner that causes minimum injury to the 'double conceptual bind' between the social and the biological. This, however, is not always possible.

Writing on sexual violence inflicted on the bodies of women through the course of a 'critical event', the partitioning of the Indian subcontinent, Veena Das (1999) shows how injury to normative concepts like purity and honour of abducted women could be absorbed within the normal structures of family and marriage as long as these breaches were covered by veils of silence (Das 1995: 218). In other words, women who were sexually violated but whose condition remained publicly invisible could be absorbed within the framework of family by marrying them off 'by some tacit negotiation of the norms of affinity'. Invoking Bourdieu's (1990) idea of 'practical kinship', Das asserts:

> The complete truth of marriage, as he says, resides in its twofold truth – its official image, which is made up of rules and rituals, and the actual alliance, which results from the internal and external political functions of marriage. He gives several instances of the 'self-serving' lies to which a group may give allegiance in order to conceal from itself its failure to find honorable solutions to problem cases. (Das 1995: 219)

While Bourdieu (1990: 178 in Das 1995) refers to this mode of accommodation as an instance of 'collective bad faith', Das (1995: 219) reinterprets this ability of a group to conceal what it perceives as a (stigmatising) normative transgression as systematic misrecognition. This idea of systematic misrecognition has important implications for the way in which clinically assisted conception is both managed and contained within the realm of marriage and the family. Although the complications arising from infertility do not approach the pain and suffering of abducted women, Das's concept nevertheless provides a lens through which to view the practical and tactical adaptations of individuals and families to the normative damage of infertility and assisted conception.

Infertility affects married bodies in India, and, while this may change in the future, an overwhelming number of treatment seekers in India remain conjugally related. It is through the act of conceiving that a couple is confronted by the possibility of lifelong sterility. Infertile couples who approach assisted conception are faced with the possibility of effecting a serious breach in the normative values of Hindu marriage and family on two fronts: first, the fear of an alien input or third party – on account of the donated sperm/ovum/surrogate womb – tarnishing the perception of the invisible tripartite biological base on which the 'official' image of a marriage and the family is erected; and second, in cases where a couple's own biological material is used to induce pregnancy, the very act of substituting sexual intercourse, which is confined to the private invisible sphere, with the expertise of a clinician, a quintessential third party. These elements become a source of anxiety, as instrumentation deployed in inducing conception renders the most intimate part of marriage – making babies – visible and public. This paradox in many ways resonates with the problems engendered by the practice of niyoga and the norm of monogamous devotion of the wife to her husband (Chapter 1). At stake is the purity of a sacrosanct institution – marriage – and a public violation of its boundaries by the inclusion of a

Figure 5.1 The Double Conceptual Bind and Assisted Conception

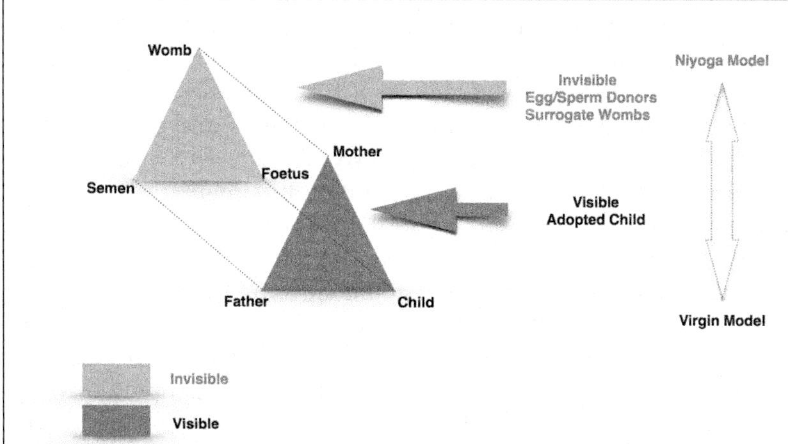

third party. On the one hand, it is acceptable to improvise to re-establish the cosmic triad of womb, semen and foetus; on the other hand, one has to count and justify the sociocosmic costs of establishing this cultural ideal.

It is, therefore, not surprising that many couples in this research sought infertility treatments either under a shroud of complete secrecy or in cahoots with family members. In all such cases the 'taboo on speech' (Das 1995) was either partial or professed with the expressed intent of maintaining it for life. In doing this, couples often lie about seeking treatment and instead attribute the birth of a child to a miracle, luck or a divine gift – the result of much penitential prayer and devotion – concepts which are easier to assimilate into the wider context of extended family and community. In this respect the social attitude to adoption becomes interesting. From outright rejection to last resort, adoption is the most difficult of solutions for infertile couples and their families because it is highly visible. Adoption is an open and public declaration of failed fertility, not to mention fears of failed sexuality (Inhorn and Bharadwaj 2007). An adopted child breaks the link between the body and the progeny and becomes a visible 'third party' in a way that makes it impossible for family groups to collude in a conspiracy of silence.

Seeking Conception and Keeping Quiet

The decision to engage with assisted conception in secret raises questions of whom to invite under this veil of discretion. This boundary is determined by the couple's relationship to the family and the wider community. The span of infertility, the duration of marriage, the family's attitude and that of the wider community together determine who becomes an active collaborator in systematically misrecognising normative infringements and the extent to which this occurs. Of all the interviewees in the 1990s cohort, approximately 40 per cent described themselves as living in nuclear family households, though a majority of these, on further probing, emerged as part of a larger unit than a notion of nuclear family communicates. This pattern persisted in all subsequent contact with treatment seekers until 2010. In the Indian context, the distinction between nuclear and joint families can sometimes be misleading. A.M. Shah (1998), for example, argues that in contemporary India, far from declining, joint families – at least in their household dimension – are on the rise. Joint living within a household is associated with rural areas. While the 'jointness' of households amongst the upper class/castes in urban areas is yielding to nuclear household living (Shah 1998), the numbers often reflected members of two elementary families living together. Thus respondents who claimed to live in nuclear households often lived with elderly dependent parents, an unmarried sibling or both. Respondents who lived in nuclear households as a result of migration did not sever contact with their extended family. Rather, the move affected only joint (household) living and not the family's relationships, including social interference and control. Regardless, the constant presence of family members in a marriage presented the couple with varying constraints or opportunities to share their treatment strategies either with, without or partially with preferred members of the family group. For instance, at an individual level couples either pursued treatment secretively or sought familial involvement to keep wider social disapproval and interference at bay. When asked about his family's response to treatment, Ram Naik replied, 'As far as my case is concerned in my family nobody knows. They only know that I am taking some treatment that's all. But the actual problem, whether the problem is with me or with her, nobody knows'.

In cases like Ram Naik's, couples often cloak the treatment process in ambiguity. Keeping family out was a way of managing stigma and the pressure to conceive. Partial concealment therefore created a degree of secrecy. Families, in cases like Ram Naik's, are happy to look away as long as the couple is seen to be taking action to remedy a continuing absence of children. The treatment could not be concealed indefinitely, however, as families soon asked about its progress. Thus couples had to resort to other ingenious ways of distancing familial or communal interference. According to Ajay, one such respondent, 'People who are doing jobs and living separately have a different atmosphere; there you can do anything. [It's not like being part of a joint family,] like in our case, we hide and come to this clinic. We don't tell anyone that we are going to the doctor. We sneak out'. Reduced to sneaking behind their family's back, the couple was clearly upset by the measures they were forced to take to retain some semblance of privacy and control. Ajay's case, above, was further complicated by the fact that he and his wife lived in a 'joint family' in a small town in Rajasthan, which meant the prying gaze of the family and the community was particularly difficult to avoid.

Middle-class business or professional couples interviewed in cities like Mumbai, on the other hand, were similarly reticent to share the details of their treatment with the wider family; at most, women took their parents into confidence while seeking treatment quietly. For Sunila, married to Ramesh, 'What treatment we are taking only my parents know. My in-laws think that we are taking some minor treatment'. Once again, partial concealment was Sunila and Ramesh's way of keeping the full truth of their efforts to secure a pregnancy localised within the marriage and within the part of the family – Sunila's parents – they perceived as supportive enough to help them keep the treatment invisible. The partial concealment meant that Ramesh's parents had an inkling of rudimentary medical involvement but remained unaware of the procedural complexities.

Forging Alliances: Couples, Families, Clinicians and Tactical Coalitions

Avoiding family pressure can be extremely problematic. The pressure to conceive compounds the anxiety that couples and individuals bring to the clinics. Couples faced significant pressure at home to seek treatment, and familial interference sometimes included active participation in the treatment process, which the couples worked hard to minimise. Dr Neeta thus recounts how she deals with mothers-, fathers- and sisters-in-law of the patients: 'They all come, sometimes the whole family comes', she asserts, which makes the initial and subsequent consultations an ordeal for the couple. On occasions at her clinic some couples observed were accompanied by family members. However, it might not be accurate to construe the family as a mere obstruction or pressure on the process of assisted conception, as family members also accompanied the couples out of concern or to show support. Nevertheless, Dr Neeta observes:

> Fifty percent are always with the mother-in-law or mother or somebody. Sometimes in [the couple's] absence the mother-in-law or the father-in-law or their mothers will call, 'Dr Neeta we just want to come and talk to you about this issue and we don't want you to tell our children that we had come here. What is the problem? Maybe they are not telling us the truth, like the problem they have' ... It is very difficult [in cases when the family accompanies the couple]. Normally I tell them, 'There is no role for all of you; if you sit outside I'll feel very happy because I am going to ask some embarrassing questions from the couple, the couple will feel embarrassed, you will feel embarrassed and because you have come to me. I have to do justice to my job, and justice to your coming. If you think you still

> want to be here it will become very difficult for the couple [and] *maybe the treatment will go wrong somewhere because they will hide some problem which they will not tell me in your presence*. So when I reach some conclusions and select the treatment I will call you here and explain everything'. That's the way I deal with difficult situations, you know. [emphasis added]

Whether out of concern or malice, the familial interference complicates the situation by adding unwarranted pressure to an emotionally charged situation. Dr Chandra spoke of the tremendous (social) pressure to conceive, which accompanies patients and family members at initial consultations:

> You will be surprised that a few days back I had a lady walk in with her daughter-in-law, and I am telling you – I mean this will tell you the kind of pressures that there are – a young girl. So [the mother-in-law] said, 'Oh! You know every month she starts menstruating'. I was really taken aback by the crude way it was put. 'What's the problem? She is not conceiving?' I said. 'How long has she been married?' That's the first question in a history that you would ask, and I'll give you a guess, what do you think it was? Just take a guess! Four months! FOUR MONTHS!! Can you imagine the kind of pressure? Just imagine the kind of pressure the poor kid was under. Her mother-in-law is watching every menstrual cycle! This is pathetic. That's the kind of social pressure there is in the country.

In India it is not uncommon for couples to seek infertility treatment early in the marriage (Mulgaonkar 2000). Severe pressure from family adds to the urgency with which married couples turn to clinical medicine for help. Thus Dr Jatin argues:

> The social pressure to have your own child is much, much higher in India. The social pressure is more within a year of marriage. People start telling the wife or the daughter-in-law, 'Why are you not conceiving? Why don't you see this doctor? See that doctor! Go to this temple, go here, go there', you know it starts within a year of marriage ... Plus there is a lot of social pressure from friends, relatives, everyone [is asking], 'Why are you not conceiving?' So [the couple] seek[s] treatment very early. You will be surprised that 19-year-old, if she doesn't conceive by a year, by twenty, she comes for treatment! Even if we say, 'We will go slow, we don't want to do laproscopy. These are operative things. We will do them after two years or so [as last resort]', nothing doing. They walk into the clinic next door. That's the kind of pressure they are under. They want instant results; they want fast treatment.

The pressure to conceive, therefore, pushes some couples, fearing further interence, either to withhold from family the truth about the treatment or to partially conceal (as seen above) as a way of silencing continuous probing. However, cases like Dr Neeta's and Dr Chandra's are difficult for couples to manage. That is, in keeping sensitive information pertaining to assisted conception concealed within the marriage and fudging the exact nature of medical involvement, the couples need more than each other (or need more help than select – sympathetic – family members can provide). In this respect the involvement of a clinician can be vital to the process of collusion as s/he often stands in a position to mediate between the couples and family interference. Through participant observation at an IVF surgery in a private Delhi hospital, I viewed cases where the couples enlisted clinicians' help in crafting 'official kinship' (mother/father/child) from more 'practical kinship' truths (donor sperm/egg/foetus) for the consumption of their families and the community. Referring to a patient whom I had briefly met on the morning of this interview, Dr Neeta said:

> The man this morning, he was really under stress. He cried a lot on the day he came to know that he doesn't have sperm; he really cried a lot and [his wife] also cried a lot, and then they again came back to me. Next day they were feeling a little better and they said, 'We are ready for the treatment (IVF) with donation', sperm-donated conception. I said, 'I am not ready today. You need some more time to talk to each other, go home'. And then they took two months, and after two months they are back and now they are happy, but this man is still going to tell in society that it is 'my sperm. Dr Neeta has taken it out with a small needle and it has been injected in my wife', and they are going to keep the secret throughout their life. The wider family doesn't know and they have told me if they (family members) phone, 'please don't say anything about our treatment and if somebody phones from our house just say that I have taken out the sperm with a small needle'.

The couple appears to be revealing only partial information about their procedure to family members, fearing that, without clear information about the procedure, family members might call the doctor for more information. The clinician is drawn into the lie that the couple is destined to live for the rest of their lives. Dr Neeta frequently became involved with her patient's domestic and personal problems as she considered it an integral part of the wider counselling process (see Chapter 8). The following are field notes from a new patient consultation on 9 June 1998:

A young couple walks in.

Woman: Dr Neeta, we called yesterday. We have slight problem. Can you take a look at these reports and tell us what is happening?

Man: We are married for two and half years, and I am in construction business.

Dr Neeta is silently reading the reports the couple brought with them.

Woman: [anxious] Do you think something can be done?

Dr Neeta: [still looking down at the reports] There is no way you can produce sperm. [interrupted]

Woman: [high pitched voice] Why this has happened? Why?

Dr Neeta: Y-chromosome genetic test [interrupted]

Man: Is there any way we can correct this?

Dr Neeta: Donor insemination…

Woman: Go for sperm donation! We are not prepared for that; what do we tell the family?

Dr Neeta: Don't tell the family [interrupted]

Woman: That's one mistake we have made! They all know about the fact that he is not producing. I am not satisfied! I want to know everything there is to know [referring to azoospermia].

Dr Neeta: We have handsome, well-educated, good-looking boys coming to us for sperm donation, and we match the patients and the donor, blood group etc.

Woman: [thoughtfully] We can also tell [the family] that now it is possible to inseminate [using her husband's sperm] or some such excuse!

Dr Neeta: I had a couple come to me who was anxious about the same thing. The man would ask me to contact him only on the cell [to fix appointments, consult on donor profiles etc.] and if I had to call him at home, because they lived in a joint family, I had to pretend to be his wife's friend. They even gave me a pseudonym, and I [or the

> assistant] had no choice but to pretend and play along this little game and give the impression that I was his wife's close friend. They went for donor insemination and passed it off as their own.
>
> Woman: [deep in thought] These tests could have been a mistake. Do you think they could have made a mistake?
>
> Man: [embarrassed smile] There can be a mistake once, twice but not after three tests. [now addressing the doctor] How to convince the family about donor sperm as they would feel their son's part is not there. Could we try parallel medicine?
>
> Dr Neeta: If this can't help [i.e. past medication] how can other things help? Look even if you can give me three or four sperms I could help you, we have such sophisticated technology here [referring to Intra Cytoplasmic Sperm Injection] but in total absence of spermatozoa I can't help you.
>
> After the couple left Dr Neeta turned to me and said, 'Did you see how arrogant the wife was?' I asked what made her say that. The doctor felt that the wife was arrogant about the fact that her husband could not produce any sperm, about her in-laws not understanding, 'The girl was angry, she was quite upset'.

The doctor's criticism of the woman's resentment reinforces the view of married relations as one in which a woman carries the burden of her husband's sterility. But this case also points to more complex dimensions of gender politics within marriage. The woman, though seen as arrogant by the clinician, is more significantly someone who is asserting her fertility in the face of her husband's 'lack'. She appears to wield assertions like 'I want to know everything there is to know', as a weapon to vindicate her normality both to her husband and his family. This is not an isolated case. Earlier in the interview, Dr Neeta referred to a patient whose in-laws (both doctors, like her) blamed her for what was clearly a case of male infertility. The woman in question has since applied for divorce and, as Dr Neeta put it, 'She says, "I will not tolerate this nonsense anymore"'. Dr Shanta, another Delhi-based IVF practitioner, similarly referred to another interesting case:

> This man came to me and broke down! He said, 'My wife treats me like a rat!' He was azoospermic. He then came to talk about donor semen and he just broke down he was so full up. This happens so many times you cannot imagine. I have so many men who come to me here, and I can see that wife is the dominating partner and the man becomes quieter and more submissive.

Each of these cases features an evident lack of passivity amongst the women who resist being held accountable for their husband's azoospermia. Though beyond the scope of this project, this aspect of infertility and its impact on the conjugal bond in relation to the wider family (including in-laws, in particular) must be further researched. It is, however, clear from the foregoing that women are occasionally able to both resist and oppose the familial practice of holding daughters-in-law accountable for infertile marriages. Also, quick and discrete conception is crucial to the survival of a marriage overburdened by familial pressure. In the case of the first couple, the practical arrangements to conceive were becoming too difficult to manage given that the entire family knew that 'he is not producing'. The couple was less concerned about sperm donation than about their family's opposition to an arrangement in which their 'son's part is not there'. Family involvement can become inevitable when couples are not careful to cover their tracks or are forced into seeking medical help by family members themselves. In either case, the process is confined to a silent enclosure of selected family members and the clinician. An interesting example of this is the case of a mother and son – Sita Devi and Rajan – who were interviewed in a Rajasthan clinic after Rajan's wife gave birth to a boy following a successful IVF by donor sperm:

> Sita Devi: Our daughter is a doctor. She had explained everything to us. Nobody in our family knows. It is either me, my husband, him [pointing to Rajan] or his wife. The fifth person to know is our daughter. Even her husband doesn't know. She hasn't told him. We are only five people who know what the reality is ... We never opened it to anyone. The moment we saw that both were of the right age, so we thought if they don't have children now then their chances would get bleak. And we tried to keep it under wraps, and we also [she and her husband] came to know because he was financially weak otherwise even parents don't come to know of it ... Besides not everyone can understand or take to or accept this treatment. Because we had the lady doctor at home, we could understand it better. The public is not capable of understanding everything; in our case we had the lady doctor in the family. If she hadn't explained us the whole thing and if it wasn't kept a secret, nobody knows.

Sita Devi's overwhelming sense of joy at the birth of her grandson is partly due to an acute sense of relief that 'nobody knows'. In the interview she repeatedly alluded to the importance of keeping the whole treatment a secret. The issues of infertility, donor insemination and clinical management, as she hints, are difficult for people to understand.

A close-knit group from within the family, therefore, colludes to keep invisible the breakdown of the double conceptual sociobiological bind. Secrecy is almost uniformly prized amongst couples and their collaborating family members. Dr Shanta described the clandestine world of such couples who create new life and obscure these details for the rest of their lives:

> Fifty percent of the patients don't tell after the baby is born that it was an IVF baby at any social gathering, in front of another lady, never. Even when they talk to someone in private they make sure they tell that person not to tell anybody that this is an IVF baby. They think there is stigma attached to the baby.

While this perceived stigma associated with IVF-conceived offspring is declining, it is true that to this day a sense of anxiety in owning up to the IVF status of their newborn compounds this 'taboo on speech'. This is even true of those whose own gametes are used in bypassing tubal damage to help them conceive. The very act of including an external agent in the process of conception compromises the entire babymaking process. Dr Shanta gave another example of a scientist who had invited her to the naming ceremony of his 'IVF daughter' with an added request not to mention anything pertaining to the procedure, especially the gamete-donated status of the child. She went along and played the part of just another guest as the happy parents had requested.

Not all tactical alliances within the familial unit or with the clinicians are this collaborative. In contrast to the couples demanding the doctor's help in warding off meddling families, one clinician described a case where the parents wanted to scheme with them to impregnate an unsuspecting daughter-in-law. Dr Neeta had been on the receiving end of such propositions from the parents of an azoospermic man. This excerpt from field notes sheds light on Dr Neeta's continuing encounters with family intrigues:

> On the way back from the clinic Dr Neeta gave me a lift in her car. She soon began to discuss the parents of a young couple who were hounding her to carry out donor insemination without the knowledge of the daughter-in-law. The man in question had two sons – twins – and wanted the elder son, who was azoospermic, to start a family. To this end he either wanted an anonymous sperm donor, a sample from whom could be used without the knowledge of his daughter-in-law, or alternatively the younger twin brother could donate as the man

> held that genetically they were from the same 'stock'. Faced with persistent resistance from Dr Neeta, the man continued to pressurise her to let the younger brother be the donor for the other twin without either of the wives – his and his brother's – ever finding out. The silver lining to this ingenious plan, according to the man, was that life would go on as normal since to the world at large and to his daughters-in-law the sperm/child would belong to the eldest son. 'The man is after my life', said Dr Neeta. 'Even when I was in England he used to call me often. He's a very rich man, one of the richest men in Delhi living in a posh South Delhi colony. He is after my life to go out to dinner with him and discuss this further over a meal. I don't know how to put this across to him that I don't operate this way, that this is so unethical!'

This case reveals how conspiratorial the 'official' truths of marriage and kin relations can be. Though still in hot pursuit of a clinician who would heed his request, it is only a matter of time before a man of his means successfully lures an unscrupulous practitioner to execute his unethical plan. The preference for 'keeping it in the family' is commonplace amongst some men and their family members, who according to some clinicians come to the clinics either on the pretext of consulting with the doctor on the appointment of an appropriate donor, or with a straightforward request to bring a family donor. Dr Shanta, when asked to comment on what people look for in a 'good donor', revealed that 'people bring family, the father of the [infertile] man, brother of the man. I don't know how it affects their personal life!'

Dr Kamraj also explained how in her years of practising in Madras, she has contended with demands from some individuals wishing to keep the source of sperm and egg donations within the family:

> Sometimes a man comes and says, 'I'll get my brother's sperm, my father's sperm'. I said, 'No way, you do that I will not treat over here'. I tell the lady a man is unpredictable. Y chromosome is very bad, [and] then they will make advances on you and claim your [sexual] rights. Are you mentally prepared for that? So I tell them I will not do it here. You can go wherever. Unidentified egg and sperm donor is best and I say the best comes to you, I will match the [blood] group. I'll match even caste community. I try and match everything and therefore I don't agree for all this. But I have sister donors, that I allow. Sperms, no! Only unidentified, but eggs from own sister is fine.

Dr Kamraj's objection can be understood as a way of keeping the identity of the donor a secret (so-called standard clinical practice), although her willingness to accept sisters in the knowledge of all the parties involved raises the question of how issues of gender and sexuality shape the donor selection process. Dr Kamraj's contention illustrates what Erica Haimes (1993) calls 'issues of gender in gamete donation'. In the context of the Warnock Report established by the British government, she convincingly argues that woman-to-woman egg donation is seen as completely asexual when compared to man-to-women semen donation. She argues that a female third party is not seen as invasive or as significant a threat to the sociopolitical stability of the family as a semen donor. In other words, family boundaries are less threatened by egg donation than by semen donation (Haimes 1993: 92). The 'dubious sexual connotations' and a sense of 'inappropriate sexuality' attached to semen donation, which Haimes identifies in the report, also reflect Dr Kamraj's fear of potential sexual misconduct threatening (patriarchal) marriage and family.

This strong personal objection to donated sperm articulated by Dr Kamraj is expressed differently by Dr Srinivas, who rejects the idea of using any gametes other than those of the couple involved:

> If it's the husband, it's okay. People don't accept, they know it's not their own child. If she is a very pious lady, then she will not accept another man's sperm at all! A couple may prefer to adopt a child than go for this option. I would consider it out of culture. What is culture? Basically everything. If you can compensate by something else, then there is no point in leading life like that. You don't know about the father. Maybe he is an outcaste fellow; probably he was a thug or a rowdy. How do you know that the sperm was not from a man from behind the bars? If he is a murderer, that thing can come in.

While Dr Srinivas's objections and fears attached to donor sperm may appear far-fetched, they nevertheless reveal something important about his personal opposition to the practice. They strongly articulate the 'yuck factor' (Haimes and Williams 1998: 141), as well as the view that the social categories of the source of biological material are significant (Daniels and Haimes 1998).[3]

The sourcing of 'life-engendering material' is contentious. For instance, the assertions made by Drs Shanta, Kamraj and Srinivas appear to push the debate towards the same conceptual complexities of the heuristic niyoga and virgin models (Chapter 1). It is evident that there is a subgroup of treatment seekers who accept the idea of donated gamete conception from only within the family. Dr Kamraj's willingness to accept egg donation between sisters also points to a prevalent trend in India where sisters help each other by either donating eggs or, as seen earlier, by surrogating their womb as a receptacle for their brother-in-law's sperm. In North India, in fact, a man's relationship with his sister-in-law is often jokingly alluded to as being semi-conjugal. This is reflected in the common Hindi adage that can be crudely translated to mean 'Wife's younger sister is half wife' (*sali adhi ghar wali*). This structurally embedded and socially tolerated joking relationship between a man and his wife's younger sister mirrors and redeploys a similar bond between a woman and her younger brother-in-law, devar (Chapter 1). Perhaps this relationship of privileged overfamiliarity is a vestige of an ancient tradition where younger (unmarried) sisters were brought up as potential substitutes for their older sisters in cases of infertility. However, although several fieldwork informants alluded to such a practice in the ancient past, this could not be substantiated, unlike the Vedic references to devar as second husband. This makes the issue of the man desiring to procure his twin son's semen to fertilise the older of his two daughters-in-law interesting. As discussed in Chapter 1, the practice of niyoga, or levirate, was a way to bypass an absence of male seed. In the context of a devar, this meant either privileged sexual access or an obligation to marry his widowed sister-in-law. This raises a vital question: in using a sibling's semen, do the family members of an infertile man acknowledge his sociogenetic death? More crucially, is the need to source semen from a brother or father an expression of intimate links that people perceive between semen and the common blood that flows through and maintains a patrilineal descent group? Dr Kamraj's opposition to intra-familial sperm donation is rooted in a kind of biological determinism that casts aspersions on the character of the 'Y chromosome'. It also hints at similar cultural concerns linked to the subtle shift from niyoga to more Brahmanical concerns with virginal purity (virgin model). Not surprisingly, therefore, Dr Srinivas eulogises a 'pious lady' who would never accept another man's sperm and presumably remains monogamously devoted to her god husband (pati permeshwara). He considers the inclusion of a third party in a marriage as 'out of culture' and shies away from what he sees as compromising the purity of a marriage. These are some of the complex issues that require further research. For the moment we can see only fragmented connections between cultural concerns, past and present, which are inflamed by infertility and its cultural management.

Couples who pursue clinical conception in relative anonymity and in insulation from their families approach the issue of alien input differently. Such cases focus more on the outcome of pregnancy than its actual source. To cite Dr Shanta:

> Our society is still not so liberated that they accept adoption. [Couples] accept taking donor oocyte. They accept artificial insemination by donor semen anything. But they want to deliver the baby so the whole world can see that she has delivered a baby. So many men have got very near normal sperm, but out of sheer frustration they say, 'Oh, use any sperm you want. I want a baby'. They just don't care! They just want to prove their fertility, that is all ... A woman at some stage in the family wants to prove it ... The man just wants to prove to the world that his wife has produced a child, that he is capable of fathering a child.

There is some truth in Dr Shanta's assertion. Barring a handful of couples, the great majority, when asked to share their views on donated gamete conception, felt it was an acceptable practice, as long as it was kept quiet. On the issue of the donor itself, couples were unanimously happy to let the doctor source a suitable donor and had no personal preferences. These couples were much less concerned about the sourcing of eggs and sperm for inducing conception than about the eventual birth of a child. Interestingly, an Indian interviewee, Ganesh, in Eric Hirsch's (1999: 121) south-east England study, insisted that in Indian culture the possibility of anonymous genetic material would not be thinkable: 'Now they want to know, if it's an anonymous sperm, will you know which caste it comes from? So it's completely out of the question, they will never accept it. Never accept it, even if they are given 100 [percent] verity it's a high caste, they still won't accept it'. When I first read this account I analysed this comment as an empirical oddity, an individual view not representative of the emerging complexity in my own data. However, Ganesh's view began to make sense when in 2005 and 2007 I interviewed non-resident Indians (NRI) seeking fertility treatment in India. It became apparent that the NRI diaspora crossed over to India for very specific reasons. An encounter in a Delhi IVF clinic is a good illustration of global 'routes' taken in search of local 'substance' and the production of evolving 'biological biographies'. Savita and Raj, a 'NRI couple', are based in Birmingham in the United Kingdom. Savita underwent fertility treatment in London where she was mainly put on fertility medication. Unsuccessful, the couple flew to Australia to try yet again. Here the doctor diagnosed egg donation as the only viable option for Savita:

> I was very concerned as egg donation in Australia or for that matter the UK would be so difficult. I had my concerns, my concerns were genetic, colouring, eye and hair colouring, face colouring, everything, to ensure the child looks like myself. Coming from obviously Hindu background and being [upper caste] Brahmin, I was clear what I wanted. The best step for me was to come to India. I was recommended by the gynecologist there, not in London, as he said it would be very difficult for him to recommend, but there were other countries like Spain and India where the legislation wasn't very clear.

The biological attributes of the baby were of paramount importance for Savita. The fact that her caste purity and religion were so inextricably linked to her biological self-fashioning made the move even more compelling, as did prevailing legislation in the West that complicated the process of acquiring a caste-appropriate donor. As Savita explained, 'Initially I was very hesitant. It's not my seed, it's not my genetic background, it's not from my ancestors, my ancestors are not in it. I am coming to terms with it now'. Like many Indian IVF treatment seekers who routinely misrecognise the 'biological truths' underscoring the conception of their donor assisted babies, the temporal depth of Savita's molecular biology and its upper caste purity was quickly absorbed by the IVF procedure. Savita's husband Raj elaborated, 'We both sat down and talked, we are educated … Yes, we are orthodox and traditional [but] in our own way we have moved, evolved with times and have a mind bent towards what's available, what we don't have, to reach it'.

Ganesh, I now think, like Savita and Raj, was responding from a mainly diasporic space in which India and one's relationship to a remote reference group gestated in the imagination rather than fashioned everyday encounters. Forging a hybrid diasporic identity in conversation with two cultures made both caste purity and origin of biogenetic substance significant issues. However, the treatment seekers in India and their pragmatism repeatedly exposed an 'invisible truth': while seemingly hermetically sealed, for centuries in India, endogamous boundaries of caste groups have remained porous and permeable.

However, an open acceptance of the 'other' in the reproduction of the 'self' is a gradual process in the lives of most couples, as Dr Sachin clarifies:

The basic idea is that somebody is violating your marital relationship, a third party, that feeling itself is not very easy to accept. If I put myself in a patient's place I understand how they would feel. Here the marriage is considered as the ultimate bond, and to have a child with donated gametes does upset a lot of couples, but then again once they reach the age of 35-36 they know they've no other option besides adoption. In adoption they get a child whose background is not known. Here, okay at least egg or the sperm, at least one of the gametes is their own, plus the woman has the satisfaction of delivery. Donated gamete is acceptable as long as it remains confidential and the husband and wife are very sure of each other; they understand what they are going in for without any cheating.

The normative injury to the double conceptual bind is first processed and accepted by the couple. As Dr Sachin explains, coming to terms with such an upheaval in the marriage can be a long process. Couples who appear not to care what sperm or egg is used to induce a pregnancy, in Dr Shanta's estimate, have often spent years pursuing conception while trying to escape increasing family pressure for results (see Chapter 2). Exhausted, some couples either eventually accept the option of a third party input or adopt, viewing a donor as an unacceptable founding component of their family.[4] After making the transition, however, couples salvage the situation by misrecognising the breach. They cut their losses by seeking satisfaction in having partial links with the child. Consider the following exchange with Ravi and Geeta:

AB: Would you prefer donor insemination to adoption?

Ravi: I'll prefer donor.

AB: Any specific reasons?

Ravi: See, with donor, the child would stay with the mother for nine months. So the affection that she will develop towards that child will be far more than what I feel when we adopt a child. It is my feeling.

AB: [To the wife] Do you agree?

Ravi: [Now explaining to Geeta] What I am saying is that, one there is adoption and on one hand there is *gift*. One child comes from your stomach and the other one is adopted. So your affection towards the one which comes out of your body and affection towards the adopted one – would you feel the difference between the two?

Geeta: A child that is your own is your own.

Ravi: What I was asking would there be a difference between the two?

Geeta: No, both will be the same. There is no difference. If nothing happens, we will adopt.

Ravi: From her side, there is no difference.

For Ravi, the connection with the mother's body is crucial to the bonding process. Geeta, however, is more open to stepping out of the confines of the sociobiological fertility triad. Ravi emphasises the visuality of fertility as central. For him, the possibility of the child coming from Geeta's 'stomach' (womb) anchors them within the biological triad.

Adoption: The Socio-Legal Domain

Adoption is not a recent phenomenon. Ancient legal codes deliberate, often at variance, the merits of adopting 'sons'. Legal codes of Baudhayana, for instance, in the words of Georg Buhler (in Müller 1894: xix), permit 'their craving for representatives bearing their name, and to allay their fears of falling after death into the regions of torment through a failure of the funeral oblations, by the affiliation of eleven kinds of substitutes for a legitimate son' (Buhler in Müller, 1894: xix).

Laws of Apastamba, on the other hand, forbid adoption although the institutes of Vishnu and recognise twelve kinds of sons, of which the adopted son (*dattaka*) was one. The practice of niyoga or male surrogacy was widely practised, and most legal codes including Manu approve of begetting sons by the appointment of a surrogate male to a widowed woman or wife of an infertile man. A plausible explanation for this may lie in the fact that the resultant child would remain peripherally connected to the double 'conceptual bind' of the mother (womb) and child (foetus) even though the absence of father (semen) injured the ideals of purity. This perhaps also explains the need for secrecy in the present-day context, where children born of donor insemination can still be legitimately absorbed in the mother (womb)/father (semen)/child (foetus) configuration in a way that adopted children cannot. Ancient legal codes, while recognising unrelated adopted children, nevertheless construe such arrangements as less desirable. The legal codes of Vishnu, which acknowledge the adopted son as the eighth of the twelve, go on to assert that 'amongst these (sons) each preceding one is preferable (to the one next in order)' (Müller 1894: 64). Not surprisingly, the first son listed as lawfully begotten is one born of marriage, followed by the son born through niyoga, and third by the son of an appointed daughter. The laws of Vishnu state that a son of a daughter who is given away by her father with the words, 'the son whom she bears be mine', can act as the 'son of the body'. Thus female children become vehicles for grandsons who can act as de facto sons. There is a clear sense, with the first three preferred sons, of a shared proximity to the familial triad of mother, father and child. This bond weakens as the list goes on, with the twelfth son – 'son begotten by any woman whomsoever' (Müller 1894: 63) – being the least desirable option. Kautilya's Arthashastra (150 AD) numerates twelve categories of sons. The ninth class of son in this schema was *datta* or 'an adopted son, given away by formal ceremony' (Kautilya 1992: 385), such a son inherited from only the father adopting him and not from the family of the adopted father. While the first listed son, *aurasa*, is biologically related and born by 'a wife [the father] had married in accordance with all rituals' (Kautilya 1992: 385), the second son in order of preference is *putrikaputra*, a son of a nominated daughter. Significantly, such a son was deemed equal in rank to an *aurasa*. The third son, *kshetraja*, was 'born to a wife by an authorised person' [other than the legal husband] whether he is of the same *gotra* (clan) or not. Adoption was low on the list of twelve modes of acquiring heirs. The ninth option, adoption or *datta*, was succeeded only by *upagata*, one who offers himself for adoption, *kritakai*, a son appointed in that capacity, and the twelfth son, *krita*, who is bought. Not unlike modern-day IVF-mediated conception, these modes of acquiring sons could fit into normative folds of conjugality, conventional fostering from next of kin or improvisational domain of donor assisted conception. My intention is not to draw parallels between these far removed perspectives but rather to show that there is a long cultural tradition of accommodating infertility or the notable absence of children/sons by orchestrating modes and codes to maintain the double conceptual bind.

The legal codes in postcolonial India, on the whole, remain parochially defined. This is primarily a legacy of the British colonial administration, which sought to codify laws in India on the basis of various religious communities. As noted in the Introduction, the East India Company codified social observance and customary law into Hindu law: 'The Manu Dharmasastra, for example, which was basically part of Brahmanical smrti was taken as the law of the Hindus and presumed to apply universally' (Thapar 1989: 218). Similarly, legal codes in British India were constructions derived from Sir

Henry Maine's reading of classical Roman law in light of Dharmasastric texts and nineteenth-century British observations on Indian customary law (Uberoi 1993, 1996: 186). The discourse on personal law actuated by the British resonates with contemporary socio-legal thinking, spilling into the contentious issue of a common code of law for various Indian communities. The postcolonial adoption law amply demonstrates this. In India, only Hindus are legally allowed to adopt a child under the Hindu Adoptions and Maintenance Act of 1956. Other religious communities, like Muslims and Christians, whose personal laws do not sanction adoption, can only take in a child in guardianship under the Guardians and Wards Act of 1890. Foreign adoption also falls under the jurisdiction of this Act. The Act only confers guardianship on the persons taking a child in their care, and this status ceases to exist once the child reaches maturity (Howell 2006).

Data from a ten-year period in Bharat's (1993) study shows that more than two-thirds (67 per cent) of the total number of adopted children were placed with foreign parents. The fact that a sizeable number of Indian-born children were placed in foreign homes augmented public concern about issues such as 'baby selling'. This led to demands for streamlining adoption procedures, which culminated in a series of Supreme Court judgments between February 1984 and 1991. In the absence of a uniform adoption law, the judgments outlined exhaustive directives and procedures to process adoption under the Guardians and Wards Act. The court directed that a child should have the opportunity to be adopted by Indian parents and that, only failing that, could adoption by foreigners be considered. The Indian government was now enjoined to provide recognition certificates to agencies in India and abroad which would permit them to work towards international adoptions. This intervention by the Supreme Court was translated into the creation of the Central Adoption Resource Agency (CARA), an autonomous body of the Ministry of Social Justice and Empowerment with an express mandate to control in-country adoption and to regulate, as well as facilitate, international adoption. CARA placed some 5,951 children in foreign homes between 1995 and 1999 (Government of India 2001). The figures show that 5,693 children were placed in in-country adoption arrangements in 2010, peaking at 5,964 in 2011 and 4,694 in 2012; in 2013–2014, 3,924 children were settled in Indian homes (CARA 2014). Inter-country adoption for the same period stood at 628 (2010), 629 (2011), 308 (2012) and 430 (2013–2014) (CARA 2014). The sharp decline in international adoption indicates a strong 'anti-transnational adoption' policy sentiment in India, a knee-jerk response to public concerns about malpractice (EPW 2001; Howell 2006). In large part, legal provisions in India seek to limit overseas adoption by promoting the view that no Indian child can be adopted overseas unless another child is adopted by an Indian couple – 'the so-called 50/50 rule' (Howell 2006: 190). Worryingly, moves are afoot to change the 50/50 rule to 80/20 with the view to encouraging in-country over transnational adoption (Agnes 2011; Thomas 2013). While the Indian state's intent to oversee child welfare is noble, the 'misplaced objectives' underscoring official policy are derailing the state's very goals (Anand and Chandra 2002: 3,893). For example, the proposed readjustment of in-country and transnational adoption ratio to 80/20 risks making adoption altogether unattractive given the burgeoning rise of gestational surrogacy in India. This alternative allows individuals and couples, both local and global, to craft kinship encored peripherally in the 'double conceptual bind' and anonymously create visuality of biogenetic relatedness between the child and biosocial parents. Moreover, a bill pertaining to adoption that would allow individuals to freely and legally adopt children regardless of their religious faith has met with persistent opposition since 1972 from communities that view it as anathema to their religious beliefs. Given the strong feelings on this that exist among religious minorities, the political will to advance the bill is weak, and as a consequence, a large number of willing, non-Hindu couples are unable to adopt children legally (Bharat 1993; Damania 1998). This is particularly unfortunate given that most Hindu couples choose to adopt from within the family, thus remaining free of legal involvement (Bharat 1993). Hence, Hindus who openly adopt children remain a small minority while non-Hindu adopting families find their access to legal adoptions severely curtailed on account of the Guardianship Act. The lack of 'open adoptions' amongst Hindus must, however, be understood in the wider context of the cultural constraints described above. In what follows the book shows why adoption is viewed as an unattractive family founding alternative.

Adopting a Stance: Reluctance towards Adoption and Overcoming It

Reluctance to adopt, or grudging acceptance as a last resort, is appreciable. Dr Mankar contends that in India, 'It is the question of male ego they wouldn't mind having a donor insemination done without anyone else apart from the couple knowing because the other option is to adopt a child, which everybody would know'. Protecting the male safeguards the image of a marriage, which could – as seen in some cases above – crumble in the face of a woman resisting being made accountable for her husband's sterility. Adoption in such cases deals a further deathly blow to the entire project of concealment that fuels and propels the misrecognition process. A publicly visible child who is incorporated into the family without any corporeal connectedness with the family unit makes the child and couple vulnerable to a more severe level of social ridicule and stigma than that caused by infertility.

Rekha and Sudhir had not given any thought to the idea of adoption, as Sudhir had immediately dismissed it because of social stigma:

> AB: Would you consider adoption?
>
> Sudhir: No!
>
> Rekha: I have considered.
>
> AB: What is your objection to adoption?
>
> Sudhir: There is no objection to it as such, immediately on the face of it I have said no. I have not even given a thought to it. Basic instinctive reaction! Maybe over a period of time I will change. I don't know, maybe, I'm not yet! The biggest problem in adoption over here in India, and it's going to stay until people don't mature in their thinking – that an adopted child is a bastard child! It's the future of the child [interrupted]
>
> Rekha: How much can they protect themselves [interrupted]
>
> Sudhir: That is the problem with adoption – the stigma attached to the child. Parents can understand because they are of particular age. They are mature enough to think; they have taken their decision for adoption. But what about the kid?
>
> Rekha: Why should you make a child suffer? Why should we make another human being suffer for us?

Sudhir and Rekha were voicing a widespread fear. This 'bastard child' is seen to contaminate the family formation in the eyes of the community, so couples fear that adoption would condemn the child to live a life of jibes and ridicule. The transgression is, yet again, a visible violation of the 'double conceptual' bind; the idea of a bastard child suggests a reprehensible union of semen and womb, beyond the institution of marriage. To absorb such a child into the fold of marriage doubly perpetuates the process of delegitimation (Chapter 2) due to the physical proximity of an infertile marriage to a bastard child. It is interesting how the invisibility of a child's origin marks him or her as socially deficient. Children given up for adoption come from a variety of backgrounds ranging from teenage pregnancies, to orphans, or children whose families are too poor to look after them. However, many of these children are born out of 'wedlock' and are invariably viewed as a product of illicit sexual union. Bharat's (1993) study of sixteen adoption agencies located in five cities or towns in Maharashtra State found that, of a total of 4,526 children given up for adoption, 74 per cent were abandoned by their biological mothers because they were born out of premarital or extramarital relationships (Bharat 1993: 55). This also links with adoptive parents' wider concerns about the issue of the 'quality' of the invisible 'background' of a child. In the present-day context, this anxiety is articulated by questioning the genetic credentials of the adopted child. Such a presentiment is in consonance with apprehensions surrounding the invisible bloodline, clan and caste origins of an adoptee.

A couple – Shanker and Sumita – dealing with secondary infertility are amongst a vocal minority of respondents who objected to adoption on the same grounds as they objected to donated gamete assisted conception, namely because of alien genetic input. Such couples either reluctantly adopted from a close family member 'if all else failed' or remained childfree for the rest of their lives. Shanker and Sumita had this to say:

> AB: Have you ever considered adoption?
>
> Shanker: [long pause] I am thinking we will have a child otherwise. If it gets too prolonged then we will adopt … Sometime back we did toy with the idea of adopting, but you see the problem is that the child should also be proper.
>
> AB: What do you mean by 'proper'?
>
> Sumita: The parents' genes are bound to show up in the child, so even if we adopt one, how do we know what kind of genes does the child have and what if our genes don't match and we don't get along at home and what if as a result it brings us bad name? So what is the use of such a child?

Shanker: It has happened like this couple of times; there are instances. Otherwise there is no problem with adoption if the child is very young.

AB: Your objection to donor insemination is also based on similar concerns?

Shanker: Yes!

AB: What do you mean by 'genes'?

Shanker: Gene *Sutra*! Certain qualities in an individuals.

Sumita: Qualities are always inherited by the child.

AB: What do you mean by 'qualities'?

Sumita: The ability to adjust in the family.

AB: Don't you think qualities are a product of upbringing?

Sumita: Upbringing does make a difference and also the environment around the child [interrupted]

Shanker: Chromosomes [interrupted]

Sumita: The child will learn from his surrounding, too.

AB: What were you saying about chromosomes?

Shanker: It's in it [laughs]. Anyway I was just saying like that. I still believe we will have a child ... and if not then we will adopt. There are a lot of children in my family.

This couple has constructed a folk model of genetic relatedness that, according to them, lies at the heart of amicable domestic adjustments between parents and children. There is an important subtext in many of Shanker's assertions. The first of these is that an adopted child from another gene pool may not readily blend in their familial environment. The source of this anxiety, though manifestly attributed to a biological incongruity between the adoptee and the family, is at least as much located in the fear of social disapproval. Consider the following exchange with another couple, Arvind and Parul, on the issue of adoption:

Parul: In the family people say [interrupted]

> Arvind: Suppose if something happens, then people would say, 'Someone else's child they adopted; that is why it happened like this'. If it's your own, anything can happen. It would not make a difference.
>
> AB: Does it mean if the societal pressure was not there you would have considered adoption?
>
> Arvind: Absolutely!

The very idea of society allowing a child of one's own a degree of freedom that is denied to an adopted child offers insight into the deep angst that infertile couples experience in dealing with the question of adoption. An adopted child's failings and achievements can in such an atmosphere run the risk of being explained away as a feature of unknown parentage.[5] An adopted child in other words runs the risk of being condemned to carry the burden of his unknown parentage as the only possible explanation of his failings or achievements.[6] Dr Srinivas's archaic views on donor insemination, reported earlier in the chapter, also substantiate the tendency to attribute character flaws and even criminal behaviour to genetic properties in semen, transferred anonymously to fertilise the wives of sterile men.

The second intriguing subtext in Shanker's assertion is his passing reference to accepting an adoptee as long as it is 'very young'. An obvious reason for this may lie in a perception that it is much easier to weave a relatively younger child into the fabric of its new family. There is, however, another far more important consideration that surfaced in an interview with the head of a Mumbai-based adoption agency:

> A case which happened recently was of this lady who came with the plea that she's tried all the treatments and wanted to adopt a young child ... She said she is going to pass it off as her own child. She's a teacher, a working woman, and this is her attitude. This is what she told us that, 'I'll pass it off as my own' ... She was even ready to say to the people, I mean, her relatives and husband's relatives, that she is having a surrogate mother, that was acceptable rather than adoption. I couldn't believe it, should be more tough to talk about a surrogate mother but she was ready for that ... [People looking to adopt children] want the youngest child that they can get ... We tell them, 'Of course zero year we can never give because zero to three month we have to keep the baby in our care because that is the reconsideration period for the (biological) mother to come back and ask for her child, but they would like to have three and half to four month old, as young as possible.

The only way an adopted child can be accommodated in a marriage is by misrecognising its origins both within and outside the family. As in the case of donated gametes, the 'visual' respectable image of a marriage can remain untarnished only by concealing this truth. In the adoption agency's estimate, educated middle-class professional couples adopting children were least likely to keep such secrets.[7] On the other hand, individuals who cannot keep an adoption a secret prefer to source the baby from within the wider family as, first, it neutralises the stigma of adopting from an unknown source, and second, such a move ensures the 'respectable' credentials of the baby in the eyes of anyone privy to the truth. This also becomes a logical extension of keeping family formation close to the 'agnatic blood', an idea echoed in the need to source gametes from within the family. Whether intra-family adoptions remain socially invisible is an issue that needs further research. That is to say, what kind of alliances are forged within families in these cases, and what kind of parameters are drawn, beyond which the truth is not permitted to travel?

Conclusion

Marilyn Strathern (1992b) argues that to talk about kinship is to allude to the basis of social arrangements and to provide a cultural context for the natural process of procreation. This process, according to her, is seen (amongst the Euro-Americans) as belonging not to the domain of society but to the domain of nature, with kinship connecting these two domains. Strathern (1992b: 17) writes, 'In the case of kinship, what is at issue is the social construction of natural facts. At the same time, established critiques, including those from anthropology, make it evident that what are taken as natural facts are themselves social constructions'. Her contention has an important implication for the 'doubly complex' task that kinship performs in the face of reproductive crisis within a family in India. Kinship, as culturally perceived, not only connects the two domains of biology and society but also, more crucially, bestows legitimacy upon the intimate link between these two domains. What is constituted as natural is thus certified by the rules of kinship. Procreation – seen as belonging to the domain of nature – becomes curiously social by rendering the 'facts of life' permeable, malleable and open to manipulation, as long as they can be reconfigured legitimately in the language of kinship and relatedness. Kinship thus authorises – and authors – the process of conception.

This chapter depicts how the practice of systematic misrecognition enables parties to collude in re-crafting biological and social links. The purity and honour associated with this biosocial bind is not compromised as long as such transgressions can be tacitly reconfigured into a legitimate kinship unit. The silence that subsumes this process of accommodation is central to its success. Moreover, while infertility is a stigmatised condition, so is its clinical management. Some respondents in this research were open about seeking treatment, though most pursued medical intervention in complete secrecy. This implies that improvisations in establishing the mother/father/child triad are acceptable only as long as some minimum connection with the 'married body' remains in place. The need to keep it a secret, therefore, becomes more pronounced in the case of an 'alien biological input' because, should it become known, the visible result (baby) would have disastrous consequences on the couple: a public violation of the sacred triad. A visible violence to the norms of kinship, therefore, cannot be reabsorbed within a family and the community to which it belongs without stigmatising individuals caught in the public gaze. In silently accepting donor egg or sperm, couples and their kin strived to socially mark their offspring as biologically related even though the 'biological credentials' of the child would be known only to them and not to the community at large. Faced with a crisis, the 'natural' biological base is overridden in favour of the social arrangements. Kinship structures are resilient enough to contain such violations only when they are invisible. Given these complexities, adoption emerges as a problematic alternative for couples seeking assisted conception to salvage their fertility. Situating a child within a marriage or family that visibly departs from the conceptual sociobiological bind makes the task of misrecognising an adoptee's origins extremely difficult. The stigma associated with infertility and adoption must therefore be read as a social response to the breakdown of a conceptual bind that conjoins the sacrament of marriage to the task of producing offspring. The fact that children secretly conceived with donated gametes remain partially connected to their parents in this conceptual framework makes adoption even more undesirable. There are interesting parallels in the ancient legal codes, now subsumed under the rubric of Hinduism, where the practice of male surrogacy provided a similar partial connection; thus, the preferred type of adopted son remains peripherally hooked into the familial unit. The socio-legal domain of adoption once again clarifies and emphasises how religious personal laws in their modern day context continue to influence access to adoption, as well as options and choices. In brief, this chapter argues that, when reproduction goes awry, couples would rather secretly resort to accepting donated sperm than adopt, an option that evokes widespread fears of making infertility permanently 'visible' and irreparably upsetting the sacred social and biological triad of mother (womb), father (semen) and child (foetus).

Notes

1. While Bharat mentions some earlier studies, most notably Chatterjee, Singh, and Yadav (1971), Ahmad (1975) and Billimoria (1984), they are nevertheless dated and limited in scope, thus confirming the continuing paucity of research in the area.
2. Catherine Kohler Riessman (1996: 168), however, rightly contends that Bharat's study suffers from staying 'very close to the data, and the reader must bring political and theoretical contexts to bear on the discussion'.
3. According to Haimes and Williams (1998: 143), an instinctive repugnance, or the 'yuck factor', has the most force in the connections between the child and the source of that child's genes.
4. Couples and individuals interviewed for this research were mainly interested in a child that was biologically related to them and had turned to assisted conception in that hope. It is critical to understand that not every infertile couple needs donated gametes to conceive. In fact, in most cases, the biological continuity between the couple and the embryo is complete. Whether the act of bypassing blocked tubes in a woman materialises into a successful pregnancy and childbirth is another matter as the success of assisted conception depends on a number of other physiological and medical parameters. In cases where, on account of ovarian failure or chronic azoospermia, it is not feasible to use the gametes of the couple, donor input is necessity.
5. It is perhaps important to recall Leela Dube's (1986) contention from Chapter 1, suggesting that the metaphorical importance of semen in rural Andhra Pradesh can result in society casting aspersions on its source. Similarly, compare this attitude towards adoption to the ancient laws of Manu, where the male seed (semen) is held to produce the qualities in the resultant offspring: 'That one (plant) should be sown and another be produced cannot happen; whatever seed is sown, (a plant of) that kind even comes forth' (Müller 1894: 334).
6. It is important to note that while couples interviewed for this study were unanimously reluctant to adopt, they nevertheless did not pose

their opposition to the practice in terms of caste or class origins of the prospective adoptee. The interviewees were more concerned with societal disapproval that may use the unknown parentage of an adopted child to further stigmatise them and their child.

7. Bharat's (1993) data suggests that adoptive parents were fairly well-educated, with 60 per cent or more possessing college-level or higher educational qualifications. Nearly two-thirds of the adoptive couples were dual-earner couples. They were mostly engaged in either private jobs (husbands: 47 per cent, wives: 36 per cent) or in government jobs (husbands: 17 per cent, wives: 12.5 per cent). However, such couples remain in the minority.

Chapter 6

SUPPLEMENTARY CONCEPTION

THE OTHER MOTHER

Indian women offering commercial gestational services to a range of local and global consumers of assisted reproductive technologies (ARTs) have received unprecedented attention around the globe (Gentleman 2008). Actors and institutions as diverse as the mass media, academia (notably, anthropology and sociology), fertility clinics, law firms, brokers and national governments have come to focus on surrogates for a myriad of political, intellectual, ethical, legal and commercial reasons.

The notion of the surrogate carries many meanings: substitution, replacement, proxy and stand-in. The conflation between the act of surrogate substitution and motherhood is well established in the scholarly imagination (Ragoné 1994). This chapter further interrogates this conflation in the larger context of transnational surrogacy arrangements involving Indian women. In large part, it explores the existential predicament of Indian women who are seldom surrogate or substitute mothers but almost always an addition – supplement – to a transnationally located mother in waiting.

Thus far, my encounters with surrogacy in India remain confined to altruistic arrangements between family members who routinely seek out specific private clinics to arrange a quick surrogate pregnancy. I use the term 'surrogate' here to signal the role of kinship in achieving conception through substitution or proxy. This mode of non-commercial family forming creates distinct but equally important sets of relations of exploitation, piety, kinship and support.

However, the rapid proliferation of commercial gestational services and global fertility travels in the new century demonstrates how swiftly the Indian fertility industry has assumed a transnational dimension. Since 2005, scholarly accounts of global reproductive travels in search of surrogate wombs and the gendered commercial underbelly of surrogate conception in India have emerged (Pande 2010b, 2014; Rudrappa 2012; Unnithan-Kumar 2013; Vora 2009). While ongoing empirical research on commercial surrogacy – most notably, that led by graduate students and scholars in the United States, Europe, and India – continues to provide rich data on gender and kinship, science and technology, labour markets and processes, global travel and local sourcing, and ethically fraught and dubious practices in India and beyond, there is an urgent need for more theoretical conversation, conceptual analysis and, above all, political debate.[1]

This chapter lies on the cusp of conceptual elaboration and political critique. It attempts to unravel tentatively the issues critical to the local politics of supplementary wombs in India. I believe that moves to accomplish political mobilisation and cultural critique require conceptual and semantic (terminological) clarity. Adriane Rich (1995) rightly observed that in the interstices of language lie powerful secrets of culture. Thus, I turn to Jacques Derrida (1998) to produce a conceptual separation between the figures of a surrogate and a supplement. I further reflect on early feminist scholarship, which I describe as the 'radical feminist challenge', to sketch out the contours of the exploitative relations of (re)production at the heart of transnational gestational arrangements in India. This is achieved mainly through a sustained critique of normative and ideological processes that shape the experience of gender and its present day consequences for supplementary women in India. I conclude by interrogating the role of the Indian state. In brief, I ask: a) What is it to be supplementary, or rather, what is it to exist, persist in a state of supplementarity? b) What are the sexual genealogies and gendered ideologies (even archaeologies) of surrogacy in India? And, c) Where is the state: is it absent or surrogate?

The Supplementary 'Other'

The poor around the world inhabit biologies routinely construed as waste, as disposable and dispensable (Scheper-Hughes 2000). In many parts of the world, wombs, embryos and kidneys – to name a few commodities – exist in states of exception, as 'bare life' (Agamben 1998).[2] Who and what gets defined as 'waste' in any given society, argues Scheper-Hughes (2002), often has a bearing on the lives of the poorest in countries with a ready surplus of 'unidentified unclaimed pauper bodies'. Extreme forms of this notion can be found in specific totalitarian contexts throughout human history. In the postwar twentieth century, a less severe and reformed relationship to waste and disposal emerged in capitalist social formations, one predicated on ethics of limitless cycles of demand and supply. From the end of the twentieth century to the closing years of the first decade of the twenty-first, this modality has given way to newer forms of exploitation and ethics of consumption that demand a different relationship to disposal and waste. This new formation can be conceptualised as the 'neoliberal mode of production'. The poor in a neoliberal world inhabit biologies that are not so much construed as 'waste' but rather as 'going to waste'; this notion, I further argue, gains traction only when those going to waste can be recycled in a tangible, meaningful and above all profitable sense. Charis Thompson (2005: 264) argues that in the 'biomedical mode of reproduction', unlike the capitalist mode of production, waste is seldom a political or logistical problem but rather an ethical one of how to designate life material (embryos) as waste. In the neoliberal mode of production, the problem of how to designate life material as waste is frequently addressed by resorting to recycling socially/ethically defined waste or surplus that cannot otherwise be gainfully accumulated. For example, innovative theodicies consider surplus embryos to be better utilised for research or adoption as opposed to being wasted. Questions of ethics and morality in this respect become commercial decisions where ethical deliberation only facilitates the recycling of entities going to waste (Bharadwaj 2010a). So, what would formerly have been discarded is now made available for maximum accumulation, recycling and perpetuation. The shift is both semantic and material: waste becomes displaced/supplemented/supplanted by what is 'going to waste'. One can say that 'going to waste' now stands in a relationship of supplementation with twentieth-century waste. Neoliberal citizenship demands that waste be supplanted and become viable through cycles of ethical, preferably legal, and above all optimal recycling (Bharadwaj and Glasner 2009). We must therefore ask, what kind of supplement is the so-called surrogate? Do the poverty and material circumstances of some women in India turn their reproductive vitality – otherwise going to waste – into a commercially viable proposition? Most importantly, what is it to live a supplementary life, not so much in lieu of or in the position of (an)other but rather as an additional other?

Derrida (1998: 199) tells us that 'substitution distances from birth, from the natural or maternal origin'. While Derrida addresses and deconstructs a different semantic context, I appropriate his notion of the supplement to suggest that a surrogate is better conceptualised as a supplement, especially given her temporal positionality vis-à-vis the biosocial mother as (an)other. To achieve this, let us first understand how Derrida invokes supplementation. 'Supplement', for Derrida, harbours two important cohabiting significations: 'The supplement adds itself, it is a surplus, a plenitude enriching another plenitude, the fullest measure of presence. It cumulates and accumulates presence' (Derrida 1998: 144). For example, writing, for Derrida (1998: 144), 'substitutes the plenitude of a speech whose deficiency and infirmity it nevertheless only supplements'. A surrogate, in this respect, is not only a substitute for the mother as a biosocial signifier, but she also, through recycling her pauper body into an innovative new permutation, becomes the tool and trope for bypassing a 'deficient infirmity', a pronatalist inflection on the body of the biosocial mother, albeit via a circuitous and supplemental detour. 'But the supplement supplements', warns Derrida. It adds only to replace (although its destiny is temporal and fixed). It intervenes or insinuates itself in-the-place-of; if it fills, it is as if it fills a void. If it represents and makes an image, it is by the anterior default of a presence.

Compensatory [*suppléant*], the supplement is an adjunct, a subaltern instance that takes-(the-)place. As a substitute, it is not simply added to the positivity of a presence; it produces no relief as its place is assigned in the structure by the mark of an emptiness. Somewhere, something can be filled up of itself, can accomplish itself, only by allowing itself to be filled through sign and proxy. 'The sign is always the supplement of the thing itself' (Derrida 1998: 145).

The surrogate becomes a mother by supplementing. This transactional motherhood is achieved in the semantic and the enunciatory realms. A surrogate knows her place in the patriarchal, pronatalist structure as compensatory, as both brought in and bought to fill the empty, womb-like void, and delegated to supplant this void left unfulfilled by the biosocial mother. The dual quality of supplement is replacement and addition. That which is deficient and replaced by the supplement is not merely substituted but rather is added to; in so doing, a new structure is produced that cannot be reduced to the entity being replaced or supplanted. According to Derrida, this second signification of the supplement cannot be separated from the first. But the inflexion varies from moment to moment. Each of the two significations, by turns, is effaced or becomes discreetly vague in the presence of the other. Thus the first erasure is that of the biosocial mother, followed by the eventual erasure of the surrogate or the supplement. And, occasionally, one mother becomes discreetly vague in the presence of the other. But their common function is shown in this: whether it adds or substitutes itself, the supplement is exterior, outside of the positivity to which it is super-added, alien to that which, in order to be replaced by it, must be other than it. Unlike the complement (the biosocial mother), the supplement (surrogate mother) is an 'exterior addition' (Derrida 1998: 145). In other words, a supplement is always doubly articulate: it fixes a fault, deficiency, absence or something missing and in so doing it adds something that is different and cannot be reduced to that which has become supplanted. A supplement in this respect cannot be a surrogate as that presupposes mere proxy, ignoring the addition inherent in supplementation. A supplementary woman, like the surrogate, substitutes only the missing, absent gestational potential of the biosocial mother. But in so doing, the supplement substitutes also the mother by adding her gestational fecundity for the duration of the contract to enrich and enhance the social career of the biosocial mother. A supplement therefore remains an addition replete with her own biographical structure, thus allowing new readings and interpretations of what it is to be the other mother.

The 'Other' Mother: Sexual Genealogies, Gendered Ideologies

The title of this chapter, 'The "Other" Mother', is a provocation. It is an invitation to question and (re)locate the figure of 'the mother' in transnational surrogate transactions. 'Mother', therefore, is a misnomer. The conflation of mother and surrogate is a fine illustration of the gendered cultural imprints that saturate thinking across a spectrum of institutions, such as biomedicine, state, law, family, marriage or religion in a stratified global reproductive topography (Ragoné and Twine 2000). Marilyn Strathern (1998) argues that, for Euro-Americans, a surrogate mother makes explicit the relationship between gestation and other factors in childbirth. She, the surrogate substitute, is 'acting on behalf of another woman, she represents a facet of motherhood but is not herself the real mother' (Strathern 1998: 185). This 'stand-in' function, 'metonymically occupying' the place in reference to another person, who, by implication, is always the 'real parent', is how the 'modernist Euro-American' sees this relationship between the complement and the supplement (Strathern 1998). However, the category of 'real parent' or 'real mother' – even in the modernist 'ethnoscape' (Appadurai 1996) of Euro-Americans – needs cautious conceptualisation. The so-called real biosocial mother's erasure from the process of gestation – her privileged Euro-American position notwithstanding – remains poorly understood and articulated in transnational surrogate transactions. This temporal slippage of the imagined real parent into the realm of 'other mother' needs more nuanced empirical and conceptual elaboration.[3] Nevertheless, this process ensconces the substitute womb in the domain of fictive kinship that designates the supplanting womb 'as if' that of the real mother.[4] Strathern (1998) argues that what makes the surrogate 'like a mother' and not the real mother is that she helps the real mother to achieve motherhood. In the case of transnational gestational surrogacy, for instance as currently being practiced in India, where the biogenetic connect with the parents of an evolving foetus and the biogenetic disconnect with the supplementary womb is almost always complete, a surrogate's nine-month-long motherhood is often figurative, a simple figure of speech that is routinised, normalised and naturalised in media, policy and clinical discourses. These 'stratified reproducers' (Ginsburgh and Rapp 1995) seldom become 'like a mother', given the racial, class and ethnic differences between the supplanted mother and the other mother.

Throughout the twentieth century the 'cultural' penetrated deeper into the realm of the 'cellular' (Keller 1995). From metaphoric postulations about women's bodies as ancient sites for/of reproduction to the gendered inscription of reproductive tissues,[5] motherhood could not only be objectified as preordained, encrypted natural destiny, but also 'enterprised up' to fulfil the fecund remit.[6] In this respect, the feminist critique, especially the radical feminist challenge of the early 1980s, is not only noteworthy but also accidentally prophetic. Long before invocations to the manifesto of the cyborg and techno-feminism became commonplace amongst feminist activists like Andrea Dworkin (1983), Gena Corea (1985a) and many others were (re)drawing the battle lines.[7] These early political encounters were largely received with guarded caution as either untenable in a globalised world or too Eurocentric to be useful in 'other cultures'.[8] However, this critical distancing would only ring true if the radical feminist challenge of the 1980s were viewed from a discursive universe that equates the empirical with the experiential, epistemological positioning and ontological spectating as generative of the real and truthful. Thus viewed, arguments around agency, structure and resistance can displace these early feminist concerns. However, the radical feminist challenge was always unashamedly located on the boundary between producing rhetoric of persuasion and manifestos for rebellion. Its vitality was of a different order; it was confrontational; it spoke in the projective future tense and re-conceived the world order in a different gendered configuration. It idealised the purity of a revolutionary: naive but infectious, shrill but sincere, sensational but trite. It was passion out of control and anger devoid of discipline. A good illustration of this genre of politics can be found in what Dworkin (1983) and Corea (1985a) passionately described as the 'reproductive brothel'.

Agitating against male control over women's reproductive destinies, Dworkin (1983) predicted a shift away from the 'farming model applied to motherhood', where men plant seeds and harvest the crop (a metaphoric postulation very much alive in India to this day), to a brothel model where women are collected together and held, thus reducing a woman to what 'she sells'. The diatribe goes on to conjure horrific scenarios that liken the latter model to animal farming. However, when describing possible future permutations of surrogacy arrangements, Corea almost predicts an uncanny and now familiar face of international surrogacy, albeit in 1985. Quoting social commentator Vance Packard, Corea argued:

> If the 'mercenary mother' were to gestate an embryo conceived with another woman's egg, the job should not require much of the surrogate 'in the way of education, family back-ground, good looks, or even skin color. If the woman is simply to be an incubator, the price would certainly be lower than if she contributed half the baby's heredity'. In south Texas, he wrote, 'pleasant conscientious Mexican-American girls might leap at a fee of 5000 dollars for bearing a child and girls (sic) south of the border might leap at half that fee. 'If lawyers can arrange Mexican divorces for Americans', wrote Packard, 'they surely can arrange Mexican gestations'. Fees paid to 'host mothers' would probably vary with the country, as several commentators have suggested. Mexican women would do it for less. When it becomes possible to transfer human embryos routinely from one women to another (and it has already been done experimentally), then the way opens to use Third World women to gestate babies for wealthier Westerners. The president of a US foundation which helps arrange surrogate

> pregnancies told me: 'If we could cross international lines, then 1000 dollars is a significant sum of money, whereas (in the US), it's just a week or month's wages'. Asked what countries he had in mind he replied: 'Central America would be fine'. It is 'inevitable' that the United States go to other parts of the world and 'rely on their support' in providing surrogate mothers, he thinks. Comparing United States to the city and Central America to the country, he pointed out that 'the cities are always supported by the country'. (Corea 1985a)

What seemed plausible in 1985 has become an empirical reality. The possibility of arranging 'Mexican gestations' has given way to the surety of acquiring Indian gestational surrogacy.

What are the implications for India? In India today, assisted conception is a visible, viable and veritably thriving industry. It is within this commercial context that the global extent of India's burgeoning surrogacy industry has become well-known, if not terribly well understood.

However, let me trace these developments in the context of India's fertility industry and the many cultural patterns that frame its spectacular rise. My point of departure is yet again conceptual. Let us return momentarily to a 'critical event' in India's history, the partition of the subcontinent into India and Pakistan that left scores of women violated, abused and abducted (Das 1999). In fact, the nature of the violence and its focus on women's bodies was tantamount to violating and polluting the source of reproductive purity. Not surprisingly therefore, thousands of women were left unclaimed by families and networks of kin as what I conceptualise and politicise as patriarchal waste. When such tainted bodies were claimed, as Veena Das (1995: 215) shows, the injury to normative concepts like purity and honour (of abducted/sexually violated women) could only be absorbed within the normal structures of family and marriage so long as these breaches were subsumed in silence. Das begins her account with the voice of Mitro, a character in Krishna Sobti's novel *Mitro Marjani*. Mitro articulates the strangeness of a world in which the sexual act is seen as a religious deed when a woman is impregnated by her husband and a sin if the man is a stranger (Das 1995: 212). The strangeness of this world lies not so much in the sacred and sinful nature of the impregnation, but rather in Mitro's inability to comprehend why this is indeed the case when in either situation she had no role in consenting to the brutal consummation. The difference between the consecrated 'seed' and the sinful 'weed' has a long cultural history on the Indian subcontinent (Dube 1986). Women are at best seen as 'barren' fields incapable of bringing the planted seeds to fruition but by the virility of the seed itself, which is never questioned. In certain communities in India, surplus and dispensable bodies of women range from 'barren' bodies conceived as empty vessels incapable of bodying forth life to bodies of widows reduced to a life of 'living death'. The normative solutions sought in order to contain/discipline such transgressing/unyielding bodies are even more harrowing. An archaeology of these problematic bodies takes us back thousands of years to the customary laws that enjoined women to remain under male control and supervision, ranging from the father to the husband and, eventually, in old age, the all-important son (Bharadwaj 2003). Here we encounter another pattern borne within the domain of patriarchal semantics. In parts of North India, the term used to denote a widow and a prostitute remains the same to this day. Like a prostitute, a widow threatens control and ownership entitlements. Condemned to lead an austere life of self-denial and religious contemplation in the memory of a dead husband, young widows are sometimes literally recycled as prostitutes or forced to lead lives punctuated by sexual violence, social exclusion and exploitation.[9] The normative and ideological reception and understanding of surrogacy arrangements in India exhibits a similarly fractal pattern, and the story of Nirmala is a good example.

On 11 June 1997, long before India gained notoriety as a commercial surrogacy destination, India woke up to a startling piece of news. Nirmala, a thirty-year-old woman from Punjab in the northwest of India, had decided to rent out her womb for 50,000 rupees to an infertile couple. The media frenzy was unprecedented. Overnight Nirmala became a household name, a woman who was renting out her womb so that she could pay her paralysed husband's medical bills. What shocked people was not her decision to rent out her womb, but the terms of agreement with the couple – a retired Air Force officer and his wife, for whom she worked. Nirmala was to have sexual intercourse with the husband, conceive a child, and, after it was born, hand over legal rights to the couple. The fear of being prosecuted under the Suppression of Immoral Traffic Act forced Nirmala to turn to the legal system to legitimise and recognise her right to rent out her womb. The subjudge in Chandigarh, the capital of Punjab state, issued requests to the government of India and the union territory administration to decide if the renting of Nirmala's womb was legal and constitutional. Her lawyer, in turn, openly declared that because she was Hindu, he would seek sanctions from the scriptures for her stance and called for testimonies from religious leaders like the four *Sankaracharyas* and the *Arya Samaj* on whether a woman could become a surrogate mother.

The outrage surrounding Nirmla's willingness to have sexual intercourse for money, with the intent to procreate for an infertile couple, is largely a reaction to an arrangement perceived to compromise cherished ideals of purity and sacredness. The surrogacy arrangement renders public the inclusion of a third party in the process of procreation and commercialises the process of conception that cannot simply be assimilated within the rubric of 'Hindu marriage'. In addition, the episode challenges the acceptable limits to improvisations in resolving infertility within the parameters of a (Hindu) community. Most importantly, Nirmala's ability to use an instrument of the state – the legal system – to assert her 'cultural rights' as a Hindu by drawing on a shared cultural memory (niyoga) to challenge her potential criminalisation under the law exposed yet another instance of 'creative tensions' underlying the relations between individuals, communities and the state in contemporary India (Das 1999).[10]

In reporting the common prevalence of surrogacy in India – in the wake of the Nirmala episode – some media accounts successfully identified the bone of contention at the heart of this controversy. An excerpt from the *Sunday Times of India* (28 September 1997) is instructive:

> Artificial insemination is 200 years old. Surrogacy is as old as the Mahabharata. And infertility specialists in Mumbai reveal that they have handled several cases of surrogacy, with legal contracts involved. So what's all the fuss about Nirmala? It's just that she's the first to have made public her desire to rent out her womb for 50,000.

The criticism that bombarded Nirmala was not merely focused on her willingness to have sexual intercourse in order to conceive for the couple, nor even in her acceptance of money for such a service, but more crucially on account of her daring public pronouncement about such an arrangement, thus rendering visible that which should have (ideally) remained private. More crucially, the past that Nirmala's defence invokes by alluding to the practice of niyoga provides extremely fractured evidence, even in the realm of myth. As discussed earlier, surrogacy in the Hindu worldview was never a preferred solution for female infertility but rather a cultural accommodation of an absence of the male seed. How common it was as a historical practice is unclear, but there is growing anecdotal evidence of this, and also hearsay evidence of its practice to this day as a means of bypassing infertility within the private realm of the family. In counter distinction to the historical practice of niyoga, informal surrogacy arrangements between sisters or sisters-in-law within a family are reportedly common in India. A woman either conceives a child with her partner for an infertile sister to adopt, or, more recently, women resort to Intrauterine Insemination (IUI) or IVF using their brother-in-law's semen to conceive a child for an infertile sister. In the summer of 2005, I met a twenty-four-year-old pregnant woman who had undergone an IUI using her father-in-law's semen. The fertility expert at the Delhi clinic where I encountered the pregnant daughter-in-law and donor father-in-law 'couple' told me how very common this was, particularly in the Jat community in the neighbouring state of Haryana. Insemination or donor IVF allowed them to practice the ancient custom of levirate. Unlike with Nirmala, sexual intercourse in the present-day variant of 'Jat levirate' was substituted by intercourse of a clinical kind. While Indian media is replete with reports of surrogacy arrangements, Nirmala's case stands out as unusual due to its non-clinical nature. To drive home this point, media accounts drew on popular culture by establishing parallels between the Nirmala story and a film, *Doosri Dulhan* (The Other Bride, released in 1983), based on a true story of a couple in the Dadar Hindu Colony in Mumbai who paid their maid to bear them a child. In the film, however, the couple hires the services of a prostitute who is impregnated by the man, resulting in further emotional complications. Similarly, in 2000 another 'Bollywood' film, *Chori Chori Chupke Chupke* (Secretly and Quietly), addressed the same theme. The protagonists – a married couple – hire the services of a prostitute to conceive through sexual intercourse. The reference to prostitutes in these films is interesting, as it likens such surrogacy arrangements to prostitution, a link that Nirmala sought to challenge. The interference patterns these diffracted dimensions produce highlight the lives and bodies of women – both normatively compliant and transgressive – within the highly charged ideological zone of sexuality, reproduction and control. In this zone the hierarchy and distinction between the Madonna and the Whore is continuously under threat. The Whore in this worldview epitomises the absence of male control; she represents the market and invades the Habermasian male public sphere with impunity (Habermas 1989).[11] Diffracted interference patterns of the Madonna and the Whore similarly compromise the attendant binaries of control and its absence, public and private, and fertile and barren. Both prostitutes, who are depicted in popular culture as surrogate wombs, and Nirmala, whose subjugated subject position challenges such cultural conflations, not only confront the patriarchal sense of control but also force the use of one's pauper body and fertility as a 'commodity of last resort' (Scheper-Hughes 2002). Other subject positions include the fertile young brides inseminated by their infertile husband's brothers and fathers or the emasculated existences of such infertile men. In this context it is also important to note that Marcia C. Inhorn (1996a), in her book *Infertility and Patriarchy: The Cultural Politics of Gender and Family Life in Egypt*, reminds us of the 'classic patriarchy' model, where within the context of patrilineal, patrilocally extended households the senior male has authority over everyone else, including younger men.

Surrogate women in India on the other hand often voice their concerns about the social and media conflation of prostitution and surrogacy (Pande 2010a). Perhaps this anxiety emerges from within this broader cultural pattern that views weak or absent male supervision as the reason for illicit and unauthorised pregnancies. The protestations and theodicies of these women, who hold up the scientific and clinical modality of their conception as proof of purity, are yet another kind of substitution, one between the phallus and the surgical syringe (most graphic and noteworthy in ICSI procedures). However, these attempts fail not because these women cannot disprove that surrogacy has nothing to do with prostitution, but rather because their substitution places them in the space occupied by similar subaltern subjects, some of whom are indeed prostitutes. The pollution, stigma, dirt and aspersion of illegitimate sexuality are not the delegitimating causes in themselves; rather, it is the very process of supplementation itself, the process of becoming the 'other mother'.

The State: Absent or Surrogate?

What role has the Indian state played in the rise of transnational surrogacy in India? I wish to ask: is the state absent or surrogate? Lawrence Cohen (2004: 167) argues that to be 'supplementable is to be able to receive a gift from the sovereign state in the form of another's body'. Cohen's work describes in vivid detail how citizenship in India is (re)made through the trope of surgical intervention. The gift from the state is mythic; it is predicated on the creation and harnessing of diverse populations on the margins of society: populations imagined as endowed with passion but not reason. The supplementability becomes the price of citizenship itself, whereby in renouncing a part of one's body, a redemptive, modern and ethical contract with the state is forged. These imaginary subject citizens are supplementary in the state's calculations; their supplementary bodies in effect become their saviour. Commenting on organ transactions, Cohen observes:

> The bureaucrat-physician [an extension/representation of the state itself] identifies with the buyer's need and alternatively ignores the seller or – particularly if the seller is female – imagines the sale of an organ as the minor exception preventing her from the more traumatic violation of prostitution. Again and again, nephrologists on and off the committee suggested that if people were not allowed to sell their kidneys, they would have to sell their entire bodies. (Cohen 2004)

Surrogates are captured in the slightly different supplementary logic of the 'neoliberal calculus of the Indian state' (Bharadwaj 2010a). Whereas a surrogate is purchased for the contracted period of time, it is more than her womb that is owned for the contracted period. Amrita Pande's (2010b) study of surrogate women in Anand, Gujarat, shows that women's labour becomes an exploitable resource, the creation of the perfect mother-worker, and her autonomy and control over her body are selectively suspended for the duration of the contract.[12] She, the substitute, is now continuously enjoined to eat, take medication and sleep while confined to the surrogate hostel, a holding facility that oversees and surveys surrogate pregnancies and (in)valuable gestating life. The prevailing legal vacuum in India restricts the whole process to the private commercial sphere, where the surrogate workers are enveloped not so much in an ethic of care but in concerns dictated by commercial profit and enterprise.

Guidelines, such as those of the ICMR, on surrogacy and assisted conception technologies demand, perhaps necessitate, interpretation. Even the proposed law falls in this gray zone of legal interpretation (ICMR 2010). For instance, Kaushik Sunder Rajan (2008: 179) shows how clinical trials in India are not conducted in the absence of ethical framing but rather in a space of 'hyperethicality', where trials are tightly regulated under some of the strictest clinical trial laws in the world. The structural violence in this scenario is not embedded in a lack of regulation, enforcement or oversight, but rather in the ethically informed and 'merely risked subjects' partaking in a gold-standard, clinical research organisation-sponsored, ethically monitored and legally supervised clinical trial (Sunder Rajan 2007). Such displacing effects of legal oversight render the intention of the state open-ended and supplemental. The state in this respect becomes either absent, silent or expressed through surrogate organs, constituents and intermediaries. The state, in Das's (2004) words, comes to have a 'spectral presence'. Through the disciplinary modality of guidelines, for instance, the state optimises the use and harnessing of the reproductive vitality of the surrogate wombs. Clinical mediations, brokers, semen banks, law firms and middlemen all step in as the state further withdraws from regulating, controlling and morally defining the contours of the commercial exploitation of its citizens. The discursive mediation facilitated by physicians, law firms and semen banks through tropes and incantations of 'the ethical', 'legal contract' and the 'invocation and interpretation of ICMR guidelines' further invokes the 'spectral presence of the state' (Das 2004: 234). The visible presence of the physician or lawyer is not merely relegated to the register of a middleman/broker between commissioning couples and supplementary wombs; rather he is the mediator between the state and the local and global citizens. The clinical space, for example, as the purveyor and surveyor of these 'surrogate hostels' (Pande 2010b), therefore becomes a substitute for the state by assuming the function of defining, interpreting and enforcing surrogacy contracts: a veritable state of the surrogate state.

The recent ICMR (2010) ART draft regulation bill proposes setting up ART banks registered as independent entities. The bank is expected to source, store, handle and keep records for gametes, embryos and surrogates. All screening and provision responsibilities for these entities would remain with the banks, which would operate independently of any ART clinic in the country. Each ART bank should have 'standard, scientifically established facilities and defined standard operating procedure for all its scientific and technical activities' (ICMR 2010: 20–21). In a manner of speaking, these surrogate banks would be responsible solely for advertising, procuring and supplying surrogates to clinics and their clients. Such a facility would replace the surrogate hostel with a surrogate bank, a veritable mirror-opposite, albeit metaphoric, holding space for supplementary wombs. The bank, privately set up under the provisions of the act, would supplement the clinic as the site of optimal control, circulation and accumulation of reproductive tissue and bankable supplementary wombs. What happens to the actual surrogates carrying precious cargo remains largely unclear. Will they continue to be interned in surrogate hostels within clinics, or would a different facility replace these spaces? In the event that the surrogates are 'liberated' by the new enactments to enjoy a greater degree of freedom and return home to some semblance of normality, what implications, if any, would this have on the surrogacy business in India? This is crucial since any such moves could create conditions where, as precious 'cargo', embryos of commissioning couples would gestate in a state where clinics cannot exercise optimal control, surveillance and scrutiny. This state of the surrogate state becomes possible in precisely such contexts where 'the state becomes illegible' (Das 2004). Rules and regulations become open to interpretation as they are diffused further through surrogate intermediaries, organs and institutions. Inevitably, oscillation between the state and surrogate state becomes the defining feature.

These developments have become suffused with even more uncertainty since 2015 when the Indian state imposed a moratorium on gestational surrogacy involving foreign commissioning couples. The Indian government, while seeking to regulate the burgeoning fertility tourism in the country, is ironically taking these ad hoc steps in the absence of any clear-cut laws overseeing fertility clinics in India. As per the directive issued by the Indian Council of Medical Research in October 2015, surrogacy services can only be used by married Indian couples. The stated motivation behind this move is to protect poor and vulnerable women from exploitation. It remains unclear how precluding foreign couples and allowing Indian 'married couples' access to surrogacy arrangements is going to protect vulnerable supplementary women. As further critical attention is directed at this sudden turnaround, it is safe to speculate that the proposed regulation will further galvanise the call for instituting ART banks. Ironically protection of vulnerable subject citizens from 'foreigners' does little to change the predicament of supplementary wombs that remain bioavailable for commercial liquidation at the behest of the state for more privileged heteronormative Indian citizens.

Conclusion

It is doubtful that India's ongoing tryst with technologies of procreation and transnational fertility travels in search of gametes, wombs and technicians, delivering conception and gestation at a fraction of the global prices in a highly stratified, competitive, and buoyant global market, will ever be truly elucidated. The problem is one of both scale and limit as to what ethnographic production can achieve in a rapidly globalising market. Herein lie the true implications for knowledge production and political activism. How do we critique and resist that which escapes the ethnographic gaze? I only sketch in broad strokes some crucial issues in need of conceptual and empirical unravelling and urgent political mobilisation. Other concerns lie scattered in the transnational terrain of supplementary gestations. The potential for exploitation and coercion by family members, brokers, middlemen and now, increasingly, 'ex-surrogates' acting as brokers – alone or sometimes in cahoots with other interested parties – can severely impact women's ability to choose, agree or challenge the terms of gestational agreements. Global media reports on 'surrogacy in India' (currently a staggering 134,000 returns on Google's search engine alone) often narrate accounts of financial hardship, of women stepping in to pay off familial debt or to bail out their husbands' bad debts or investments. Just how such a state of social, familial and financial depredation can become the basis for a liberal contract with the neoliberal state under the sign of informed choice and consent remains both deeply problematic and untenable.

Elsewhere I show that a 'moral economy' is on the ascent in India (Bharadwaj 2010a).[13] I argue that the unprecedented ethical quagmire created by emerging life forms under the neoliberal formation also creates states of exception where capital, profit, accumulation, production, consumption and circulation by (market-dictated) necessity become aligned to local and global ethical and moral registers (Bharadwaj 2010a: 242). The search for ethical and moral standards is in turn inextricably linked to the creation of standardised research, assembly and production protocols, routinised manufacturing practices, the purchase and procurement of raw materials and the expertise contained in standardised supply chains around the globe. Although research practices, manufacturing processes, labour markets, quality controls and moral, ethical and governance protocols are mobilised to create a standardised entity (e.g., a human embryo, surrogate womb, stem-cell line, or a pair of shoes!), political formations and businesses are seldom able to achieve the 'ethical end products' without invoking states of exception. I describe this neoliberal condition as a 'moral economy', which allows us to witness what kinds of regimes of exploitation, tropes and technologies of obfuscation and processes of unproblematic, guilt-free consumption are facilitated if one literalises the moral in the economic calculation of new invention, experimentation and globalisation. For the moral economy to flourish, the state of exception must either remain systematically misrecognised or become a feature of the autonomous, rational, informed and freethinking ideological calculus of neoliberal citizenship (Bharadwaj 2010a: 242–44). Thus argued, the Indian state can recycle the pauper bodies of its many millions of citizens and reinvest the 'reproductive viability' of its formerly going-to-waste citizens in the service of a booming neo India (Bharadwaj 2010b).

The enactment of laws in India to control surrogacy would only have a displacing effect. As argued earlier, under the new proposed ICMR-sponsored law, surrogate women would find themselves removed from the clinical context and 'held', surveyed and supplied through dedicated facilities with legal recognition. This oversight renders moral and ethical any procurement of supplementary wombs alienated from the real person and her biological and social experience of pregnancy. While the focus stays on the gestating life in the supplementary womb, legal control remains on the entire body held which is under contract for the duration of the pregnancy. The structural violence and material circumstances, not to mention a woman's ever-depleting agency and control for the duration of the contract, remain in a state of exception. The body of the supplement can now be imagined as relocated and held in a 'symbolic' private bank. Under the proposed new law, these new facilities or surrogate organs of the state curiously perform the necessary work of making the entire process legal, moral and ethical. The legal context bestows and restores much more than commercial gestation, as now supplementary wombs become legally accessible and guilt-free. The moral 'taint of commerce' (Hirsch 1993: 88) is removed by the fine print of the neoliberal, legally enforceable contract, and the very modality of 'stratified reproduction' – via the supplementing detour – is thereby misrecognised. However, these developments compel us to reflect further on the decisions that surrogate women take in a market where their fecundity is commercialised through a moral economic sensibility. As we move forward, perhaps we should ask: what kind of agency is at work? How, in a stratified global reproductive sphere, does the market both ingeniously shackle and liquidate a woman's corporeality? Like the organ trade, where systemic failure of the welfare state leaves paupers with little else other than their bodies, can we argue that a pragmatic investment in one's body and the selective liquidation of one's 'corporeal possession' (I see corporeal here as both biogenetic and commercial) becomes a legitimate survival strategy? Or, like 'stratified reproducers' (Ginsburg and Rapp 1995) who leave their un-nurtured children behind to nurture others in the global labour market, are surrogates too making the best use of a commodity of last resort: a viable womb?

The margins of the state in India appear frayed and unclear. At these margins the state is made and unmade, added to and withdrawn from, or, as Derrida would remind us, forged in a relationship between the complement and supplement. In this analysis there are two key entities in the transnational topography of fertility travels: the Indian state and the 'other mother'. The two are hugely different in scale, power, agency and ability. Nevertheless, the surrogate state and supplementary wombs curiously underscore the everyday, mundane generation of gestating life in a state of moral, ethical and legal exception.

Notes

1. For a notable political critiques see Gupta (2006), Unnithan-Kumar (2013), SAMA (2012) and Qadeer (2009, 2010).
2. Agamben (1998) resurrects the figure of the *homo sacer* as the one allowing the sovereign to resort to a state of exception in which the bare killable body becomes situated as one lying before the law; thus it cannot be sacrificed, as this positioning renders it outside the purview of divine law. In other words, certain bodies become killable as they become positioned as lying before the very institution of law.
3. A recent ethnographic account by Elly Teman (2010) produces just such a nuanced narrative of a very specific case of 'surrogate bodies' in Israel, where surrogates and intended mothers negotiate and cooperate in bringing forth new life that produces both a deep and lasting bond between the surrogate and biosocial mother.
4. I borrow the formulation of fictive 'as if' kinship principally from the work of Judith Modell (1994), who in the context of American adoptive kinship shows how bonds created through adoption are made 'as-if' genealogical and natural.
5. Both of these aspects are brilliantly described by Emily Martin (1987, 1991).
6. See Becker (2000), Franklin (1990, 1997), Franklin and Ragoné (1998), Greil (1991), and Strathern (1992b).
7. Donna Haraway's (1990) article, 'A Manifesto for Cyborgs' and the radical feminist critiques were in fact contemporaneous; Haraway's 'Manifesto' was first published in 1985, and then republished in 1990, when it rose to global prominence.
8. For example, see Stanworth (1987).
9. For more on the status of widows in India, see Chen (1998) and Reddy (2004).
10. Veena Das (1999) shows that the relations between the state and (religious) communities in India are fraught with creative tensions on the issue of cultural rights. She draws on the case of a divorced Muslim woman – Shah Bano – who appealed for maintenance under Section

125 of the Code of Criminal Procedure in India, addressing how state involvement conflicted with the Muslim community and the assertion of cultural rights to practice its personal law. The second case she examines is that of a Hindu woman – Roop Kanwar – who in 1987 was forced to ascend the funeral pyre of her husband to commit *sati*. The state intervention was met with resistance from a section of the Rajput community asserting the cultural right to practice its religious customs. In both cases, the breakdown of the private and public distinction is crucial to the way in which communities asserted their 'rights' as lying separate (and hence private) from the public domain occupied by the state. The definition of the community itself in both these cases came to centre around the 'organisation of memory' (especially the glorification of *sati* in a mythic/historical mode), thus memory becomes, as Das (1999: 115) puts it, 'both an archive and a history'. The Nirmala case is an interesting site to witness how reference to a 'cultural memory' (niyoga) recreates tensions between Hindu ideals of procreation as sacred and confined to the institution of marriage and its commercialisation that Nirmala is seeking to legitimise by turning to state institutions.

11. See also Benhabib (1995) and Fraser (1992).
12. See also Vora (2009).
13. See also Thompson (1971).

Part IV

The cultural domain of ideas that treatment seekers and treatment providers simultaneously inhabit intimately informs an engagement with the technologies of procreation. In making sense of infertility treatments, clinicians and their patients routinely situate the rigours of day to day encounters with assisted conception within these domains of ideas that formulate and articulate their experiences. Part IV addresses the paradox that lies at the heart of assisted conception by situating the process of 'making sense' of treatment seeking and its provision within the same quasi-sacred conceptual cultural frame that produces social suffering and stigma in the first place. Perhaps this is indicative of a wider cultural facility to enable and disable, to shackle and to free the human agency. The chapters that follow reveal that, while treatment seekers sometimes hold the clinicians responsible for eluding conception, mounting expenses and lacking a 'human touch', they persist in seeking the possibility of clinical conception. Ironically, this uncertainty and tentativeness reroutes them and the clinicians back to the same meaning-giving cultural domain of religious and quasi-religious ideas that delegitimises infertility.

Chapter 7

Long Road to Conception

Emotional and Financial Costs

Infertile couples bring to a clinic not only dissatisfaction with a harsh and judgmental society (Chapter 2) but also disaffection for their bodies and failed attempts to salvage their fertility with medical help. The experience of secretly circumventing and accommodating the normative constructs of relatedness while seeking treatment (Chapter 5) further strains a continuous search for conception. While on this long road to conception, couples face disappointment and struggle with 'failure'. The situation is further exacerbated by high financial costs that mount with every unsuccessful attempt to conceive.

This experience of seeking conception contrasts with emerging evidence from Britain, where women undergoing IVF, 'despite its costs and pains', not only endorse the technique but even feel 'it has "made something of them" as women' (Franklin 1997: 165). Sarah Franklin argues that this enabling aspect of IVF helps to explain why women pursue it despite very high failure rates, physical demands and high financial, emotional and psychological costs. According to Franklin (1997: 165), 'As a "way of life", IVF was something [women] coped with ably and knowledgeably, an appreciation that must be borne alongside the very justifiable concerns about IVF as a means of alleviating infertility'. The experience of infertile couples in this research seems vastly different from that of Franklin's interviewees. A possible explanation, apart from cultural differences, may lie in the fact that Franklin's couples had endured in the past different kinds of reproductive health care interventions. However, there is a valuable theoretical implication in Franklin's position, i.e. that in order to understand why people endure assisted conception – given the high financial and emotional costs – it is important to appreciate different ways in which the infertile 'make sense' of such treatments. More recently Franklin shows that:

> Few people go through IVF, in other words, without experiencing, either temporarily or permanently, and to a greater or lesser extent, a degree of ambivalence about this procedure – a view that is widely shared by IVF clinicians and nurses, who know better than anyone the potentially high costs of IVF. This ambivalence indexes the difference between the norms that IVF belongs to, and the extent to which it also challenges or contradicts these very same conventions. (Franklin 2013: 7)

Therefore, how people experience, understand and explain their underlying ambivalence towards reproductive struggles becomes a matter of perspective, a way of 'making sense' of their situations. Assisted conception in this respect becomes both enabling and disabling, bound up with the material circumstances and cultural location of 'experience' that informs how the infertile – whether British women or Hindu couples – understand medical management of infertility.

The following narratives in this chapter are full of expressions of disappointment, anger and helplessness. The emotional and financial burden of assisted conception has turned the experience into one of mistreatment and exploitation. The way in which these couples make sense of their long haul on the road to conception is by mounting a critique of the way their treatments were and are being handled and the ensuing financial burdens. The wider context of familial expectation and pressure and societal stigma adds to their sense of urgency. While no corroborating evidence substantiates their claims of medical mistreatment, they can nevertheless be viewed as explanations of elusive conception, failed expectations and anger at the way promised outcomes of specific interventions have not materialised. In pursuing this line, the chapter resists the temptation to narrate these experiences as 'objective and truthful' instances of exploitation. While there is no evidence to suggest that these experiences are 'mere fabrications', they must be considered within the context of a long, harrowing search for conception often at a high emotional and financial cost.[1] As Byron J. Good (1997) argues, in medical anthropological accounts the 'critical' distinction between power, domination and exploitation is sometimes lost when inequity of power and knowledge in a doctor-patient interaction (or even a patient's experience of such an engagement) is analysed as a straightforward case of exploitation.

The chapter opens with accounts of infertile couples and individuals and their experiences with medical interventions. It goes on to examine the financial costs they bear in order to persist with treatments that some can ill afford. The chapter concludes with a short discussion of how the clinicians perceive (and make sense of) the critical stance adopted by treatment seekers.

The Long Road to Conception

For the better part of their married existence – ranging from three to twenty years – these infertile couples had been in search of conception. Deeply touching and disturbing accounts reveal a clear and well-delineated trajectory of treatment-seeking behaviour underlying their quests. The predominant response was, 'We got married, and then nothing happened'. This usually entailed seeking an appointment with the family doctor or a local gynaecologist, thus setting into motion a long and harrowing journey which was still awaiting its logical conclusion at the time of these interviews. In the absence of clear information and proper diagnosis, these couples reveal a pattern of drifting from clinic to clinic, frequently changing doctors, who in turn pursued different lines of treatment, tests and even medications. Lack of proper referrals to specialists (Chapter 4) resulted in untimely treatment and at the same time loss of crucial childbearing years. An absence of information on how to seek proper guidance for their conditions also means that they relied on word of mouth, recommendations from over-enthusiastic well-wishers and the highly visible media propaganda on conception technologies (Chapter 4). Couples frequently travelled great distances across the country in search of the 'right expert'. It was therefore not uncommon to meet couples from Uttar Pradesh (North India) in Mumbai clinics (on the west coast), or patients from Assam and Bihar (East India) in clinics located in Rajasthan and Delhi (Northwest India). Doctor Suman, for instance, commented:

> Well, you know, there is a woman sitting outside. She is infertile. She's been advised IVF by a doctor but when she came here ... we re-canalised her [tubes]. She is now come for a follow up of that. Her husband is in Shillong [Assam] and she comes from Shillong you

> know [for] her follow up ... She actually belongs to Rajasthan ... They are very strongly motivated and they are so cloistered in themselves. The husband and wife, they've nobody to talk to. You know, for that reason, I think they can go to any extent and anything, and I would say some doctors really take them for a ride ... They do ... They do ... They do! ... I mean they have been kicked here and there and maltreated. Sometimes you find that they have lost ... so many precious years of not being referred to the right centre, to the right place.

Nearly all accounts from couples undergoing treatment confirmed this observation. The experience of a couple – Rati and Sundar – interviewed in a Mumbai clinic is particularly interesting in this respect. Married in 1978, they had been seeking medical help since 1986. Throughout the interview Sundar kept quiet and listened to his wife pour out her rage at what she saw as shoddy handling of her treatment:

> Rati: ... local doctor, and I also showed myself [to a private clinic], took regular treatment. They said, 'Wait and watch', wasted two to three years there. He couldn't set it right so we were told that another doctor is good. He also said everything is normal, reports, etc. Likewise took treatment from two to three very prominent doctors [in the city of Ahemdabad] ... Afterwards we came here. The doctors I initially consulted kept saying everything is normal...
>
> AB: Do you have a proper diagnosis now?
>
> Rati: Madam said that you are very late. If you had come earlier, it would have been much better. But then all the doctors kept saying, 'Don't worry, you will conceive, might take some couple of years'. So we kept waiting ... In Ahemdabad I showed to all the best doctors, but they kept saying, 'It will happen, it will happen!' These doctors delayed me ... I used to think and say, 'Just say it to me! Let me stop the treatment, wherever you will say I'll go' ... But they said, 'Everything is normal. It is in the hands of God; you will have something'... Whatever they said we did. We never said, 'We won't do this' ... The main thing is the doctors misled me. They should have told me to go to a good doctor, to Mumbai elsewhere ... They said, 'Why do you go to Mumbai? We will do good treatment here'.

An acute feeling of betrayal compounds Rati's anger towards her doctors. Feeling misled and mistreated, Rati and her husband struggle with the thought of having lost crucial years on account of medical incompetence. They are not alone. Kavita and Suresh, interviewed in a North India clinic, were in treatment for eight years with little conclusive medical evidence on why Kavita had miscarried four pregnancies. Having undergone fertility treatment for so long – which meant among other things by her own admission enduring more than 120 injections – Kavita was at the very edge of her patience and fortitude:

> The problem is only this, that the doctors should tell us clearly as to what the problem is. For seven years we have been pursuing the treatment and we must have consulted some twenty doctors in these seven years ... This is no life! Even the doctors don't tell us what is wrong ... Here also nothing but investigations and normal reports, only investigations, no results! If this doesn't show anything try this; if this doesn't work try that...

Jeet and Sonia's experience was again one of endlessly trying doctors and medical tests with little actual diagnosis and treatment:

> Sonia: [The doctor] told us that don't worry you will have a child. So we feel, let us try him, also.
>
> AB: Did you consult other doctors likewise?
>
> Sonia: Yes! Everyone gives hope, nobody says no!
>
> Jeet: Nobody has given proper treatment so far.
>
> Sonia: We do exactly what the doctors ask us to do, but when you go to another doctor after we are completely demoralised and disheartened, he says, 'No, don't do like this; this should be done, not this but this should be done, like this', they say.
>
> AB: Have you never asked for any explanation [interrupted]
>
> Jeet: No! We just leave that doctor and move on to the next one. The last report we showed to the doctor here, I [interrupted]
>
> Sonia: The earlier doctor had asked us to do another test, but [the doctor they are currently seeing] tells us that there is no need for that. We do exactly as the doctors tell us.

It is interesting to see that both Sonia/Jeet and Rati/Sundar repeatedly maintain that they did exactly as the doctor asked them. It is clear that they view themselves as having kept up their end of the bargain by fastidiously following the treatment regime, thus further heightening the sense of betrayal as doctors failed them by either promising too much or misleading them, whether unscrupulously or not.

On the issue of misleading the patients, the case of Harjeet, a farmer from Punjab (Chapter 2), stands out as particularly bad as he was given no pretreatment counselling on what to expect from an IVF procedure or information about its success rate:

> AB: Do you know that a child is not guaranteed in this treatment?
>
> Harjeet: Outsiders, people outside are telling me this [referring to other patients in the clinic's lobby] that out of 100 only 30 percent or 25 percent times it is possible.
>
> AB: The doctor didn't tell you this?
>
> Harjeet: No! He did not.
>
> AB: Do you understand that there is a possibility that you might not have a child and at the same time there is a possibility that you might succeed?
>
> Harjeet: The doctor did not say in these many words. He didn't say like this. Doctor *sahab* [respectful way of addressing a superior] is saying, 'You will have'. He was saying, 'You will have a child, for sure'.

The doctor's virtual promise to Harjeet above that 'you will have a child for sure' can be understood as a communication gap, or even misleading and substantially misrepresentative of IVF success rates. This incident also points to a general practice amongst busy clinicians of not spending much time counselling patients (see Chapter 8).

Rekha and Sudhir, a couple interviewed in Mumbai, have been married since 1986 and within a year of their marriage decided to start a family. Their experience once again points to a trend of encountering often distressing and unpleasant experiences on the long road to conception:

> Rekha: Within a year's time [of marriage] we decided [to start a family] ... At that stage, we didn't know what was happening. We tried the natural way ... We talked to our family doctor, [and] she put me on some tablets. Later on when things did not materialise, we thought of consulting another doctor/specialist, Dr ABC ... Mentally, physically and financially in all sites we were, at least I felt I was treated like a vegetable ... The problem was ... we were not gradually treated... 'Okay, just keep on taking hormones, keep on taking tablets, keep on taking injections. If you are over-stimulated, forget the cycle. If it is alright then let's try', like you know it was not a ... I was not very comfortable with the doctor to be honest.

> Sudhir: The problem that she had was easily identified but then later on what happened was a proper line of treatment was not followed … It was trial and error method, trial and error method! It was terrible! … The mental and physical torture was more, which you could not take.
>
> Rekha: … We were having problems and [interrupted]
>
> Sudhir: 1991–92 we stopped it … After going through what she did, I mean Dr ABC is very reputed.
>
> Rekha: Very reputed!
>
> Sudhir: But her approach was very, very inhuman and [interrupted]
>
> Rekha: Probably she never had the time … You just got dragged along … Physically it is a torture, torture in the sense there is a lot of discomfort physically like you have to be mentally prepared for these things [interrupted]
>
> Sudhir: Number one, you have to go through the hormonal treatment. Then you have to come for the sonography after a particular period, number of days, then [turning to his wife] what's left? What did she use to do? The day I got angry with her?
>
> Rekha: [laughs] I think it was [interrupted]
>
> Sudhir: I told her, 'I am sorry to say you have lost track what you are doing with her'!
>
> Rekha: Yah!
>
> Sudhir: That's what I told, that's what I told her! Better not give the treatment, ya? I'll be happy living with her without any issue. I don't want to lose her [to bad medical treatment].
>
> Rekha: It's like you've wasted your ten years because we don't have any problem. It is just a basic simple common cold as we would talk about it in simple layman's language. We are not suffering from any severe problems of any kind. I mean that's what I was wondering that ten years are wasted!

This is yet another narrative of abject disappointment and anger, of precious time lost at great emotional, physical and financial cost. Like Kavita, above, Rekha and Sudhir appear to have lost crucial years. However, while resisting 'bad' medical interventions they continued, in the absence of any tangible results, to endure the 'trial and error methods' of the doctors. Resistance of this kind is not uncommon and is in no way an exclusive preserve of the Indian urban middle to upper-middle classes, who are often construed as capable of resisting more powerfully.

Hariram, a migrant from a village in Uttar Pradesh, North India, seeking treatment in Mumbai together with his wife, was forthcoming in sharing his disappointing experience of medical interventions:

> We got married twenty years ago. After one year of marriage we wanted a child. I brought her to Mumbai. She used to live in the village; I brought her to Mumbai and got medication here in Parel [a Mumbai suburb], so first the doctor said that her tubes are damaged, closed, and after that both tubes were closed ... After this we met a doctor who said, 'I'll operate on her; let me open the tubes'. We said, 'Okay, this seems alright, too'. We agreed if we can get a child this way ... Then he operated; it was not successful, after that we got medication from here and there. After that I met another doctor who said to come here ... This could have happened fifteen years ago, also ... After the operation she is in more discomfort, the doctors are at fault, something that is not needed, why do that? First doctor where we used to go used to say, 'This method is the only way possible and any other intervention will not give you success' ... Seven to eight years ago we got the operation done which we shouldn't have ... They said, 'Get the operation done; everything will be alright' ... If we had known the right thing to do eight years ago, none of this would have happened!

After a twenty-year struggle, Hariram's wife was finally pregnant. On the day of the interview, she and her husband had come to the clinic for a follow-up after a successful embryo transfer. Their main grievance, however, was how past doctors had erred by recommending tubal surgery as the only option (they could have conceived, as they now had, with recourse to IVF, which is less invasive than surgery). It appears that, like many gullible patients eager for an early resolution of their infertility, Hariram and his wife put all their faith in the doctor's diagnosis and proposed line of treatment.

Yet another interesting case was that of Seema and Vani, from the town of Kota in the northwestern state of Rajasthan. Seema, who was undergoing treatment in a Jaipur clinic, had come, chaperoned by her sister-in-law, to see the doctor on the day of the interview. The sister-in-law, Vani, did most of the talking and gave a detailed history of Seema's long and ongoing struggle with infertility. This is an excerpt:

AB: When did you get married?

Seema: 1987

AB: When did you plan on starting your family?

Seema: Right from the very beginning.

AB: What happened [interrupted]

Seema: Nothing in particular but when I couldn't conceive ... I went to the doctor

AB: What was the initial stage like? Whom did you consult and what was the diagnosis?

Seema: Gynaecologist at the hospital

AB: How long did your treatment last before coming to this clinic?

Vani: Continuously for two three years. We even got her operated, but she showed no sign of recovery.

AB: Where have you come from?

Vani: Kota

AB: Did you consult someone at the local hospital?

Vani: There's a private clinic [in Kota]. She was quite a good doctor, and I think she is in London these days. After three years of marriage when we showed her she said tubes are blocked. She opened the tubes. After that we felt everything is okay. Even then nothing happened. For about two to three years, we were under her treatment since there was nobody better in Kota to turn to. She said, 'This treatment is the best, and you leave the rest to God'. Whatever has to happen will happen. Otherwise you are physically fit. We spent two to three years like this. Then we heard of Jaipur...

AB: When you were undergoing treatment in Kota did the doctor refer you to any specialist?

Vani: They consistently maintained that we have removed the blockage from your tubes and now you should have a child. After that, the doctor went off to London for two years for further training programme or something. She on her part had closed the chapter. As far as she was concerned, [Seema] was completely fit, [and] we couldn't meet her as she left Kota. For the two years that we were with her she said, 'You should have pregnancy and ... are physically fit'.

Seema and Hariram's wife are among a number of female patients who underwent surgery as the first line of treatment. By invoking surgery – which is usually understood by lay persons and professionals alike as a last resort – the doctors appear to be following the only option available to them. Gynaecological interventions can do little more than surgically open blocked tubes, a procedure that is sometimes less effective than IVF, where the fallopian tubes are bypassed altogether.[2] Recipients of such needless surgical procedures – like Hariram, who clearly benefited from IVF – rightly question the decision.

Hormonal therapy was yet another problem some interviewees faced. Sumita and Shankar were struggling with secondary infertility since the death of their only child – a daughter – in 1976.

> Shakar: [In] 1981 the treatment started. We went to Ahemdabad and lots of other places. We went to a lot of places in Gujarat. They gave us hormonal treatment but no result. Nothing came of it!
>
> AB: What do the doctors have to say about your case?
>
> Shankar: A lot of doctors used to say, 'You don't make ova', while the other lot said that the cycles are not proper.
>
> AB: What kind of treatment was prescribed?
>
> Shankar: All were hormonal treatments.
>
> AB: Did you experience any side effects?
>
> Shankar: Yes! She put on a lot of weight, cysts in the ovaries [interrupted]
>
> Sumita: Twice I had cysts in the ovaries!
>
> AB: Any other complications?
>
> Shankar: More cysts all because of these hormones!

For over sixteen years, Sumita's body was at the receiving end of hormonal therapy, inflicted on her by the very doctors to whom she and Shankar turned for help. Her narrative paints a story of medical mismanagement and a total absence of proper guidance and information, resulting in the loss of crucial childbearing years at great physical and emotional cost.

Neelanjana, a woman interviewed in a Jaipur clinic, was evidently upset at receiving substandard medical intervention. Here is a long excerpt from that interview:

> Neelanjana: It is not only the gynaecologists. I think it is the entire medical profession itself. They have mystified the whole thing. They ... the technical information. This person is an ignorant person; even if we try to explain they cannot understand the whole thing. They don't have time; they don't have the inclination or the patience to explain what is happening. Sometimes the patient feels, 'Okay, my God! I am being treated like a guinea pig'. I mean it is so specialised; there is no individualistic treatment. I think it's just like, 'Okay stand in a line, all of you have infertility – tac! tac! tac! ... that's the treatment you get' ... I went to a gynaecologist ... The first instance was to do a D&C [Dilation and curettage] for me [sic]. I asked her, I said, 'Why do you want to do an invasive kind of thing?' She said, 'I want to know what is there', and then she told me, 'You go for HSG'. So I asked her, I said, 'Looks like what little I know [if] suppose my tubes are blocked that you would have come to know through HSG. Why didn't you do HSG first and DNC later?' HSG, somebody was doing it outside, and DNC was okay, it is her power she would have made money. It might be a wrong decision; it might be a right decision. But somehow the answer couldn't convince my logic. You think like, 'Okay, they treat you with hormones, okay you take hormones, you take "fertile", you take this, nobody did ... the hormone profile for me!' It wasn't done earlier. It is here; I did it [at the clinic]. My first hormone profile, it was a little low. You know, like there is some kind of a bias also, like all of them have, it's the female who needs to be treated. Whereas if you look at what is being said in the reports about sperm count, why don't they treat the male? You know? Okay, [if] the male can't be treated or something there are various options, but I feel there is definite gender bias. Okay, even ... leading infertility treatment specialists ... think that [only] the female body ... has to undergo some kind of invasive treatment. The first thing is that a male, you don't require any invasive thing. All you need to do is a semen analysis. In my case like semen analysis was incidental, you know like they said, 'Okay, there is a little count but not so low. Let's do a DNC on you!' And every gynaecologist you go to, okay, they don't criticise the other. I think there is a little professional ethic or something or they are not, but you can make out from their body language that okay probably somebody else has made a mistake. I believe when you are treating a person for infertility the patients are paying through their nose. They are probably pushing all their savings into this. I think there is some responsibility on the part of these people at least to explain to the patients what is happening. You know, I have a little bit of biology

> background. I try to read sometimes. I don't understand [but] I have access to text books. What about the other person who doesn't even know about fertilisation, who doesn't even know what an embryo is? How can you treat a patient like this? Don't you think your patient needs psychological support?
>
> AB: way! No way! No way … They treat you like [laughs] … any animal ready to be slaughtered. They don't explain to me. I said, 'Why are you doing a DNC under GA (general anaesthesia)'? There are patients who can't tolerate pain [but] for simple surgery they made me undergo GA. The only thing is you have to come fasting because you will be operated under GA. How long you will be hospitalised, what will be the after effects, what kind of preparation, no preparation. Even like, okay, 'You don't have to worry. [It's a] small surgery'. They don't explain. They don't have the time. And then also if you ask for information, the information is so incomplete that you realise it's useless asking them. I might as well refer to some other source. I don't think any female who [is] probably going through treatment is not perturbed by this. When you don't understand what is happening, that kind of support is not existing.

Neelanjana's outburst encapsulates most graphically the torment of past medical interventions in the infertile lives of most couples in this research. Like Seema and Hariram's wife, Neelanjana has undergone what appears to be needless surgical intervention. She registers her protest like Rekha – who reflected, 'I felt I was treated like a vegetable' – in terms of feeling like a 'guinea pig' and an 'animal ready to be slaughtered'. Neelanjana is also unique in that she is the only individual – amongst those interviewed – who was critical of the gender bias built into the treatment procedure, which is focused on the surgical exploration of female anatomy. She is aware that male infertility can be treated with recourse to no (or minimum) surgical intervention, but she uses the simplicity of a mere semen analysis to challenge the tendency amongst doctors to operate on the female body as the first line of treatment. She critiques the sensitive issue of pretreatment counselling and its absence, which renders her predicament similar to that of Harjeet. Though rural/urban, farmer/professional, uneducated/educated, working-class/middle-class, man/woman polarities appear to separate them culturally and spatially, it is clear that as infertile individuals they experience the same impersonal treatment, stripped of all social markers and subject to a medical regime that appears to them (and to other treatment seekers) to be a crude trial and error approach in the name of assisting conception.

The Cost of Conception

These emotional and physical costs are exacerbated by the financial costs. These struggles were evident from the very beginning in this research and remained a constant source of anxiety in the lives of treatment seekers encountered in subsequent years. On the morning of 5 April 1997, two men accompanied by their wives accosted me right outside the clinic [in Jaipur]. I had spotted them in deep animated conversation from quite some distance as I approached the clinic. On closer inspection I recognised one of the two couples – Sumita and Shankar – whom I had interviewed the previous day. Shankar, visibly upset, took me aside and asked me in a hushed tone to come to his hotel room sometime later in the day to tell me something about the doctor. At this point the other man joined us, shouting, 'The doctor here is after money, money and more money! There is no humanity. Show some humanity at least!' As I pondered possible reasons for this new diatribe against the doctor, the man exclaimed, 'Look at the national culture of money making. Look at our Prime Minister! Can anything go right in a country whose leader is so incompetent?' At this point, Shankar chipped in, 'There is no humanity and no nationality [*sic*] (I think what he meant was a feeling of nationalism) in the country. The doctors are interested only in your money!'

Later that day I visited their hotel to learn more about what was on Shanker and Sumita's mind. 'The doctor doesn't give us a clear estimate ever on how much it is all going to cost', they griped. Initially, his complaint seemed mild compared to the severity of the morning's outburst, but soon the chat revealed the depth of this financial and administrative struggle. Shanker and Sumita had been coming to this clinic since 24 October 1996 and maintained that they still, to that day, had not been offered a realistic estimate on the overall treatment cost. Given that they had to travel an enormous distance to the clinic, it was impossible for them to travel back and forth to retrieve more money, which they mobilised in their hometown of Dungarpur, on the northwestern tip of Gujarat State. While they acknowledged that the doctor permitted them to pay the balance due on subsequent visits, the person responsible for collections was not as accommodating. This communication gap between doctor and staff was the cause of undue harassment. That morning, when the couple requested to pay the balance on their next visit, the cashier reportedly said something 'obnoxious and rude' that triggered the emotional outburst outside the clinic.

Paying for an expensive medical intervention they could ill afford was in their case partly a function of conforming to social expectations and definitions of socially responsible behaviour. Shanker had been hit by personal tragedy earlier in 1996 when he lost his father. They had to rush back home, abandoning the treatment midway. Continuing to explain his present financial struggle, he spoke of how meeting the expenses of his father's last rites added to his financial worries. 'The society expects it', he ruefully added while emphasising that any compromises or economising in the proper discharge of last rites would invite social disapproval and ridicule. He likened this to society's disapproval of individuals who do not make an all-out effort to secure a child should natural conception fail. Both husband and wife saw social change as a law of nature, suggesting that 'everything in nature changes including the customs, traditions, attitudes but to stand up against the contemporary norms is impossible, you have to conform'.

The couple had pulled numerous threads from the world they inhabit to make sense of their long-drawn financial drain. The other man's earlier rants against India's materialistic national culture and the prime minister's incompetence resonated with the couple, testifying to the money-grabbing and impersonal inclinations of clinical medicine. Though they were reasonably happy with their doctor's accommodation of their financial needs, they nevertheless held him responsible for the inhumane attitude of his staff. In doing this, they drew parallels between the widespread desire for material gain and the political culture that sustains it, seeing the commercialisation of clinical medicine as but one feature reflecting in microcosm the state of the nation. Shanker had weaved a tangled web of complex ideas that he later summed up in an ancient *Sanskrit* proverb (*yatha raja taha praja*) that alludes to subjects reflecting the virtues of the king. The couple highlighted how the need to conform to socially defined expectations respecting birth and death obliged them to go beyond their means.

Similarly, Ajay and Shanti were spending money they did not have, and after two failed attempts the anxiety was mounting. According to Ajay:

> I did not know [how] much it will cost. I said [to the doctor], 'We are not very moneyed people. We are working class people, so we have to have an estimate [as] we will have to arrange the money from somewhere'. He said that it would cost about sixty thousand rupees, thirty thousand is the clinical charge and medicines, etc. are extra … You

> see, the expense is enormous. It is outside our budget, beyond our capacity, but for a child we are trying everything humanly we can do. We told the doctor that our budget is over; he reduced a little for us. The fifteen thousand he charges for IVF I asked him to charge less as my budget for IVF expense is over. I am mobilising money from here and there on interest. You see we live in a family. To make the full picture clear to them as to what is involved here is not right. People talk unnecessarily, so what we are thinking even if it is expensive and if we succeed then in front of the society it would be a major face-saving. So from here and there I am borrowing money on interest almost double the amount I have spent, sixty thousand was the target. I have spent one lakh twenty thousand [120,000 rupees].

Ajay and Shanti were very anxious after two failed IVF cycles, since with each failure they dreaded facing family back in their hometown. Yet IVF remained a potential face-saving device which they continued to endure in the hope that success, even at a great financial cost, would secure them a new lease on social life.

Apart from the pressure to conceive, the exact scale of the financial costs was not entirely clear to some couples. Jeet and Sonia were totally unprepared for the expense entailed in IVF:

> Sonia: Even we have our limits. We can't go on like this [referring to various tests]. We can't afford, we are from service background and it is very difficult for us. Here it is too much expensive.
>
> Jeet: We have done A to Z all the tests here, and the estimate they have given is around 15,000 rupees.
>
> Sonia: When we started from home with 2-3,000 rupees, we had our earlier treatment estimates in mind and we have to go back also. We simply don't have the money! We are here from past three days we are staying in an *ashram* because somebody gave us a written recommendation. Otherwise just imagine if we had to stay in a hotel.

On her way out after the interview, Sonia suddenly turned around and said, 'We find this treatment backbreaking. Can you suggest somewhere cheaper we can go?' The anguish in her voice was palpable. She and her husband were in a no-win situation, as they were subjecting themselves to a treatment regime that they could neither afford nor ignore. Kavita, seething with anger at the progress of her treatment, saw little point in wasting any more money on tests that were yielding only inconclusive results: 'Waste, money is definitely being wasted! I always have this tension whatever income is there almost the entire amount is going towards meeting the medical expenses. We can't live for ourselves except medicines and the expense. This is no life! Even then the doctors don't tell us anything. What is wrong?' Kavita sees little point in a fruitless 'wild goose chase' that is affecting only the quality of her married life. Pursuing a baby at any cost is therefore not an acceptable solution for her. Individuals like Vani (Seema's sister-in-law), on the other hand, viewed the treatment expense as the corollary of a tradeoff between fertility and infertility. This was significant as Vani stood as a visible symbol of familial approval to an act of assisting conception clinically, in place of other more normative alternatives like remarrying their son. Treatment cost plays a vital role in Seema's case, as the 'purse strings' are under the joint familial control, and willingness to spend on an infertile daughter-in-law as a consequence translates into a subtle progressive shift away from traditional conservative thinking. Vani says:

> Actually we belong to the middle-income category so we can't really afford private treatment ... It is no doubt expensive, but if the result is positive then money is no consideration. When we earn money, we are in a job, okay we will think like for two, three years we did not make any money, that we simply sat at home. If the result is positive, then as far as money is concerned I don't think you should give it much importance. If you can afford, I agree it is very expensive and everyone cannot afford it especially middle class thinks a lot before going for it but in this cost if you get the satisfaction [of having a child] then one feels that maybe I didn't pay so much after all. But if the result is not positive then definitely you feel that you have lost everything. You are physically upset, mentally you are upset, even economically you will become weak. But if the result is positive, okay when a person works so hard and earns money why does he do it? For his family, for himself!

The over-expenditure of money on private treatment is explained away as worthwhile as long there are positive results. Failure to conceive is a shattering blow to couples, who often pursue the treatment by gambling their life savings or borrowing at further expense. Even couples who could bear the financial burden of seeking treatment – including some upper-middle-class professionals interviewed in Delhi and Mumbai – wondered how people of limited or no means must struggle to pay for the treatment. Shakher, interviewed in a North Indian centre, whose wife had undergone an embryo transfer on the day of the interview, was astounded to see large number of people coming to the clinic from the countryside:

> Fortunately I am well provided for, substantial ancestral property and personal property to sustain this. But I marvel the number of poor people who come here who literally have nothing to eat, who are pursuing this because of the Hindu mythology and the myths that unless you have a son your forefathers in heaven, some stuck-up sort of philosophy is there about how they don't get *moksha* (deliverance) something like that.

While the force of religious conviction cannot be entirely dismissed, this aspect never emerged as the sole motivating factor in assuming such a huge financial commitment.[3] The gruelling poverty that he alludes to was in part a feature of his urban upper-class bias, which essentialised people from the hinterlands as uniformly poverty-stricken. Although they were disadvantaged compared to the educated upper- and middle-class clientele of the clinic, most had modest financial savings and small property holdings that they often mortgaged or sold to fund their treatment. Rekha and Sudhir, who could afford to pay for the treatment, were quick to point out how difficult it was for some people to cope. Sudhir reflected, 'I talk to other patients, other people, these are people who come from ... a very, very poor background ... Money in such cases is not essential. People will sell themselves to get a baby – this is India! It's too important to have a baby'. Sudhir speaks for a sizeable number of patients in treatment for infertility. Harjeet, for example, had sold part of his agricultural land to fund IVF cycles and was prepared to spend even more money if the need arose:

> I did not ask anything from [the doctor]. I only said one thing – that we should have a child and do what you like; we only have to spend money and that we will go on spending. Then the doctor said that 'you will have a child' so we are getting the treatment done from him on this assurance.

Harjeet's brief to the doctor is clear: he wants a child. He has not only surrendered his and his wife's bodies to medical manipulation (he had already undergone testicular surgery) but has pledged full financial support. One can only extrapolate that he will continue to part with his farmland on a piecemeal basis as the treatment costs mount. 'Scientifically' there is no way to foretell how many IVF cycles it would entail to deliver the promised child, and the doctor's 'guarantee' contravenes available medical evidence on successful IVF outcomes, making Harjeet and his wife vulnerable financially and medically. (His wife was in great discomfort on the morning of the interview as she was hyper-stimulated.)

Making Sense of Treatment Seekers: Clinicians Speak

Patients forced to bear these physical, social and financial burdens eventually begin to externalise their disappointment. Unassisted emotionally, it is not uncommon for some patients – as seen above – to blame the doctors for failing them. Dr Chandra summed up this emotional distress:

> When they come in, they think, 'Now this is the answer and it's going to happen', despite the fact that you tell them it's going to happen to only 25 to 30 percent of patients – the carry home baby rate is only maybe 15 to 20 percent – but they still feel they are going to fall in that category ... When the patient does not conceive, it's almost like a personal failure [of the doctor]. The patient now feels that everything now has become the doctor's fault. Despite the fact that they were explained that this is the rate of success in the procedure, they don't see it like that anymore. They feel something is wrong with this doctor, let us move on to the next. So whatever their feelings are they want to find a focus, a feeling of disappointment that they try to explain in their own way: it happened because of such and such doctor...

Hoping against hope, couples believe they will become part of the 20 per cent of the projected success statistic. When this does not happen, they blame the doctor as a way of coping with the failure. Dr Suman has had similar experiences:

> First day you are a god and third day you are a thief. Despite the fact that you [tell them], 'You are going to spend so much and it may not end up in pregnancy and you may lose all that you've spent'; despite the fact that you tell them, 'You are going to have a lot of emotional trauma' and everything, they turn around and tell you that you didn't do your job properly, you are not good enough!

Dr Suman is not alone in experiencing such an emotional backlash from patients struggling with assisted conception. Dr Kalakar – heading an IVF unit in North of India – in return blamed patients for lying:

> A lot of patients lie even after they have been told what the treatment would involve. Very often I get patients cursing and badmouthing other doctors. This is a trait of most infertility treatment seekers; they move from doctor to doctor, and when they say anything bad about another doctor I am on my guard because possibly I will be next, when they go to the next doctor.

However, the doctor does not account for how disconcerting and incapacitating the experience of seeking treatment can be in light of what are experienced as late referrals, misdiagnoses, failed treatments, false promises and adulatory media accounts of the miracles of assisted conception, growing familial pressure and deepening social stigma. For example, Ajay and Shanti's case illustrates that, in the face of evasive success, patients find themselves trapped between the dwindling promise of clinical conception and unsympathetic probing from family:

> Shanti: [Family members] ask, 'What happened about your treatment, you've shown yourself in such a big hospital, what happened?' What answer should we give them? …
>
> Ajay: We tell the doctor that first you were reasonably hopeful. Now after two failures, you are not so hopeful. We can only say rest. We can't do anything!

As a result, couples look for ways to manage anxiety and explain failure, as Dr Chandra suggests, by turning the potential source of conception – the clinic – into the cause of failed conception. Beyond this, when the clinically acknowledged need for active stress management of patients is unmet (Chapter 8), patients seek further support from the very clinicians they blame. However, there is another explanation for this cycle of resentment, one that originates from within the ranks of clinicians themselves.

Unrealistic expectations are engendered in treatment-seeking individuals not only by media narratives on ARTs, but by clinical encounters themselves (Bharadwaj 2000). A clinical setting can be geared to produce subliminal messages on the effectiveness of assisted conception (see Chapter 8). This, coupled with assurances from the doctors on the positive outcomes of technologies such as IVF – as, for example, in the case of Harjeet – further disillusions patients when promised outcomes do not materialise. The resulting despondency that engulfs a couple accentuates the sense of being let down by the clinician, of a breach of trust and a loss of faith in his or her ability to produce results. This is predominantly the case when patients are needlessly subjected to medical interventions or given unrealistic accounts of the potency of assisted conception techniques. Thus Dr Sukumari asserts, 'Success of any clinic depends on how many of your failed IVFs come back to you [for more cycles]!' Such a measure of success in medical circles is often attributed to comprehensive pretreatment counselling that alerts a patient as to what to expect (see also Chapter 8). Many clinicians strongly believe that couples have to be told that IVF is not always successful at the first attempt and that many first-time failures do conceive in their second or third attempts. For example, Dr Jatin feels that:

> the importance of counselling is to emphasise to [patients] that this is going to be a long process. It's not going to get over in one month unless you are really, really lucky – that is the idea of counselling, and they accept it well because they can cope with failure much better. If they fail they are strong enough. They don't just go into a hell again and stop treatment for one year; they are mentally prepared. Okay we predict [depending on the case] ten cycles, six cycles, one year, two years, ten years, that kind of counselling is done right at the outset...

How common such candid counselling is remains unclear. No evidence suggests that IVF clinics uniformly pursue such a line of pre-treatment counselling. On the contrary, clinicians often criticise rival clinics for making extreme claims vis-à-vis the success accruing from ARTs. Dr Mukta asserts that the carrot of new technological breakthroughs is dangled in front of expectant patients to enroll them on IVF/ICSI programmes:

> All these new techniques, initially when they are brought into the market people are lured. Okay, ICSI [is popular] because it's recently brought into the country. Everybody thinks that ICSI gives them the ultimate solution. But slowly time will come; they will realise that ICSI only improves IVF success by 25 percent, which is not the real picture which is given to the patient. What the patient is told is that 'we've brought this equipment, this is going to give you more success'. What more success? From 15 [percent] we may go to 18 [percent], it is not told to the patient clearly. [Patients] see the equipment, they see T.V. and [hear it on] radio, they immediately think this machine is really going to produce them a baby.

On a number of occasions, doctors alluded to a common tendency amongst clinicians to fabricate their IVF success rates to lure patients, but the evidence in the main remained anecdotal. Dr Neeta, for instance, spoke of how in India:

> Everybody is having a success rate of 45 percent, 50 percent, 90 percent. I cannot be dishonest, that is my stress. I tell them [patients] my results are 20 percent, 25 percent if I stretch myself too much, but I still say a figure of 22 percent in IVF. In ICSI I'll give you figure around 30 percent, and then when they go out and come back and say, 'Doctor *sahab* he said that 90 percent of [his] patients get

> pregnant'. [Other clinicians] talk in consultations like that, and their secretaries sitting outside [in the waiting area], the first thing they tell patients, 'At our clinic a lot of patients get pregnant'... I hate dishonesty, and these patients when they suffer for two to three months they come back to you again.

Without naming individuals, many clinicians similarly stood by the contention that, apart from a handful of 'good clinics', most doctors were simply not doing high-quality work and were making claims pertaining to the effectiveness of fertility techniques that were inconsistent with the scientific evidence. This phenomenon explains how patients come to have such unrealistically high expectations from the treatment process. As Dr Shanta contends, it is mainly members of the medical profession who put such ideas in a patient's head, a point further corroborated and expanded on by Dr Mukta.[4]

Conclusion

The lived experience of infertility is so disconcerting and incapacitating for most infertile couples in this research that waning hope of conception on account of repeated medical failures registers as the failure of an individual practitioner. The paradox at the heart of this quest for conception is that, while the infertile critique medical interventions as unsatisfactory, they continue to endure them in the absence of any tangible alternatives. The long-drawn out pursuit of conception, therefore, perpetuates the vicious circle of simultaneously blaming and believing the clinicians (more on this in Chapter 8). The critique in these narratives, therefore, can also be read as one directed not only against the medical (mis)management of infertility, but rather against its inability to deliver the desired resolution – a baby. The absence of this anticipated outcome results in individuals and couples 'making sense' of this failure in differing ways. For instance, the experience of Neelanjana, Rekha and Sudhir embodied resistance and feeling dehumanised. On the other hand, couples like Rati/Sundar and Jeet/Sonia had actively collaborated with the disciplinary modalities of the treatment process by doing 'exactly as the doctors asked'. These couples (Rati/Sundar and Jeet/Sonia) clearly see the clinician as a 'gatekeeper to the delivery of services', and as a consequence the clinician's 'decisions gain authority emanating from a medical setting and prove difficult to challenge' (Price 1999: 30). More generally, treatment seekers appear to be simultaneously resisting and pursuing medical intervention. Ultimately, it is their only recourse of escape from oppressive familial and societal pressures, which explains why these individuals are prepared to make an enormous financial commitment that some simply cannot afford. Sudhir's contention ('Money in such cases is not essential. People will sell themselves to get a baby. This is India! It's too important to have a baby') encapsulates the torment of couples, as successive failures contribute to their financial drain and ruin.

The predominant concern faced by clinicians in their practices, in countries like Britain, for instance, is the 'pressure of time passing by' that the patients bring with them to the clinic (Price 1993). On the other hand, in India treatment seekers bring many stressors to the clinic (also see Chapter 8). Clinicians in this context make sense of their patients' tribulations as a way of accommodating failure and as a feature of unfulfilled expectations. However, some clinicians (like Dr Kalakar) do not recognise the sense of anxiety and desperation that patients bring to the clinic, after years of experiences with infertility; nor do they consider the unrealistically high expectations set by the media, even though some clinicians disparage their colleagues' misrepresentation of the potency of assisted conception. Further research into the potential charges of unscrupulous misrepresentation of treatment outcomes is needed.

The next chapter extends the experience of treatment seekers and providers into the realm of the clinic. Overall, the chapter examines how these agents make sense of assisted conception from within the clinic, and how such encounters further unfold the process of living with and treating infertility.

Notes

1. It is worth recalling the methodological quandary, flagged in the Introduction, of whether to treat interview responses as providing 'access to actual experience' or as 'actively constructed narratives'.
2. Throughout the course of this research I came to understand from various ART conferences and scientific symposia that assisted conception practitioners and gynaecologists alike consider surgically opened fallopian tubes (recanalisation) as an inhospitable environment for fertilisation to occur. In this respect, bypassing the blocked tubes altogether was often agreed to be the best solution.
3. A very few individuals from the rural areas agreed to talk about their infertility, though informal discussion with them on occasions pointed

to familial and community pressures as primary motivating factors to see treatment. On the question of religion, there was surprising unanimity in attributing infertility to God's will.

4. Commenting on the stresses of setting up an IVF unit, Dr Sachin (Chapter 4) was quoted as arguing that new clinics have a 'growth phase of 1,000 days', and in this phase it is very difficult to source 'young patients'. Many clinics (in this research) stood accused by their competitors of being selective in recruiting young and promising cases who would have conceived regardless. It seems that young couples, who are easier to get pregnant, are preferred over those who have been in the pursuit of conception for several years and may even have 'clomid resistant ovaries'. These young couples, as a consequence, are viewed as better placed to improve the statistical success of a clinic.

Chapter 8

In Search of Conception

Clinicians, Patients and Clinics

In approaching a physician for help, a patient brings not only a physical problem but also a social context that is seldom critically addressed during a medical encounter (Waitzkin 1991). Thus, drawing on C. Wright Mills (1959), Howard Waitzkin further argues that during a medical encounter, patients bring to their doctors a variety of personal troubles often rooted in social issues that transcend the individual (Waitzkin 1991: 11), rendering medical problems simultaneously social and biological (somatic). In short, Waitzkin argues that since patients and doctors do not examine critically the contextual sources of personal distress – seeing little scope for basic change in context – they talk about adjustments instead that might help patients continue to function in their customary social roles. As a result of this, 'potentially relevant modifications in social setting do not arise as topics for discussion' (Waitzkin 1991: 5).

In the context of infertility, this oversight amounts to a vast dispersal that, when collated, reveals intimate relationships between irreversible tubal damage, plummeting sperm counts, super-speciality IVF clinics and debilitating social and financial worries, among a multitude of other similar sites that mediate the experience of infertility and its medical management. As sites offering medical resolution to the biological inability to reproduce, IVF clinics in India revolve around the very epicentre of moral, social and medical dilemmas, as well as the ensuing conflicts. The doctor/patient relationship as a result sometimes stands transformed, in that the classic – textbook – doctor/patient model does not completely apply to those within these IVF clinics.[1] For instance, patients routinely brought the social context of their infertility to the consultation rooms, but, contrary to Waitzkin's (1991) assertion, social issues and their wider ramifications on the treatment process sometimes received critical attention in conversations between individuals seeking (infertility) treatment and the clinicians.

This chapter presents an account of how wider 'cultural issues' are sometimes addressed in clinical settings, while on other occasions a lack of critical attention – as also seen in Chapter 7 – perpetuates the 'social sources of distress and suffering' (Waitzkin 1991: 5). In doing this, the chapter focuses on the paradoxical nature of clinic/patient interaction that both reinforces high expectations and deepens the ambivalent feelings treatment seekers have about their past and present medical encounters. It deals with core issues that the infertile bring to the clinic and how the clinicians respond to them, and also makes the case for viewing the broader cultural context, in which assisted conception is both understood by the clinicians/patients and explanations for success and failure of treatments are sought.

The Clinical Space

The focal point of an IVF clinic is its lobby or waiting area, where the infertile take refuge away from the world outside the clinic. To many, this clinical space is the first introduction to the 'world of conception'. A clinic's lobby appears to respond to the infertile quest for conception in two broad ways: first, by reinforcing their sense of impending conception; and second, by providing an element of informality that allows patients to normalise key aspects of their treatment procedures. These themes are examined in turn.

IVF clinics across India are remarkably consistent in their structural organisation. The clinical space reflects a predominantly urban and upper-middle-class ethos. This is significant, given that clinics often service, in addition to the urban middle class, a cross-section of rural and urban working-class infertile populations. Drawn from different social backgrounds, the infertile patients gravitate to these urban centres in the absence of 'affordable alternatives'. The clinic interiors reflect accurately the class position of the doctors who own them rather than the sum total of the client base that makes up their practices. Given the upper-middle-class locations of the ART experts (not surprisingly the clinics are mainly located in affluent neighbourhoods), their interior layouts correspondingly oscillate from smart to ostentatious. The level of ostentation varies, however, depending on whether the clinic is part of a large privately owned hospital or an individually run centre. For example, clinics in private hospitals in Madras and Delhi closely resemble five-star hotels in India as plush, centrally air-conditioned and chandeliered granite lobbies of the hospital – together with coffee, book and flower shops – welcomed visitors into state-of-the-art clinics. Smaller clinics were comparatively understated but included as part of their decor similar embellishments on a much more modest scale. The entrance to these clinics was mostly through a small foyer that opened into a lobby or waiting area – usually the largest part of the clinic – where patients waited to see the doctor. This waiting area is particularly important, as it is in this space that the 'core' interaction in the clinics – both amongst the patients and between the patient and the clinical bureaucracy – unfolds. This waiting space is also a junction where the inside and the outside of the clinic intersect. Routes to the doctor's chambers, the laboratories, sonography room, culture rooms, rest rooms, patients' wards and semen collection rooms, etc., all pass through the lobby or connect with this waiting area in some circuitous way. In this sense waiting areas in IVF clinics occupy an ambiguous place. While lying at the very heart of the clinic they appear to be outside of its clinical bounds. This liminality is peculiar to this space as it mediates the outside world and the clinical world within. Given this unique vantage, the waiting area also serves as an introduction to the clinic and the clinical expertise. All settings researched for this study used this space to make a bold statement about the state-of-the-art credentials of the facilities and the expert at the helm of the ART programme. This usually meant that a waiting (potential) patient was exposed to as much information about the facility as his or her captive audience status allowed.

A clinic located in the north of India stands as a particularly good example of this method. It had a lavish lobby with expensive marble flooring and elaborately designed glass and wood-panelled partitions separating the waiting area from the rest of the clinic. The walls were replete with paintings and photographs of the doctor taken with influential people (mainly politicians) and important clients. The sitting space consisted of smartly upholstered settees along the walls, interspersed with tables featuring magazines and strikingly bulky photo-albums full of newspaper clippings about the clinic and the clinician, along with pictures of couples and their newborn babies. On several occasions couples were observed flicking through these albums with much interest and fascination. Field notes reveal that a particular woman waiting at this clinic was so overcome by some of the pictures in the album that she tightly clasped her husband's hand and her facial expression became visibly contorted with the effort of fighting back the tears. Another clinic in the city of Mumbai – possessing more than the usual indicators of a successful clinic as reflected in the interior layout – boldly displayed more than a dozen beautifully framed membership certificates and citations of various national and international medical bodies. In another clinic in Mumbai, the walls of the waiting area were adorned with similar pictures, certificates and newspaper reports. One newspaper report (duly framed and hung) unabashedly proclaimed, 'City Doctor Proclaims The End Of Male Infertility – Any Man Can Have A Baby'.

One significant fixture is the preponderance of baby pictures, a graphic display of babies conceived in the clinic and the faces of proud parents and happy doctors. While at one level unsurprising, it is also clear from Chapter 3 that ART-conceived babies are much more than a simple medical resolution of infertility; they are highly prized medical trophies for which doctors compete (and in this case display) as a sign of their achievement. These baby pictures are either solo shots or simple pictures of the doctor holding the baby. Rarely do parents appear in these pictures, emphasising the primacy of the medical expert. Many successful parents in media reports attribute the outcome of the treatment to the medical experts, with assertions such as 'This baby is given to us by Doctor Sahab', or 'It feels like the baby is more his/hers than mine' (implying the clinician's). These statements should be seen as expressions more of gratitude than anything else, but the primacy of the experts in the pictures further illustrates that these conceptions through medical intervention are seen as individual clinician's triumphs rather than as successes of a medical technology. Subliminal messages abound in clinical lobbies, and waiting bodies rapidly absorb them, which in turn feeds their expectations and structures their opinions, tinged by awe and hope. 'Hope technologies' (Franklin 1997) in this respect become assisted and circumscribed by material artefacts that elevate their credibility and 'hope potential'.

An IVF clinic's waiting area is much more than a mere threshold to the clinical world of conception; for some treatment seekers certain important aspects of the treatment process unfold in this space. Some of the most private and intimate moments of the treatment process are rendered openly public here, as the day-to-day rigours of seeking medical assistance culminate in the total demystification of private aspects of the treatment process.[2] The patients and the clinical staff – including the clinician – appear to gravitate towards an unspoken rule of engagement underscored by a sense of functional informality. The focal point in these lobbies is a counter or a desk from where the doctor's assistant or support staff handles inquiries, answers personal and telephone calls and handles patient records while coordinating appointments and laboratory staff. This is also the usual post where all routine payments for the procedures are made, receipts issued, test reports delivered and future appointments made. While being the bureaucratic nerve centre of the clinic, the wo/man behind the counter often develops an informal working relationship with patients and many times acts as a bridge between the doctor and waiting patients, especially during the rush hours of surgery. The sense of informality in these clinics extends throughout all aspects of clinic/patient interaction. Nurses often stroll into the lobby, call aloud the name of a waiting (woman) patient and then instruct her to visit the toilet in order to clear her bladder before a sonogram, all within earshot of others present in the lobby. Yet this evoked very little or no embarrassment on behalf of the patients. The issue of producing a sperm sample was similarly broached with surprising nonchalance. In many clinics, sperm samples were approached by both patients and clinic staff with extreme matter-of-factness.

In a Mumbai clinic, for instance, a couple emerged from the doctor's room and walked up to the counter to pay for the day's appointment only to be told by the duty nurse that they would have to return the next day for semen analysis. At this point the woman said something inaudible to the nurse, to which she further queried, 'Where do you live?' 'Bandra', came the reply from the woman. 'Okay if you want to do it at home, it's okay... we have a room here [though]'. After one or two inaudible exchanges the woman was overheard yet again, this time saying, 'He'll try here; if he can't do it we will go home and bring it'. 'Bring it within half an hour of collection', replied the nurse. 'Okay', said the woman and they left the clinic. The entire exchange was candid and conducted without much concern about being overheard in a crowded waiting room.

In a Delhi clinic, a duty nurse called out a man's name in the waiting room and, as he rose to his feet, handed him a plastic container with instructions. It was difficult to tell whether the man was embarrassed or took it in stride, but it nonetheless established a pattern of public articulation of some of the most intimate aspects of the treatment process. In yet another upmarket IVF unit in Delhi, on one occasion the doctor walked into the lobby full of waiting patients – on the way to her room – and paused to inquire of one, 'Did you give the sample?' The man simply replied, 'I was waiting for you to get here'. 'No! But you should have given the sample. I told my assistant she should have asked you to give the sample!' The doctor spoke in a high pitched but friendly voice, 'Okay, please give the sample now'. Slightly self-conscious, the man braced himself for the imminent masturbation, collected the sterilised plastic cup from the nurse and entered the collection room.

On another occasion in the same clinic, the doctor who was in consultation with a couple was interrupted by yet another couple who had seen her earlier, to ask if her husband could come alone the next day to give the sample. The doctor, in her characteristic cheerful demeanour, quipped, 'If you can produce a sample without your wife, please do come alone by all means'. Everyone present in the lobby, including the querying couple, burst out laughing. In this particular clinic, it was not uncommon for the patients to walk into the doctor's consultation room or stop the doctor in the lobby for clarifications. On this particular occasion, what was most striking was the ease with which the couple walked in, unfazed by the presence of strangers or even the doctor's possible reaction to this out of turn intrusion. On the contrary, their open approach was more than matched by the doctor's ability to invoke humour in dealing with potential inhibitions about aspects of a process such as sperm collection. This episode also highlights how permeable the clinical space could become, by allowing patients access to areas outside the clinic lobby at will, once the clinic/patient dealings has produced a familiarity that everyday interaction tends to generate.

Similar observations in other clinics indicate that whether it was the woman's experience of preparing for tests, or the man's experience of producing sperm samples, couples dealt with the day-to-day rigour and demands of treatment with a sense of understated straightforwardness and forthright frankness. The procedure became routinised, and the couples did not appear awkward about openly discussing supposedly private aspects of the treatment process. It appears that a sense of common suffering permeated the IVF settings, infusing the infertile participants with a feeling of camaraderie. The clinical space in this respect became a great leveller. This effectively translated into a space where no one hid anything, resulting in the blurring of private/personal and public distinctions. This is a significant departure from the shroud of secrecy subsuming assisted conception, as seen in Chapter 5. The couples (and sometimes select family confidants) came across as sharing with each other precious moments of respite away from familial interference and the wider prying society. Not surprisingly, therefore, the waiting area doubled as a space for sharing personal experiences, confiding and discussing the experience of infertility. Many individuals interviewed commented on how comforting it had been for them to be able to meet and talk with other people in similar situations. Experiences of family pressure, social disapproval and not least the intimidating medical procedures, along with the emotionally and financially trying search for conception, were subjects that patients reportedly discussed.

This information relates to the 'expectations' that patients bring to a clinical setting. For a first-time treatment seeker the setting goes a long way towards establishing the credibility of the practitioner. The first impression has an added dimension for those bearing longer infertility struggles. Having endured past medical interventions at considerable emotional and financial cost, treatment seekers need reassurance that on this occasion their efforts will be worthwhile. Paradoxically, while themes of credibility and success of clinicians in the waiting area of clinics may help to allay fears regarding the competence of a practitioner, they nevertheless reinforce high expectations that in eighty out of one hundred cases cannot be met (given that the clinical success rate is generally agreed to be 20 per cent).

The informal approach to assisted conception helps to normalise the treatment process, extraordinary in so many respects, to which many couples are subjecting themselves again. It also, however, addresses something far more crucial – the need for sympathetic and humane treatment. The credibility of a practitioner, in conjunction with an informal approach to dealing with patients, helps to address this issue. To many, the exhaustion of past failed attempts and the harrowing experience of stigma intensified the need for a human touch. The clinic in this respect is much more than a site for medical management of infertility for these couples. In searching for the right clinic and clinicians, patients are also searching for a refuge and a sanctuary where they can escape the pain of 'living infertility'. This explains the evident catharsis experienced in the clinic lobbies, where on occasion, patients purge themselves of pent-up emotion. Laughter at the intimate aspects of treatment, tears at the sight of baby pictures or even outbursts brought on by the high cost of treatment (Chapter 7) give vent to unaddressed social issues that together constitute the lived experience of infertility.

End of the Road? Clinicians and Patients: An Ambivalent Engagement

Having spent years searching for conception, infertile couples gradually drift towards a 'resist and persist' approach to medically assisted conception. While they are opposed to medical mismanagement, they nevertheless persist in the hope that their search for conception will eventually connect them with the right 'expert'. The 'trial and error' approach of the doctors in this respect doubles up as a 'trial and error' search for the correct medical diagnosis and treatment. Such an approach causes patients to feel deeply ambivalent about clinical medicine. This was particularly evident when couples discussed their current ongoing medical treatment, in the light of their past encounters. There was a noticeable departure from the earlier critical reflections on the clinical mismanagement of their condition, a trend pointing to either a sense of relief or a workable compromise with the standard of clinical assistance now handling their infertility. Some couples openly praised their ongoing treatment and clinician, in marked contrast to their horrific experiences of the past. Rekha and Sudhir were pleased with their current doctor:

> Rekha: Dr Shaileja is extremely busy, but when she is with you she is with you, even ten minutes of your time [interrupted]
>
> Rekha: I just recently went through a miscarriage. I conceived through IVF and GIFT [Gamete Intra-Fallopian Transfer]. It was six months of pregnancy, and then I miscarried and it was with the help of doctor I could pull along.
>
> Sudhir: [The doctor] was there for the delivery. She was there all the time, like you feel that is a part of you. She is with you all the time. She is discussing your problems, trying to help you out. She is there whenever you are around. You see all these things are necessary. Money is immaterial in such cases. People have money, they don't have money; it's immaterial. But what is required is a human approach. That is what is needed.
>
> Rekha: Or right kind of advice given to you ... for example in a cycle she says, 'This is not going to be possible. Don't try the cycle', whereas any other doctor behaves like you are just [interrupted]
>
> Sudhir: You are just dragged along ... In fact even after the incident [referring to the miscarriage] we had everything researched. We sat down with her for five days and asked her one thing. I said, 'Doctor, is it late now? Shall we go ahead with it? Or shall we forget about it?'

> She said, 'No you still have time, and [I] still can't give you guarantee', but she is there with you. It's immaterial whether we have an issue or we don't have an issue, but she is there, that human support is there. [A] human approach is very essential!

'She is there for you; she is there with you', is Sudhir and Rekha's predominant refrain. Having suffered and struggled with clinical medicine for ten years, they have found refuge, a sanctuary in Dr Shaileja's clinic.

Many couples interviewed craved a sympathetic approach and, at the same time, appeared prepared for the rigours of the discipline that the 'clinical gaze' imposed on the body, as long it was confined to the manipulation of the 'anatomical body' and did not extend to include the doctor/patient interaction. In that respect, patients sought a softening of the 'gaze', which couples like Sudhir and Rekha experienced in their doctor's 'human approach'. Neelanjana – though highly critical of clinical medicine and its 'inhuman approach' – had reached a point where she was thinking of giving up the resistance all together, in terms of 'I am also like fed up. Okay, let's get it over with, once and for all. After this, what?' However, there were reassuring moments in her ongoing treatment:

> But one thing is very good. Like, before I went for this treatment, I talked to Dr Kalakar. I was being offered some consultancy job. I don't have a regular job, so I said, 'Look, this consultancy involves travelling. Should I take it up?' And he said, 'Yeah! Why not?' That is first time. I said, 'Okay, that gave me a lot of confidence. Like, otherwise I was thinking, 'Oh God! You are going for something artificial, something which goes against your whole physiological process'. Maybe, I started feeling, that it requires special care – a diseased condition. But when I talked to him, he said, 'You don't require!' One thing he told me is, 'It's very important for you to be mentally in a healthy state. You know, it is more important that you have a rest for the night than if walk for say about two kilometres or so'. That gave me a lot of confidence. Okay let's, let me take things in a stride. And he said later, 'You can travel. Of course, you'll have to be careful' ... I think [in this clinic] there is possibility of a dialogue provided I seek information. But [clinicians in general], somehow they are too busy. They can't understand that something is bothering the patient. They will not say, 'Okay, is something on your mind? Can I talk to you? Can I help you?' You know, those kind of things. They will never allay your fears.

Once again the need for a 'human approach' in the absence of any psychological counselling is strongly articulated. This effectively means – as in the case of Sudhir and Rekha above – a clinician who lends a sympathetic ear. As a consequence, infertile couples approached new clinics or doctors with a renewed sense of expectancy and hope.

Saroj, an infertile woman from Delhi, summed up the never-ending vicious circle of 'wishful thinking' that pervaded such an engagement:

> What is stressful is you know you are going through a process, and the doctor says to you, 'Okay, let us see this month'. The moment the doctor says, 'Okay, now this month we can see if something works', then your wishful thinking process starts ... I think if the patient is well prepared – 'Okay, we are making our efforts, we are trying our best for this kind of treatment', and if the patient is made to relax during the whole process I think it will definitely help ... I am now putting all my trust in Dr Suman. This is very important. The patient has to put their trust in the doctor....

It is important for Saroj to put her trust in her doctor, in the hope that the doctor will in turn remain truthful, thus hinging the doctor-patient relationship precariously on an imagined trust-based contract.

Taken to extremes, this expectation sometimes assumes the form of blind faith in the clinician. Dr Shaileja once spoke during an informal conversation at her clinic about how, in India, there is 'a lot of hero worship', and that when people come to her, they do not come to her clinic but rather 'they come to Dr Shaileja; it doesn't matter to them where you are attached or what you do as long as you have a big name'. The publicity generated through the media can have such an effect on a patient, but blind faith or hero-worship must also be viewed as a surrogate cry for help, a beseeching supplication for a quick resolution of the social and physical suffering wrought by infertility. Dr Mukta, an IVF clinician from Madras, asserts, 'Patients accept whatever we say, [whatever] line of treatment: "It's IVF? Okay", "ICSI? Okay", and the patients also say, "Whatever doctors says". Unlike in the West, the patients blindly believe a doctor here'. Similarly Dr Neeta, an IVF practitioner in Delhi, spoke of the faith her patients place in her: 'They say, "We have faith in you", and this is something too big to say. And when they say "faith in you", it means it is something too big somebody has said and that you have to take care of it'. Blind faith is expressed in the clinician's ability to perform a miracle by a feat of medical prestidigitation, rather than in the superiority of the technologies. Interventions like IVF assume meaning only in the context of an able physician, who has the expertise to apply technology to create the desired outcome – pregnancy. In assuming the primacy of the technician over the technique, some patients place themselves in a situation where they are left to adulate and worship the expert as a last resort. It is therefore not uncommon for patients to compare past and current medical encounters and attribute their leaving a clinic to a lack of success and an absence of sympathetic counselling.

In the wider context of failed past treatments and high economic costs, a patient's search for a human touch evoked two principal responses from the clinicians. First, clinicians sporadically yielded to the patient's need for compassionate and reassuring treatment by addressing the wider social context of their suffering. Second, clinicians responded to the continuing financial hardships the treatment seekers routinely faced by making concessions towards the costs of IVF and other therapies. Both these responses reinforced the informality that underpinned the clinical settings and allowed for a degree of improvisation in formulating clinical responses to patients suffering.

Searching for the Human Touch

None of the IVF clinics covered for this research provided psychological therapeutic interventions designed to help patients manage the anxiety that often accompanies infertility and its treatments. Thus, patients effectively sought this human touch from the clinicians, who fulfilled these expectations sporadically, as they juggled the roles of counsellor and infertility expert. According to Dr Sachin:

> counselling couples is very, very less, very less, in most centres because the clinicians are too busy or they don't have enough time to counsel the patient. The patients feel that IVF is a miracle treatment. First shot, they will conceive and when they don't, they really take it as a big blow.

It is common for clinicians to witness very high stress levels, coupled with unrealistic expectations of IVF and other related technologies, in their patients.

Dr Mukta spoke of the stress produced in patients by their feelings of urgency and their high expectations: 'The level of expectation in a patient is that she should conceive at any cost. [She is/they are] not bothered whether [the doctor] is going to do IVF, ICSI or give hormones or do insemination or just give counselling. The first concern is, "I should conceive"'.

Dr Mukta is not alone in experiencing such pressure from patients. Dr Shanta, a Delhi based IVF expert, expressed similar pressure:

> From three months onwards they start coming ... They come and say, 'Oh! Doctor, please hurry up this process. We have already wasted so much time'. They will say, 'Doctor, we have done everything. Even you are saying nothing is wrong' [in cases of unexplained infertility]. Then they will start counting [their] problems ... You don't like being driven by the patient, and maybe the patient doesn't like it, you don't like it. The patient ends up going to somebody [else]!

A patient's sense of urgency, bordering on desperation, can sometimes burden the doctor-patient dialogue. This can result in their abandoning the treatment and opting for another clinic, thus perpetuating the vicious circle of continually seeking resolution and a human touch. Some doctors therefore lay down the rules of engagement at the very first consultation. Dr Lalit prefers professional distance between himself and the patients:

> When I am dealing with an infertile couple, I don't try to go into the depths of their problem. I only counsel at a technical level that there is a chance of 20 percent pregnancy rate, it is a chance you know. I never delve into the social aspects. I feel that you need to be a bit hard with them. [Otherwise] they start becoming more emotionally laid back once you start trying to relate too much with them about their infertility problems because their problems can have a lot of ramifications, you know. I am nice to them, but I don't like to go into the depths of what happens with their family. I never go into that area.

In contradistinction to Dr Lalit, Dr Neeta takes a diametrically opposite approach to counselling her patients: 'I've sat down with them from time to time, discuss with them. I have heard them cry. I sorted out all their domestic problems, and now they are very happy and they are in treatment now.' Field notes on her consultation sessions with couples reveal instances of counselling patients and addressing the wider social issues underlying her patients' experiences of infertility. The following excerpt from Dr Neeta's interaction with a young couple gives a sense of how the subject of stress, and its implications for infertility treatment, was explained to her patients:

> Dr: You have a lovely wife!
>
> M: Thank you!

Dr: [addressing the woman] How old are you?

W: Twenty-four years old, married for two years.

Dr: Do you work?

W: No. I am a housewife. No intentions of working.

Dr: [joking] Lucky! [...]

After taking a detailed case history, the doctor asks the couple how she can help:

M: I only want a baby I am prepared for everything. I am living in a joint family. My younger brother got married last year, and his wife is pregnant. I live in a joint family and find it very difficult ... I'll do anything [alluding to a sperm test].

Dr: [addressing his wife] You are twenty-four. There is a lot of time ...

Sensing the couple's anxiety, the doctor began to explain the impact of stress on the endocrinal system:

Dr: The hypothalamus orders the pituitary to begin its work. FSH and LH [hormones secreted by the pituitary gland] come down to the ovaries where eggs are already present and the FSH and LH stimulate the ovaries and the eggs are matured.

Continuing, she explains the entire process again, this time using an analogy to make it more accessible:

Dr: If the elders in the family are not good, what will the junior or younger people do in such a family? If the family elders set a bad example for the younger lot, what can be expected of the young ones? Look at our country, if our political system is so bad what will become of the country. Same way the hypothalamus has to set the right example for pituitary in order for it to be able to stimulate the ovaries. So keep tensions away as it affects the proper functioning of the hypothalamus. Please promise me you will leave all your troubles here with me. I had a patient who used to call me at 8 o'clock in the evening saying 'my mother-in-law is scolding me' [interrupted]

M: This way she will call you ten, fifteen times a day [laughs]

Dr: [smiles and continues] I told her that either take your husband and go out, or if he is scared of his mother, you cook for her and pray. She is so pretty just like you, and she is so tense. Please promise me that you will not think about these tensions anymore.

The clinician outlines how biographies of individuals can be inextricably linked to their biology and biological outcomes. Elsewhere I argue how the very notion of 'bio' can be 'conceptualised as an instance of biologically based biography, be it individual (e.g. an illness narrative or cultural/"ethno" conception of human body) or institutional (bio-science/medicine/technology etc.). A biography is inextricably inserted in any individual and/or institutional understanding of the biological' (Bharadwaj 2008: 102). In this sense Dr Neeta outlines how biographies of individuals can be linked to their biology and biological outcomes. She drives home the biomedical visualisation of the division of labour in the working of the endocrinal system by comparing it to the delicate power balance in wider society. However, what is interesting about this approach is its ability to invoke the metaphor of hierarchical familial relations and their accompanying rights and obligations. The analogy of a family patriarch setting the right example for the 'juniors' to follow, in the context of counselling, doubles as a subtle reference to the couple's predicament – which is loaded with undue family pressure to conceive – as irresponsibility on the part of the elders of the (joint) family in allowing the burden to conceive to add to the couple's stress. Sensing anxiety in the man, the doctor appears to deliberately take up the example of one of her other patients, obliquely alluding to the importance of a husband supporting his wife in the face of hostility from the mother-in-law by suggesting that a woman who is unable to enlist her husband's support can do little other than cook to please her in-laws or pray. Dr Neeta, in other words, addresses one of the core biographical subtexts underpinning the cause of stress in the couple's life, by splicing it with explanations which are more biomedical in nature. She does this surreptitiously – by urging the couple to leave all their troubles with her, thus encouraging them to tackle the source of stress in their lives – as openly confronting these sensitive issues may be considered outside of her professional remit.

Not all clinicians, however, saw the merits of counselling patients. In Dr Shanta's experience, counselling worked for only 50 per cent of the cases:

> For a lot of people, the counselling goes to a total waste because they are not interested in knowing how a test-tube baby shapes what really happens. Even if I make a diagram of the treatment process, it doesn't work because at the end of the whole lecture you hear just one sentence: 'Doctor, what medicine do we have to eat?' You know, so pretreatment counselling works for few people. [For a] few it just

> doesn't work. In the private clinics, a lot of educated people are coming, a lot of people who are otherwise very well-off, but they don't want to work their brains at all and they don't want to understand the logic. On the other hand, there are fifty percent of patients who feel very happy because they've been explained something. They really understand the logic, and they are the ones who really stick to the treatment.

These three different observations indicate how individual clinicians approach the subject of counselling and address the issue of the social context of their patients' predicaments. They give a sense of differentials in doctor-patient dialogue across clinics and the value attached to such a dialogue. While Dr Lalit stays aloof from all social aspects of his patients' condition, Dr Neeta encourages her patients to tackle such issues, as a means of balancing the stress of treatment and growing family impatience. There are also some important clues as to what is understood and construed – differently by different clinicians – as effective pretreatment counselling. These differences are also a feature of the individual personalities of clinicians rather than a clinically endorsed criterion of counselling.

Monetary Help

Many patients struggle to cover the high cost of treatment and are forced to gamble their entire life savings. The clinicians respond to such patients by either reducing fees or letting patients pay owed bills in succeeding visits. This gives assisting conception an altogether new meaning. A sizeable number of clinicians admitted to reducing fees or accommodating requests to pay later for specific treatments, as in the case of Shanker and Ajay (Chapter 7). In a Mumbai clinic, for instance, the counter clerk was often busy counting wads of currency notes and answering inquiries pertaining to payment procedures and receipts. One man, in particular, was asked to pay part of the sum involved (6,000 rupees) with the balance due on a later date, to which the clerk explained that he could either pay the entire sum on a later date or he could put 5,000 rupees as a down-payment and the balance on his next visit, as this would make it easier for her to manage the records and issue receipts. In one North Indian clinic, patients were observed haggling with the clerks about how much a specific intervention was worth. On the day of our meeting in their hotel room, Sumita (Chapter 7) complained about the steep insemination charges (5,000 rupees), given that the procedure was simple and took less than ten minutes – the doctor simply injected the sperm into her cervix. Many patients pursued this line of reasoning with the clinic staff when paying for specific interventions.

Clinicians, on their part, maintained that they were particularly concerned with the financial burden some patients undertook and therefore felt morally obliged to assist them financially in every way possible. Dr Suman appeared genuinely worried about this aspect:

> I keep trying to figure out how to keep their costs low to manage them so that they don't have to shell out extra money and at the same time try to keep their stress levels low by giving back results as fast as possible and to try and bring cost down. This is the single most difficult problem for us in India.

In trying to minimise the stress levels of the patients by managing the cost of assisted conception, various clinics were found to use innovative methods to deal with patients who could not afford the treatment.

Dr Kamraj developed an interesting way of discriminating between patients at her Chennai clinic:

> Patients who have already been abroad can obviously afford, and patients who come to me for a long time and they have failed due to unforeseen cause I treat them free, I don't charge them. And patients who are mediocre, we do come down and give concessions because we identify them as the couple walks in. My people, I have taught them to identify: do they have a gold chain or are they wearing yellow thread? You know, I say yellow thread give free, so all the antibiotics, medicines we give free. The patient doesn't know that we identified her, and automatically we try to give maximum concession. Knowingly or unknowing we do it. But once the patient tries to exploit us in that way, then we become very strict. Then I change everything, then we are very careful. Even some rich patients sometimes I go out of my way to help them. I feel sorry for them, and we mostly work like a huge family not doctor-patient relationship. It's more like friends or relations, like that we behave.

The doctor's ingenious way of identifying patients in need of financial assistance is based on a reading of symbols in Hindu and particularly South Indian Tamil culture. Married South Indian Hindu women wear a gold chain – *tali* – around their neck as a mark or representation of their married status, but individuals who are too poor to afford a gold tali often make do with a simple yellow thread. This absence translates into a commentary on a couple's financial situation, since individuals of even limited means do allocate resources if at all possible to invest in such a marker, given its religious and social importance. Additionally, Dr Kamraj claims to reject conventional 'clinical' distance between her and her patients, although use of metaphors like family and friends is more a description of the informality present in IVF clinics (in India) than an accurate account of the doctor-patient relationship.

Several other clinicians considered their patients' economic circumstances. Dr Mukta similarly reported that, in her centre, hormonal administration was carried out free of charge, although patients had to pay for the hormones as they were quite expensive to subsidise. In addition, ultrasounds were performed at a nominal rate of 150 rupees per scan, and disposables were supplied to the patients at international prices, which worked out much cheaper than the prevailing domestic rates (as import duties made disposables more expensive). On the issue of consultation fees, she had this to say:

> As far as consultations are concerned, I tell them, 'You can pay the doctor after you conceive'. If they don't conceive, I don't take anything. There are patients who don't pay. I have a couple who is from Vijaywardha; they conceived and even six months after the pregnancy they've not met me or paid me, but I am not unhappy. It's okay, there are patients who paid me 8,000 rupees and there are patients who have paid me 2,000 rupees.

Two other clinicians in South India claimed that forgoing part of the consultation fee or reducing the price of various procedures was common. One confirmed that if patients request, he is willing to drop the 5,000 rupee charge for consultation. Another spoke of the financial burden most patients undertook by selling their properties and borrowing from financiers, which led her to routinely drop various charges, though, like Dr Mukta, she faced repeated bad debts. Clinics in North India also, such as Dr Kalakar's, purportedly faced similar problems, with some patients either refusing to pay in the case of failed cycles or simply not returning after a successful pregnancy. Clinicians like Dr Sachin had a more systematic approach to patients with financial difficulties, in contrast to the ad-hoc accommodations made by the clinics above: '80 percent of our patients still cannot afford ARTs; only 20 percent can afford. We have charitable schemes and we do one or two free IVFs per month. The donation fund comes from patients who have conceived and the money is utilised for treating including drugs'.

Dr Manker had established a similar system:

> We have made a foundation that allows for one or two cycles per month. We don't charge. The patient pays only for the drug cost, and the foundation subsidises the treatment. So we can do one or two cycles at the moment a month at almost about 50 percent of the cost. Some of the patients who have conceived and delivered, many of them we have found like to donate money towards this, and we can utilise that money for doing IVF. The moment we tell them, 'Since you have had a baby and many patients who really cannot afford this and who need it', so they are extremely willing to help out. So it's not a big number, but we can do one or two cycles at a much, much lower rate.

These clinicians are, however, not unique in establishing mechanisms to manage the high cost of treatments. Naomi Pfeffer (1992) showed, in the case of Britain, how in some hospitals patients are asked to make voluntary contributions, while in others the patients' support group raises money to buy equipment. Some consultants even operate what Pfeffer calls a 'Robin Hood system' – that is, 'robbing' better-off patients in order to provide free treatment for people who cannot afford it. However, such arrangements are restricted to private/public partnerships in Britain, where, according to Pfeffer (1992: 67), gynaecologists have successfully attached IVF clinics on to existing National Health Service facilities, thus avoiding the large start-up capital costs of an independent unit. The 'Robin Hood' model in the Indian context does not so much entail 'robbing' well-off patients but rather offering pro bono treatment subsidised by well-off domestic and international patients who routinely fund IVF cycles as a gesture of good will and gratitude for a successful IVF treatment outcome. On occasion, well-off patients subsidise cycles in exchange for gamete donation from a less well-off treatment seeker.

However, not all free treatments are motivated by pure altruism. As discussed elsewhere, in the burgeoning context of embryonic stem cell research, fertility treatment-seeking patients are also offered ethically problematic 'free IVF for spare embryo donation' arrangements (Bharadwaj 2010b). Again, the stem cell treatment domain is as mixed as the IVF treatments on offer. There is much evidence to suggest that well-off domestic and international stem cell treatment-seeking patients are charged for therapies while less well-off or returning patients are subsidised or treated pro bono (Bharadwaj 2013a, 2013b). In the Indian context, such IVF and stem cell clinics are exclusively confined to the private sector, with substantial 'personal' financial investments made by individual clinicians. Their sense of urgency in making treatment affordable is therefore markedly different from the British case, where personal investment predominantly takes the shape of raising funds. In the past this meant developing quasi-private clinics, using staff, equipment and drugs paid for by a mixture of the NHS, research and drug company monies, and charges to patients (Pfeffer 1992).

Not surprisingly, therefore, the high cost of interventions and their patients' general incapacity to afford treatments leads some clinicians to argue that running a successful centre is not as lucrative a proposition as it is made out be. Dr Shanta was disappointed by the attitude and rate of return of the patients, despite putting long hours into managing infertility. In her assessment, IVF offered at the hospital where she heads the clinic is one of the cheapest in the country, since the consultation fee is split between the embryologist and the gynaecologist. 'I can make more money doing a caesarean section than what I get doing IVF', she stated. Dr Kamraj maintained that '[People] think [IVF practitioners] make a lot of money, but you can have a test-tube baby lab only if you have an outpatient. Otherwise you go for tremendous loss.'

There was substantial unanimity amongst the clinicians on the importance of having a daily routine gynaecological out-patient inflow to make the IVF programme financially viable. There are a number of factors involved in understanding the spread of assisted conception in India, given the high investment and uniformly high cost that is consequently passed on to patients. As is clear from Chapter 4, a rift between gynaecological and infertility specialists has set in motion not only a struggle for credibility to manage infertility, but also a rush to hold on to one's patients, destroying in the process the referral chain vital to appropriate and timely infertility treatment. This also means an aggressive marketing of infertility techniques hitherto unavailable to the majority of the population. The need to subsidise IVF, therefore, can in part be viewed as lying at the cusp of altruism and the need for commercial gain. While clinics accommodate poorer patients out of a sense of magnanimity, such an approach also provides an opportunity to undercut the competition. Where genuine altruism ends and commercialism begins is difficult to ascertain. It is not easy to say whether the need to make assisted conception more affordable and straightforward is born out of a need to simplify an agonising wait for conception, or to capture the fertility market (Chapter 4). However, it does significantly alter the face of medical engagement between clinicians and patients by suspending the contractual approach to buying and selling medical care that underpins medicine in the private sector.

Despite the informal arrangements between clinicians and patients, treatment outcomes remain uncertain. The success of a procedure like IVF is not bound up with a clinician's expertise nor located in the technology itself. The elusive pregnancies are subject to a number of other critical parameters (both technical and biological) that together produce 'results'. This uncertainty, and the accompanying lack of results, at once places clinicians and treatment seekers in a cultural paradigm that helps to rationalise and accommodate 'failures', 'failings of clinical medicine' and the 'perpetuation of suffering'. This explanatory frame is religion.

End of the Road or Dead End? From a Clinician's Hands into God's

The suspension of 'scientific rationality' – the hallmark of clinical medicine – is at its most prominent in a clinician's ability to explain the unpredictability of assisted conception outcomes by resorting to rationalisations more metaphysical in nature. The success or failure of any treatment was partly acknowledged as a product of scientific and technical intervention, beyond which lay the unexplored realm of the unknown that was best understood by resorting to spiritual and cosmological explanations. In the clinicians' understanding there were definite limits to what could be achieved through scientific expertise, beyond which the work of God played a role in creating human life. Ironically, if assisted conception was 'man's' way of assisting when nature failed – as routinely described in medical literature and popular media accounts – then the process of assisting nature itself needed assistance, which drew back on the conceptualisation of 'nature' as 'God'. Rati and Sundar's assertion (Chapter 7), for instance, refers in passing to how, in their earlier clinical encounters, they were repeatedly told by the doctors that, 'Everything is normal. It is in the hands of God; you will have something', an experience not dissimilar from Seema's who was (according to Vani, her sister-in-law) told by her doctor that her 'treatment is the best, and you leave the rest to God' (Chapter 7). Leaving 'things' to God emerged as routine clinical practice as couples were repeatedly told by their clinicians, after the most sophisticated interventions to bypass their infertility, that their cases now rested with a 'higher court of appeal' that would determine the eventual outcome of the clinical efforts.

This explanation places the tentative nature of science and the technological management of the human body in sharp relief. Without exception, all the clinics studied were favourably predisposed to the idea of divine intervention in the process of clinical conception. This was most discernable from pictorial and iconographic displays of various Hindu gods and goddesses, as well as patron saints, in the clinic lobbies and inside the clinician's consulting rooms. One clinic in South India is named after a local goddess whose name literally translates in English to mean 'the mother goddess who protects the womb' (*Garbba Rakhambigai*). Infertile couples in search of conception congregate at her temple from all over India. This juxtaposition situates an IVF clinic in relation to divine blessings associated with reversing the scourge of infertility. Religious beliefs, therefore, emerge as playing an important role in routine clinical practice. A further example was encountered in a clinic in the north of India where a large signboard, conspicuous by its bold display, occupied a prominent part of the clinic's waiting area. The display was entitled 'IVF/GIFT Patients – Instructions'. A long list of dos and don'ts for patients while in treatment was succeeded by one last instruction: to 'not think too much of the results and leave everything to God or your destiny; your treatment was carried out to the best of our ability'. This approximate translation from Hindi offers a sense of how uncertain or unwanted treatment outcomes are explained by destiny (*bhagya, niyati*) and God (*ishware*), rather than by empirical and 'objective', 'clinical' facts (such as the 20 per cent chance of success). Accounts of couples and individuals substantiated this tendency. Shanker, for instance, when asked whether he was prepared to face the high failure rate of the treatment, said, 'Doctor was saying that [the failure rate is high and that] it is all up to God. Whatever we can do, we will'. Similarly, Ram Naik, a patient whose wife had undergone an embryo transfer on the day of the interview, had this to say: 'Right now ET is going on the operation is in XYZ hospital. So far the response is good, even the doctor has told us so that the result is with The Almighty'. In both Shanker and Ram Naik's case, it appears that the clinician – having done his or her best in trying to induce a pregnancy – was simply awaiting a supernatural verdict on his/her efforts.

The reasons for such reliance on spiritual and religious explanations are complex. While clinicians may hold firm religious convictions that help them make sense of treatment outcomes, they also turn to God as a way of managing the anxiety that typically accompanies the running of a successful IVF programme. There is a great stress to continually produce results and remain financially viable by recruiting newer patients to the programme to ensure its commercial feasibility (Chapter 4). Dr Sachin is one clinician who attributes his clinics' success to cosmic forces and sees no harm in turning to complementary therapies alongside the assisted conception process, as he firmly believes that, despite all the advances, ARTs continue to be a 'partial science':

> I believe a lot in God, in astrology, palmistry. I believe in *Vastu* science [ancient craft of positioning like *Fung Shui*] – you know, position science. All my four centres are designed as per *Vastu*. The culture room is situated in the corner that is supposed to be best for producing new life, OT tables are in the right direction to aid conception, magnetic fields whatever, whatever, whatever! These are all now turning out to be good sciences so we don't go blindly by it but [also] ART is incomplete science. In whatever we do we are not exceeding 32 percent. That means we are not good enough. Today I find so many sperm counts improving with *aruyvedic* treatment, so many sperm counts improving with homeopathic treatment. My first pregnancy, her husband's mother was a good homeopathic in Jabalpur and two IVF cycles we had done for her in Bangalore before. First cycle she came here (Mumbai); she was the eighth IVF here. Her endometrium was very thin, just six mm; go through any literature, endometrium on the day of ET has to cross eight to ten mm to get a pregnancy. Three beautiful embryos, I told her that you don't have much chance because of six mm endometrium. Without telling me she took homoeopathic pills before and after the embryo transfer that her mother had given her – she conceived and delivered! That means ARTs are an incomplete science. When our books say eight mm is the cut off, most Western literature says endometrium less than eight mm, cancel the cycle. So all my failed ETs, I send them for homeopathy you know as a contributory medicine because it doesn't really harm. It might only do good! *Vastu* and all that was done three years ago. Having made those changes, the success rate jumped, the economic picture jumped, financially we have jumped, everything changed. Astrology – you won't believe this – but couples, if they go to a good astrologer, they are told that, 'Okay, this is the best month for you to conceive', and almost 70 to 75 percent of cases it works out if you correlate. We are not a complete science. Okay, if we can say 100 percent guarantee for IVF cycle fine, then all these other sciences have no meaning, but where is the 100 percent guarantee? Where is even a 50 percent guarantee?

The doctor's faith in complementary medicine and what he describes as parallel 'sciences' reanimates clinical practice in a way that assumes the shape of a potent critique of the tentative character of clinical medicine. His predominant concern is conception rather than a broader ideological commitment to scientific rationality. The eclectic combination of the clinical and the non-clinical, therefore, helps the doctor to answer questions that biomedicine leaves unanswered. His spiritual beliefs, in this respect, fill the vacuum of uncertainty that clinical medicine has failed to fill with so-called rational explanations. The engagement with divine or cosmic forces therefore becomes a mechanism to make sense of the unknown in the working of the human body. Nowhere is this need more pronounced then at the stage of embryo transfers. Clinically, it continues to be a grey area, as the exact conditions that contribute to the success or failure of an embryo implant remain relatively unknown. Dr Neeta also invokes divine assistance in the process:

> I am a great believer in God, greatest believer on earth! When I put embryos in the uterus I keep praying, I keep praying. I tell my patients, 'Please tell God to leave everything now and come and be with me just for half a second only. You don't need God more than one second, just tell God be here for just half second, please God come here!' I am a great believer in God!

The doctor's cry for help, and the patient's participation in summoning God's help to assist conception, goes beyond creating a fleeting intimate bond between the clinician and the patient struggling and praying from within the definite limits of science. More importantly, it highlights an acknowledgement of having traversed the scientific terrain only to arrive at a frontier where one encounters the great 'unknown' in the absence of any persuasive explanation. God, therefore (in the context of the clinic in India), stands in for an absence of rational explanation and is invoked for guidance and success. Dr Suman also believes in a higher power to bring forth a pregnancy. When asked whether she believed in God her answer was quite simply:

> I do! Of course! Oh! Ah! Of course! Of course! I believe in God very firmly! In the sense that whatever I may do I can try my best. Like I go through their entire case history, trying to do my best, to make my correct judgment and yet she doesn't get pregnant. After the embryo has been transferred it all depends on God or nature. You may call it nature or God. In medicine anywhere what is faith healing after all? When the patient comes to you, what are you doing for him?

> Basically the faith that is going to play a major role. We are talking about anxiety and stress. When the patient is doubting you, when the patient doesn't get confidence or faith in you, then the results are not going to be good because her stress levels are going to disturb the endocrinal profile. That is what God is. There is a saying that 'Doctor is God'. They are going for the treatment cycle. We are gods for them, so it's a cycle. I have to believe in something in order to perform. Therefore I believe in God!

In approaching religion, doctors make sense of the uncertainties of clinical conception but also echo how patients approach clinical healing. Dr Kamraj, in a 1998 autobiographical account, reveals:

> My mother said, 'You should have a Guru to follow'. I thought a superhuman being was better than a human being. I do not trust human beings – each one has a drawback. You have to be a super being to be perfect, clear and right. I chose Lord Vinayaka [Ganesha the Hindu Elephant God of good luck and prosperity is known as Vinayaka in Tamil Nadu, South India]. He has always been my guru, my guide and my best friend! He is someone I look up to, someone from whom I can ask for anything, scold, fight, pour out my despair and frustrations, and yet he never chides me or gets angry with me. Isn't that just great! He has been my most faithful and best friend. He has not ever harmed me. He has always done the best for me and will continue to do so! Even if something negative happens, there is sure to be a hidden reason which will surface later. Lord Vinayaka is one I trusted, I trust and will trust till the last breath of my life.[3]

This excerpt provides a glimpse into how some Hindus approach the idea of the divine and the otherworldly. The relationship between the deity and the disciple is forged in the spirit of a parent-child relationship with accompanying allowances that such a relationship affords a child. Individuals may choose the metaphors of parental bond, friendship or even mutual love to create such a relationship. Thus complaints, demands, even occasional tantrums are means of attracting the benevolent attention of the parental figure. An accommodation such as this undermines the possibility of a devotee turning blasphemous, or into a plain heretic, as routine displays of anger against an unyielding deity (which in its extreme can amount to questioning the divine credentials of the deity) are explained away as those of a child who would eventually be placated with parental love and reasoning.

This conceptual framework also appears to inform the doctor-patient relationship in the Indian context, as doctors are conventionally viewed and revered as life-giving, sustaining gods – a point to which Dr Suman obliquely alludes. In this context, it may be worth recalling Mani Chadwa's assertion in a media report (cited in Chapter 3) on the birth of 'her' and 'India's first scientifically documented test-tube baby':

> Anchor: The Chawda couple has a special place for Dr Hinduja in their heart:
>
> Mani Chadwa (Mother): I was never ... I was not meant to have a child ... but madam did the test tube and gave me a baby. We consider Indira Hinduja God. She is our God. Madam made it possible, everything she did, I feel [Harsha] is her daughter...

Media renditions – such as Mani Chadwa's – on the 'experts' can assume a quasi-sacred iconographic dimension and result in the projection of these 'demigods of fertility' as the only beacon of hope. Paradoxically, like the Hindu trinity, as well as giving and sustaining life (*Bhrama* and *Vishnu*), a doctor can also play the part of life destroyer (*Shiva*). Equally, like the gods and goddesses in the Hindu pantheon who may be critiqued from time to time for failing their devotees, doctors too are construed as failing their patients. This may elicit protestations from those let down, but an eventual resolution and return to the deity/doctor becomes the only source of comfort and healing. I am not suggesting that the infertile couples in this research perceived the clinicians as quasi-divine but rather that the healing professions – including clinical medicine – in India have for long been viewed as sacred, with medical/healing work looked upon as noble and imbued with extreme religious merit. An analogy between the sacred domain of a culture and its healing tradition – of which clinical medicine is now an integral part – enables one to see how cultural conceptualisations may reanimate social interactions, such as doctor-patient relations, to carry culturally embedded meaning. The growing cynicism with the material culture which is corrupting the medical domain, echoed by Shanker in Chapter 7, is not dissimilar from the momentary disenchantment, and even alienation, experienced by devotees when their deities fail them. Referring to the downfall of a noble profession (medicine), a couple interviewed in a Delhi IVF unit summed up their dejection as follows: 'Everywhere it's become a business these days ... Otherwise previously I remember twenty years back we use to think God is, I mean doctor and God together you know, doctor used to be the God'. Although they are consistently and individually critiqued as having fallen from grace, doctors, or rather 'fallen gods', are continually approached in the absence of any tangible alternatives. The deep ambivalence permeating clinical encounters in this respect only mirrors the Hindu engagement with the sacred domain, as in both instances, in spite of the disappointments, the devotee/patient returns to the source with renewed supplication.

The notion of theodicy as developed by Max Weber and explained by Talcott Parsons (1949: 208) amounted to a 'fundamental distinction between the significance for human action of problems of empirical causation and the problem of meaning'. Parsons posed an important problematic in arguing that whereas 'how' questions, such as death through accident, can be reasonably understood by recourse to an adequate explanation of empirical causes, 'why' questions, that is, why such things must happen, posed not merely emotional but cognitive frustration. A 'why' question therefore poses a problem that theodicy seeks to address. Anthropologist Gananath Obeyesekere (1968) clarified that while in theology theodicy generally means justification of God, as popularised by Gottfried Wilhelm von Leibniz in 1710, Max Weber used the term in several distinguishable ways. These range from Leibniz's classical description to the phenomenon of unjust suffering, which arises in any existential or social context, as well as the charter for explaining the discrepancy between hope and experience in the context of human suffering (Obeyeseskere 1968: 9). Redefining the concept, Obeyeseskere (1968: 11) proposes that 'When a religion fails logically to explain human suffering or fortune in terms of its system of beliefs, we can say that a theodicy exists'.

The rapid proliferation and assimilation of IVF in India, however, poses a different problematic – that is, when science rather than religion fails to explain human suffering or fortune, can we argue that a theodicy exists? I argue that metaphysical explanations have become culturally acceptable coping mechanisms for the clinicians and their patients, as they both struggle to make sense of the uncertain nature of assisted conception. Such a way of 'making sense' not only indigenises biomedicine (Kleinman 1995) but more crucially produces clinical theodicies that resolve the 'why' questions posed by intractable infertility. A clinical theodicy similarly helps to make sense of biomedical uncertainty so as to resolve tentative outcomes of conception technologies. This is perhaps indicative of a larger process of double entrenchment of tradition in India today, a coming-together of reconfigured traditional notions of divinity and the modern idea of clinical space. More crucially, the indigenisation of biomedicine in India demonstrates that the clinical/biomedical modalities are far more open to uncertainty and more amenable to pluralistic understandings than the 'technocratic imperative' (Davis-Floyd and Dumit 1998: 9) permeating the clinical application of science in the Euro-American contexts.

Arthur Kleinman (1995: 27) has argued that the monotheism of Western tradition has had a determinative effect on biomedicine, even as it is practised in non-Western societies, which distinguishes it in a fundamental way from Asian medical systems. He argues that Chinese and *Ayurvedic* medical traditions, unlike biomedicine, tolerate alternative competing paradigms, seem less troubled by the uncertainty of human experience, and are more pluralistic in their theoretical orientations and therapeutic practices. While Kleinman's argument undoubtedly problematises the biomedical intolerance to alternative therapeutic modalities, I argue that biomedicine, at least in the Indian setting, is becoming rapidly assimilated into a cultural worldview that is transforming the way it is both perceived and practised.

Conclusions

The clinical world of conception as seen in this chapter is deeply embedded in cultural topography. The very act of seeking conception represents – paradoxically – both an escape from and conformity to the dominant social norms regarding fertility as a logical outcome of married relations. For clinicians, the very nature of their work – treating infertility – renders them incapable of confronting critically the social and cultural sources of distress and suffering in their patients' lives (with notable exceptions like Dr Neeta). Unwittingly, clinicians continue to reinforce cultural norms about fertility (Chapter 1) and sanction the unjust treatment meted out to the infertile (Chapter 2) by, for example, colluding in the secrecy surrounding treatment seeking (Chapter 5). This reinforcement is further exacerbated when clinicians promote themselves and assisted conception through the media as 'benign' and as a 'solution' for infertility (Bharadwaj 2000). This approach may serve the purpose of promoting individual claims to credibility (Chapter 3), or even the commercial viability of a clinician's high-investment private enterprise (Chapter 4). However, these ideas are reinforced microcosmically within the clinic, where the 'promotional themes' permeating the lobbies reinforce patients' sense of expectancy while obliquely assuring them that their current investment in assisted conception is worthwhile (Chapter 8). Treatment seekers understandably view unfavourable outcomes as the personal failures of clinicians (Chapter 7). The infertile, on the other hand, can uncritically respond to cultural pressure by seeking assisted conception to 'save face', once again reinforcing the dominant cultural norms about infertility (Chapter 1).

Infertility treatment is not restricted to the 'mechanics' of offering and receiving treatment, but more crucially to the ways in which clinicians and infertile couples make sense of the cultural context. The success and failure of assisted conception, when placed in the universe of Hindu faith, becomes a powerful critique of the 'incompleteness' of the science of conception. Placed in the broader context of a clinician's faith, assisted conception conjoins the disparate domains of the sacred and the profane, the human and the superhuman, science and religion, all working together to produce human life. It is perhaps tempting to assume that clinicians invoke the divine in order to both enlist patients and to dismiss low success rates by attributing outcomes to a supernatural will. The reality, however, is more complex since a clinical theodicy implicates, in very direct ways, an 'expert's' own 'expertise'. In this respect, divine assistance in the process of assisting conception is an open admission of personal, professional limits and those intrinsic to the science of conception itself. This also points to a significant suspension of technical and scientific rationality, on which the philosophy of the clinic purportedly hinges. This enchanted version of a 'thoroughly disenchanted worldview' of biomedicine is part of a larger cultural process of the 'indigenisation of biomedicine' (Kleinman 1995). These metaphysical explanations also become culturally acceptable coping mechanisms for clinicians and their patients, as they both struggle to make sense of repeated failures, stigma, financial drain and lack of credibility. In brief, the paradox at the heart of clinical conception – one of resisting/critiquing and persisting – is in this sense extended further, where the clinicians and patients not only forge fleeting 'intimacies' and 'informalities' but also begin to accommodate 'failure' within the same religious/cultural paradigm that produces social suffering and stigma in the first place.

Notes

1. In the context of IVF clinics in India and in the light of Waitzkin's contention, it is possible to see that relationships between the doctor/patients are sometimes shaped by the wider cultural context of infertility.
2. Charis Thompson (2005) shows that in the case of infertility clinics in the United States, there is a rehearsed choreography of privacy. The boundaries between the private and the public blur in the Indian context; the vocal and candid articulation of intimate (sexual) aspects of the treatment helps to normalise this process. Therefore, while boundaries between private and public are maintained, they are equally and frequently transgressed by the informal approach of the clinical staff and clinicians.
3. Reference withheld to maintain anonymity

Afterword
Conceptions

Once anything comes to this country it only grows. Our soil is fertile, everything grows!

An IVF clinician in Delhi

Since 'cultures do not hold still for their portraits' (Clifford and Marcus 1986), I have developed a photographic image of the culture of infertility and its clinical management in India. This means that, as in all photographs, I have managed to frame and capture only a fleeting part of the scenery. Each chapter in this book therefore offers the reader a 'snapshot' of the world of infertility and its cultural milieu. Through these different points of entry into a poorly understood area of human reproduction in contemporary India, I show how infertility is both managed and dealt with as a biological and social disruption. This task has not been an easy one, as the very process of grappling with these complex issues has posed many more multilateral research questions. However, it is my intention to provide an insightful point of departure for all future research engagements with infertility and assisted conception in India. This study contributes to the neglected area of research on infertility and new high-tech conception possibilities in a 'non-Western' locale. It attempts to trace infertility and conception technologies in India in a number of different locales in which infertility is experienced and conception technologies used, contested and promoted. The location of this study within an expansive terrain of 'conceptions' reveals new insights and raises crucial questions.

***

The Indian state's support of private interest in medicine has significantly altered the face of investment in modern high-tech medical facilities. As a consequence, individuals and industries are investing in the private medical sector and are responding to the curative medical needs left unfulfilled by the public sector. Assisted conception's journey from its public sector beginnings to a private sector monopoly is indicative of a long sustained interaction between the public and the private sectors. The research thus found that in the private sector, clinicians and enterprising gynaecologists turn the very process of assisting conception into an unprecedented opportunity to enhance their professional, financial and social standing. The unravelling of the politics of conception in the media becomes one way to establish professional and scientific credibility that can potentially obfuscate peer-reviewed and endorsed credibility. Such credibility, and the ensuing financial reward, has resulted in a media/medicine interaction that has come to promote both the technologies of conception and their practitioners. While raising serious questions about the ethics of such self-promotion through the media, this admixture of science, journalism and advertising has promoted a benign image of these technologies and their practitioners (Bharadwaj 2000). The validation of conceptive techniques through media narratives therefore becomes part of a much larger private sector initiative, where clinicians struggle to run infertility clinics as financially viable and commercially successful enterprises. If one views what Price (1999) has called the 'marriage of medicine and the market', in the context of assisted conception in the West, then one is confronted by the chronically under-researched upbeat climate of investment in the private medical sector, and equally absent research on the role of the Indian state in controlling the sector's unabashed spread. This indicates a wider state of disarray within the Medical Councils in India that have failed to update profiles of qualified private practitioners in India, a situation further amplified by the under-reporting of hospitals in the private sector. It is therefore hardly surprising that no 'hard' baseline data is available on the spread and take-up of assisted conceptive techniques in India. If the reasons for the spread of assisted conception can be located in the public/private sector dialectic in health care, then the reasons for their uncontrolled and undocumented spread can equally be viewed as indicative of a much broader, uncontrolled and poorly regulated private sector expansion, under the supportive public sector gaze. With the entrance of 'corporate hospitals', India appears to be heading in the direction of the 'medical industrial complex' (Relman

1987). While this development may eventually steer health care towards a two-tier health system, like that of Britain, where only those who can afford to pay have access to superior care (Franklin 1997), it is important to keep in mind that the private sector in India is diverse and, notwithstanding the corporate hospitals purportedly offering state-of-the art medical care, in no way guarantees superior care. In this context, the lack of regulatory mechanisms and the Indian state's laxity in legislating private sector expansion become even more problematic.

More than twenty-five years ago, Patricia Spallone and Deborah Lynn Steinberg (1987) warned us that what the world in general, and women in particular, face is 'an international multi-billion dollar competitive race among scientists, pharmaceutical companies, medics, and politicians to lead in conquering this last frontier of human domination over nature'. The private sector monopoly over assisted conception, together with a series of transnational IVF collaborations drawing global players to 'soft states' like India, where there are minimal legislative controls in place, clearly indicate the urgent need for further research in this area. There is a tremendous dearth of research on the role played by multinational corporations and pharmaceutical companies and their interests in pushing for the greater medicalisation of infertility. In the Western context, early feminist contributions remain the only groundbreaking initiatives seeking to problematise the 'pharmaceuticalisation' of infertility. For example, as early as 1995, Annette Burfoot (1995) tried to show that due to the high degree of reproductive hormonal manipulation of women and ovulation assessment associated with what was then known as the New Reproductive Technologies (NRTs), pharmaceutical companies have capitalised enormously on these developments. Elsewhere, Burfoot (1990) showed how two pharmaceutical giants, Organon and Serono, nurtured substantial financial interests in the promotion of IVF technology. Particular attention needs to be paid to this in the Indian context, as ARTs have received unprecedented media attention, particularly since 1991, with the so-called liberalisation and opening of the Indian economy to foreign direct investment. My limited interactions with medical representatives of various pharmaceutical companies – including Organon and Serono – in India, revealed that these companies routinely offer incentives to clinicians for prescribing their drugs. This encouragement in India takes the shape of funding conferences, financing foreign sojourns of clinicians and rewarding them with cars for reaching certain quantities of drug prescriptions.

A long conversation with medical representatives in Chennai and Jaipur, for example, revealed the pattern of drug/hormone prescriptions followed by some clinicians. Whereas 10 to 20 per cent of clinicians were described as having rejected these incentives (invariably described as 'the ethical lot'), 40 to 50 per cent had accepted the offers. Of these, 10 to 20 per cent were described as having demanded extra inducements and help towards their expansion plans in return for repeated prescriptions. Another 10 per cent were estimated as having adopted a 'shifting position', and a further 10 per cent were described as the 'pathbreakers': leading clinicians in the country who want gifts, free samples and incentives. These pathbreakers are important clients for pharmaceutical companies as, according to the medical representatives, new clinicians imitate their prescriptions, since the hormone/drugs prescribed by these clinicians are seen as 'result-oriented' drugs.

Evidence lies scattered in stories narrated by gynaecologists and medical representatives which must be urgently researched for any credible insights to emerge. The percentage figures in these conversations were mere narrative devices and not concrete data; they were routinely conjured to paint a figurative landscape of pharmaceuticals and ARTs in India. In addition, it must be acknowledged that a probable reason for the paucity of research and information on national and multinational pharmaceutical involvement – as I myself experienced – is due to the shroud of secrecy and confidentiality surrounding such operations. In a significant move, the Indian state recently banned all 'freebies' for doctors from pharmaceutical firms (Mukherjee 2014). The code, first promulgated in 2011 (Mukherjee 2011), is to remain voluntary in its implementation and will come up for review in mid-2015.[1] The code bans all gifts, hospitality, medical samples and grants from pharmaceutical firms or their agents to doctors (Mukherjee 2011). A large segment of doctors who will be impacted by the ban are working in the fertility industry. It remains to be seen how doctors and pharmaceutical companies will react to this new directive and what, if any, measures will be orchestrated to sidestep a blanket ban on 'freebies'.

Against this backdrop, the internal functioning of IVF clinics in India needs to be scrutinised, especially the need to run private practices at an optimal level to maintain economic sustainability and viability. This necessitates a wider examination of the self-promotion of clinicians through the modern media channels, rendered even more crucial in light of purportedly unrealistic success claims and charges of medical mismanagement. Moreover, there is very little social science research on the contentious claims of IVF success rates, save a few notable early feminist interventions. Françoise Laborie's (1987) data, for example, suggests that at a large number of IVF centres in France the success rate, in terms of live births, was almost zero. Similar research in the 1980s looking into the efficacy of IVF concluded that the procedure leads to the birth of a baby only 5 to 10 per cent of the time (Klein 1989). Likewise, Renate Klein and Robyn Rowland (1988) showed that the failure rate of IVF in Australia and the United Kingdom in the 1980s was 92.6 per cent and 91.4 per cent respectively. In an article in the official journal of the American Fertility Society – *Fertility and Sterility* – Dr Michael R. Soules (1985), an associate professor and director of reproductive endocrinology, clearly stated that 'the widespread practice of exaggerating the IVF pregnancy rate appears to be a marketing ploy to lure prospective infertile couples into becoming active IVF patients'. In 1987, an article in the same journal, titled 'Are We Exploiting the Infertile Couple?', drew attention to the inappropriate use of credentials to lure patients (Blackwell et al. 1987). These arguments, especially those put forward by feminist researchers, are more than two decades old. There appears to be a near total absence of research looking at the success rates of interventions like IVF in the twenty-first century. At one level, this can be read as indicative of a broader, less critical shift in the feminist and social scientific thinking on assisted conception as outlined earlier. The low success of technologies, therefore, does not invite the same critical scrutiny as it once did in the feminist scholarship of the 1980s (Arditti et al. 1984; Corea 1985a, 1985b, 1987; Klein 1989; Stanworth 1987b). In fact, in the 1990s, the low success rate of technologies did not discredit them as a treatment option. As Sarah Franklin showed (1997: 83), 'a very high percentage, 95 per cent, of the women interviewed were well aware of the low success rate of IVF before they decided to attempt it'. These shifts in the West notwithstanding, feminist studies on IVF success rates from the 1980s can help to formulate an agenda for the subsequent exploration of assisted conception in India, especially in the light of conflicting claims by clinicians in this research. And while there is sporadic concern over exaggerated claims of clinical success rates in social science, journalistic and biomedical accounts, what we now need is a more concerted and focused look at the success claims of ART assisted conception in India. In this respect, the incongruous disjunction between the public image of assisted conception and the private acknowledgements of its tentative nature becomes a valid point of departure for future research on success claims.

The Indian state has also woken up to the rapid spread of assisted conception in India. In the last decade the Indian Council for Medical Research has formulated several iterations of what it describes as the 'Guidelines for Assisted Reproductive Technologies in India'. The most recent version, if ratified by the Indian lawmakers, is likely to become legally enforceable. However, in the past, moves to monitor and regulate the steady growth in the number of IVF clinics, as well as egg and sperm donation in private sector practices, created a furor in the Indian medical community (Bharadwaj 2011). The publication of these guidelines and their eventual ratification and consolidation into law, once introduced in the Indian parliament, are anticipated to further stoke the question of the controlled application of assisted conceptive techniques. As in the past, this resistance will re-merge in the public domain and be hotly debated via the various media channels. Future research should consider the ongoing governance and proposed legislative developments, which may effect a fundamental change in the way in which infertility treatment is offered in India.

Though seemingly worlds away from the 'modern' biomedical politics of conception, the 'traditional' realm of ideas and norms about fertility remain central to understanding the biomedical management of infertility. In choosing to assist conception through modern high-tech conception technologies, clinicians also inadvertently choose to reinforce these concepts. While the ancient sources explored in this book testify to the quasi-sacred nature of human fertility originating in ancient texts, law codes and myths, they also reverberate in contemporary Indian settings, as the anthropological and sociological studies amply demonstrate. The stigma attached to infertility is one crucial manifestation of the strength of these conceptual ideas. The very process of delegitimation can implicate the couple despite the overriding tendency to blame women for failed conception. The stigma and ostracism is born out of an open violation of the 'rule of patrilineal marriage' that is clearly instilled in ancient legal codes such as the *Manu Smriti*. However, the fact that traditional normative solutions, like abandoning barren wives, are not invoked draws attention to the experience of infertility within the context of a strong conjugal bond. Equally it draws attention to the inferior status of women in Indian society. The very fact that the patriarchal structure allows men to abandon 'barren' wives, whether or not they choose to exercise this option, perpetuates the gender asymmetry. Give that women exist in this state of 'institutionalised disempowerment', one can further read the experience of a 'married infertile woman' in the broader context of being 'lucky' enough to have a supportive husband. This, however, poses a far more complex question which is especially important in the context of conjugal treatment seeking. Does this make assisted conception an important component, or even a 'natural filter' through which only the strongest of conjugal unions can pass? The fact that these couples persist in seeking treatment in the face of the widespread practice of abandoning women/wives in infertile marriages necessitates more research in this area.

This research also complicates the nature of stigma in the Indian context. This phenomenon can no longer be analysed as a mere case of spoilt identity but rather as a 'contagion' leading to the delegitimation of the infertile couple. The nature of patriarchy also emerges as fundamentally complex. For example, in Harjeet's case, the fertility competition between his wife and sister-in-law in the face of vocal support for adoption from the wider family in rural Punjab poses complex questions about how patriarchy speaks through the bodies of indoctrinated agents. The daily squabbles between two sisters-in-law has in this case forced Harjeet to press ahead with expensive treatment by selling his agricultural land with the unconditional backing of his brothers and mother. Agricultural land is a highly prized commodity in rural India and the backbone of patriarchal (unilineal) social reproduction, making sons crucial to the transmission of land rights. The fact that Harjeet and his family are willing to sell 'fertile land' to treat a replaceable/substitutable 'barren field/wife/woman' shows that urgent research is needed to explore the complexities inherent in gender relations in India.

These cultural norms and ideas about conceptions also manifest themselves in treatment-seeking strategies that infertile couples employ to make their fertility visual. I argue that the practice of systematic misrecognition enables interested parties to collude in re-crafting natural/biological and social links in a bind that is conceptualised as immutable. The purity and honour associated with this biosocial bind is salvaged by tacitly recapitulating any transgressions into a legitimate kinship unit. The silence subsuming this process of machination ensures that the couple, or the colluding unit (i.e. family members), succeed in crafting such practical kinship even though it remains partially connected to the married body on account of donated gametes. The whole process is deeply affected by the fear of openly (visibly) violating norms and ideas about relatedness and sacredness, which lie at the very heart of the contemporary Hindu worldview. This explains the reluctance towards adopting from unknown sources, as it strikes publicly at the very core of the 'double conceptual bind'. In this respect the Indian case departs significantly from Euro-American concerns that view the concept of nature and culture as dominating the model of biological reproduction and kinship structures (Strathern 1992b). As the research shows, when faced with a reproductive crisis, the social arrangements of kinship take precedence over an imagined 'natural biological' base within the double conceptual bind, thus authorising the process of conception by silently authoring it within the kin domain. However, the process of systematic misrecognition permeating the treatment-seeking strategies of couples and their families needs further attention, as it remains an inaccessible and difficult issue to research. Hence, a number of questions that arose throughout the course of this research – largely pertaining to the preferred 'agnatic source' of donated gametes and adoptees – need particular attention. Women's growing resistance at being made accountable for their husband's infertility emerged as another important dimension for future research, which poses bigger questions about subversion and even open defiance of patriarchy. Hearsay evidence suggests that the role of caste in sourcing gametes is appearing in certain clinical contexts. While no evidence of caste-based preference for sourcing gametes was encountered in the past twelve years, it is feasible that some enterprising clinical entities have begun offering 'caste matched' gametes to their client base. A recent media report suggested that 'Brahmin sperm is in high demand among childless couples' (Choksi and Ram 2012). While the journalistic hyperbole cannot be dismissed out of hand, expert testimonials in the media report merit further investigation.

Coping with such normative prescriptions is emotionally and financially debilitating for some treatment-seeking individuals. Research shows that the waning hope of conception and constant pressure from families and society registers as the failure of an individual practitioner to many treatment seekers. The long-drawn out pursuit of conception perpetuates the vicious circle of blaming and believing the clinicians. Couples make sense of their treatment and elusive conception by focusing their critiques on the finer processes of their past and present treatments. Such criticism, despite its manifest focus on the medical (mis)management of infertility, or even a lack of sensitivity on the part of clinicians, seems to be directed against a clinician's inability to deliver the desired resolution of their infertility, often at a very high financial cost. Ironically, faced with an absence of tangible alternatives and a mounting urgency to conceive, treatment seekers persist in seeking conceptive technologies. Clinicians, on the other hand, while blaming their profession for instilling unrealistic expectations in their patients, do not critically revisit the positive renditions of assisted conception in the media, making them partly responsible for such high expectations. These are themes that clinicians reinforce microcosmically within their clinic lobbies, thus instilling a sense of impending conception in treatment seekers and an oblique assurance that their current investment in assisted conception is worthwhile. The criticism of colleagues merely reinstates the same professional rivalry and competitiveness that underlies the contest for credibility and the need to hold on to their respective patients. Within the clinic, however, both treatment seekers and clinicians appear to struggle with infertility within the definite boundaries of the clinical science of conception. The very act of seeking conception, as argued earlier, becomes both an escape from, and conformity to, the dominant social norms about fertility. The success and failure of assisted conception, when placed in the universe of the Hindu faith, becomes a powerful critique of the 'incompleteness' of the science of conception. This means, in the context of a clinician's faith, that assisted conception conjoins the disparate domains of the sacred and the profane, the human and the superhuman, science and religion, all working together to produce human life. This accentuates the paradox at the heart of clinical conception, where clinicians and treatment seekers critically evaluate each other, as well as forge fleeting intimacies and informal accommodations towards the costs of the treatment. Most important, the absence of 'results', or 'failure,' is contextualised by the clinicians within the same religious/cultural paradigm that produces social suffering and stigma in the lives of the treatment seekers. The IVF clinics in India need to be more systematically examined. To do this, researchers will have to surmount the difficult task of gaining access to these institutions for some length of time. This is crucial if new insights into the reconfigured face of IVF clinics in their cross-cultural avatar are to emerge.

***

The management of infertility in India lies at the threshold of a culture that not only views fertility as quasi-sacred, but as connecting the worldly and otherworldly domains. While the pursuit of conception in the lives of treatment seekers in this research appears to be entrenched in more worldly concerns, like managing accentuating stigma and societal pressure, the power of science to bypass infertility is partly located by the clinicians in an otherworldly realm. This conjoining of two widely separated domains is intimately related to the double entrenchment of tradition in contemporary India. In exploring these conceptions, this book examines the domain of assisted conception and those that assist and sustain it. Further research might reveal more open and divergent approaches to seeking conception. At the risk of sounding essentialist, my experience in India thus far compels me to assert that for any given situation, an exact opposite instance can be discovered. It is the task of ethnographers to collate and analyse this diversity to reveal the multiple trajectories of lives and institutions, with surprisingly similar goals and intentions. There is no correct or incorrect depiction, but only difference that manifests and saturates our line of vision. The world of infertility and assisted conception is ontologically complex and multiple. It seems to me that parallel worlds coexist, come into being and pass away. The ethnographic task is to jump nimbly between these worlds as they pass each other by, to look for an opening, a door or a window that lets one move effortlessly between terrains of analysis, unexamined routes of inquiry and unexplored ethnographic fields, revealing multiple meanings of the same experience or same underlying meaning tethered to multiple experiences. It is hoped that future research will add new insight into how assisted conception in India is being promoted, used and understood. In this respect this book is both an invitation and a commitment to future research.

Note

1. There is no indication whether this review has taken place since the code of conduct came into force from 1 January 2015.

Bibliography

Agamben, G. 1998. *Homo Sacer: Sovereign Power and Bare Life*. Stanford: Stanford University Press.

Aggarwal, A.K., et al. 1999. 'Community-Based Study of Reproductive Tract Infections among Ever Married Women of Reproductive Age in a Rural Area of Haryana, India', *Journal of Communicable Diseases* 31(4): 223–28.

Agnes, F. 2011. 'Bringing Home the Child: The New Adoption Guidelines do Not Go the Last Mile', *Indian Express*, 21 June. Retrieved on 30 August 2014 from https://indianexpress.com/tag/bringing-home-the-child/.

Ahmad, I. 1975. 'Adoption in India: A Study of Attitudes', *Indian Journal of Social Work* 36(2): 181–90.

Altekar, A.S. 1959. *The Position of Women in Hindu Civilisation*. Delhi: Motilal Banarsidass.

Anand, A.A. and P. Chandra. 2002. 'Adoption Laws: Need for Reform', *Economic and Political Weekly*, 21 September, 3891–93.

Anand Kumar, T.C. 1997. 'Architect of India's First Test Tube Baby: Dr Subhas Mukerji 16 January 1931 to 19 July 1981', *Current Science* 72(7): 526–31.

Appadurai, A. 1996. *Modernity at Large: Cultural Dimensions of Globalization*. Minneapolis: University of Minnesota Press.

Arditti, R., et al. 1984. *Test Tube Women: What Future for Motherhood*. London: Pandora.

Bajpai, V. 2014. 'Challenges Confronting Public Hospitals in India, Their Origins, and Possible Solutions', *Advances in Public Health*. Retrieved on 15 January 2015 from http://www.hindawi.com/journals/aph/2014/898502/.

Banerji, D. 1974. 'Social and Cultural Foundation of Health Service System', *Economic and Political Weekly* 9: 32–34.

Bang, R. and A. Bang. 1994. 'Women's Perception of White Vaginal Discharge: Ethnographic Data from Rural Maharashtra', in J. Gittleson, et al. (eds), *Listening to Women Talk about Their Health: Issues and Evidence from India*. New Delhi: Har-Anand Publications, pp. 79–94.

Bang, R.A. et al. 1989. 'High Prevalence of Gynaecological Diseases in Rural Indian Women', *The Lancet* 1(8629): 85–88.

Baru, R.V. 1998. *Private Health Care in India: Social Characteristics and Trends*. New Delhi: Sage.

_______. 2008. 'Blurring of Boundaries: Public-Private Partnerships in Health Services in India', *Economic and Political Weekly*, 26 January, 62–71.

_______. 2010. 'Inequities in Access to Health Services in India: Caste, Class and Region', *Economic and Political Weekly* 65(38): 49–58.

_______. 2012. 'A Limiting Perspective on Universal Coverage', *Economic and Political Weekly* 67(8): 64–66.

Baru, R.V., I. Qadeer and R. Priya. 2000. 'Medical Industry: Illusion of Quality at What Cost?', *Economic and Political Weekly*, 15 July, 2509–11.

Basu, A.M. 1992. *Culture, the Status of Women and Demographic Behaviour: Illustrated with the Case of India*. Oxford: Oxford University Press.

Becker, G. 2000. *The Elusive Embryo: How Women and Men Approach New Reproductive Technologies*. Berkeley: University of California Press.

Becker, G. and R.D. Nachtigall. 1994. 'Born to be a Mother: The Cultural Construction of Risk in Infertility Treatment in the U.S.', *Social Science and Medicine* 39(4): 507–18.

Benhabib, S. 1995. 'The Pariah and Her Shadow: Hannah Arendt's Biography of Rahel Varnhagen', *Political Theory* 23(1): 5–24.

Berman, P. 1991. *Health Economics, Health Financing and the Health Needs of Poor Women and Children in India*. New Delhi: Ford Foundation.

Berrien, R. 1987. 'What Future for Primary Care Private Practice?', *New England Journal of Medicine* 316(6): 334–37.

Bhalla, N. and M. Thapliyal. 2013. 'India Seeks to Regulate its Booming "Rent-a-Womb" Industry', *Reuters*, 30 September. Retrieved on 12 January 2014 from http://www.reuters.com/article/2013/09/30/us-india-surrogates-idUSBRE98T07F20130930.

Bharadwaj, A. 2000. 'How Some Indian Baby Makers are Made: Media Narratives and Assisted Conception in India', *Anthropology and Medicine* 7(1): 63–78.

_______. 2002. 'Conception Politics: Medical Egos, Media Spotlights, and the Contest over Test-tube Firsts in India', in M.C. Inhorn and F. Van Balen (eds), *Infertility Around the Globe*. Berkeley: University of California Press, pp. 315–33.

_______. 2003. 'Why Adoption is not an Option in India: The Visibility of Infertility, the Secrecy of Donor Insemination, and other Cultural Complexities', *Social Science and Medicine* 56: 1867–880.

_______. 2005. 'Cultures of Embryonic Stem Cell Research in India', in W. Bender, C. Hauskeller and A. Manzei (eds), *Crossing Borders: Cultural, Religious and Political Differences Concerning Stem Cell Research*. Munster: Agenda Verlag, pp. 325–41.

_______. 2006. 'Clinical Theodicies: The Enchanted World of Uncertain Science and Clinical Conception in India', *Culture, Medicine and Psychiatry* 30(4): 451–65.

_______. 2008. 'Biosociality to Bio-Crossings: Encounters with Assisted Conception and Embryonic Stem Cells in India', in S. Gibbon and C. Novas (eds), *Genetics, Biosociality and the Social Sciences: Making Biologies and Identities*. London: Routledge, pp. 98–116.

_______. 2010a. 'Assisted Life: The Neoliberal Moral Economy of Embryonic Stem Cells in India', in D. Birenbaum-Carmeli and M.C. Inhorn (eds), *Assisting Reproduction, Testing Genes: Global Encounters with New Biotechnologies*. New York: Berghahn Books, pp. 239–57.

_______. 2010b. 'Reproductive Viability and the State: Embryonic Stem Cells in India', in C. Browner and C. Sargent (eds), *Reproduction, Globalization, and the State*. Durham: Duke University Press, pp. 113–25.

_______. 2013a. 'Experimental Subjectification: The Pursuit of Human Embryonic Stem Cells in India', *Ethnos* 76(1): 84–107.

_______. 2013b. 'Subaltern Biology? Local Biologies, Indian Odysseys and the Pursuit of Human Embryonic Stem Cell Therapies', *Medical Anthropology* 32(4): 359–73.

_______. 2013c. 'Ethic of Consensibility, Subaltern Ethicality: The Clinical Application of Embryonic Stem Cells in India', *BioSocieties* 8: 25–40.

Bharadwaj, A. and P. Glasner. 2009. *Local Cells, Global Science: The Rise of Embryonic Stem Cell Research in India*. London: Routledge.

Bharat, S. 1993. *Child Adoption in India Trends and Emerging Issues: A Study of Adoption Agencies.* Mumbai: Tata Institute of Social Sciences.

Bhat, R. 1993. 'The Private Health Care Sector in India', in P. Berman and M.E. Khan (eds), *Paying for India's Health Care*. New Delhi: Sage, pp. 161–96.

Bhattacharji, S. 1990. 'Motherhood in Ancient India', *Economic and Political Weekly*, 20-27 October, WS50–57.

Bhattacharya, N.N. 1977. *The Indian Mother Goddess*. New Delhi: Manohar.

Bhatti, L.I. et al. 1999. 'The Quest of Infertile Women in Squatter Settlements of Karachi, Pakistan: A Qualitative Study', *Social Science and Medicine* 49(5): 637–49.

Bhujwala, R.A. et al. 1988. 'Detection of Chlamydial and Gonococcal Antibodies in Women with Pelvic Inflammatory Disease and Infertility: An Aid to Diagnosis', *Journal of Obstetrics and Gynaecology of India* 38(1): 96–99.

Biardeau, M. 2003. 'Hinduism: The Anthropology of a Civilisation', in *The Hinduism Omnibus*. Delhi: Oxford University Press, 16–177.

Billimoria, H.M. 1984. *Child Adoption: A Study of Indian Experience*. Mumbai: Himalaya Publication House.

Biospectrum. 2013. 'Report: India Imports 75% of its Medical Devices', 4 September. Retrieved 30 August 2014 from http://www.biospectrumasia.com/biospectrum/news/194791/report-india-imports-75-medical-devices.

Birenbaum-Carmeli, D. 2004. '"Cheaper than a Newcomer": On the Political Economy of IVF in Israel', *The Sociology of Health and Illness*, 26(7): 897–924.

Birenbaum-Carmeli, D. and M.C. Inhorn. 2009. *Assisting Reproduction, Testing Genes: Global Encounters with the New Biotechnologies*. New York: Berghahn Books.

Birke, L. et al. 1990. *Tomorrow's Child: Reproductive Technologies in the 90s*. London: Virago.

Blackwell, R.E. et al. 1987. 'Are We Exploiting the Infertile Couple?', *Fertility and Sterility* 48(5): 735–39.

Bledsoe, C. 1990. 'The Politics of Children: Fosterage and the Social Management of Fertility among the Mende of Sierra Leone', in W.P. Handwerker (ed.), *Births and Power*. Boulder: Westview Press, pp. 81–100.

Bochaton, A. and B. Lefebvre. 2009. 'The Rebirth of the Hospital: Heterotopia and Medical Tourism in Asia', in T. Winter, P. Teo and T.C. Chang (eds), *Asia on Tour: Exploring the Rise of Asian Tourism*. Abingdon: Routledge, pp. 97–108.

Böck, M. and A. Rao. (eds). 2000. *Culture, Creation, and Procreation: Concepts of Kinship in South Asian Practice*. New York: Berghahn Books.

Boerma, T. 1987. 'The Liability of the Concept of a Primary Health Care Team in Developing Countries', *Social Science and Medicine* 25(6): 747–52.

Boonmongkon, P. 2000. 'Living through Infertility: From Loss to Resolution of the Life Course of Thai Women', in F. Van Balen et al. (eds), *Social Science Research on Childlessness in a Global Perspective: Proceedings of the Conference 8-11 November 1999*. Amsterdam: SCO-Kohnstamm Institute, pp. 215–19.

Bourdieu, P. 1990. *The Logic of Practice*. Stanford: Stanford University Press.

Burfoot, A. 1990. 'The Normalisation of New Reproductive Technology', in M. McNeil et al. (eds), *The New Reproductive Technologies*. London: Macmillan, pp. 58–73.

_______. 1995. 'In-Appropriation: A Critique of Proceed with Care Final Report of the Royal Commission on New Reproductive Technologies', *Women's Studies International Forum* 18(4): 499–506.

Burkitt, I. 1999. *Bodies of Thought: Embodiment, Identity and Modernity*. London: Sage.

Central Adoption Resource Agency. 2014. 'Adoption Statistics'. Retrieved on 24 April 2015 from http://adoptionindia.nic.in/Resources/Adoption-Statistics.html.

Chakravarti, U. and K. Roy. 1988. 'In Search of Our Past: A Review of the Limitations and Possibilities of the Historiography of Women in Early India', *Economic and Political Weekly* 30: WS-2–10.

Chatterjee, B.B., S.S. Singh and D.R. Yadav. 1971. *Impact of Social Legislation on Social Change*. Calcutta: Minerva Associates.

Chatterjee, P. and M. Janwalkar. 2014. 'The Great Indian Egg Bazaar', *Indian Express*, 9 February 2014. Retrieved 12 February 2014 from Indianexpress.com/article/india/india-others/the-great-indian-egg-bazaar/.

Chaudhuri, P. and R. Iyengar. 1994. '*Chlamydia Trachomatis* Infection in a South Indian Population: A Prospective Pilot Study', *Journal of Obstetrics and Gynaecology of India* 44(4): 593–94.

Chawla, M. 1996. *Dual Job-holding by Public Sector Physicians in India*. Boston: Harvard School of Public Health.

Chen, M.A. (ed.). 1998. *Widows in India: Social Neglect and Public Action*. Delhi: Sage.

Chhabra, S. and L. Fali. 1992. 'Clinical Genital Infection in Infertile Women with *Chlamydia Trachomatis* Infection', *Journal of Obstetrics and Gynaecology of India* 42(1): 68–70.

Choksi, M. and S.G. Ram. 2012. 'Brahmin Sperm in High Demand among Childless Couples', *Times of India*, 13 May. Retrieved on 10 July 2012 from http://timesofindia.indiatimes.com/city/mumbai/Brahmin-sperm-in-hi...-among-childless-couples/articleshow/13114610.cms?intenttarget=no.

Chowdhury, S.R. 2011. 'Doc to Pay 15L Damages for Failed IVF Process', *Times of India*, 3 August 2011.

Clarke, A.E. and V.L. Olesen (eds). 1999. *Revisioning Women, Health and Healing: Feminist, Cultural and Technoscience Perspectives*. New York: Routledge.

Clarke, M. 2008. *Islam and New Kinship: Reproductive Technology, Anthropology, and the Shari'ah in Lebanon*. New York: Berghahn Books.

Clifford, J. 1997. *Routes: Travel and Translation in the Late Twentieth Century*. Cambridge: Harvard University Press.

Clifford, J. and G.E. Marcus (eds). 1986. *Writing Cultures: The Poetics and Politics of Ethnography*. Berkeley: University of California Press.

Cohen, L. 2001. 'The Other Kidney: Biopolitics beyond Recognition', *Body and Society* 7(2/3): 9–29.

———. 2004. 'Operability: Surgery at the Margin of the State', in V. Das and D. Poole (eds), *Anthropology in the Margins of the State*. Santa Fe: School of American Research Press, pp. 165–90.

Comaroff, J.L. and J. Comaroff. 1997. *Of Revelation and Revolution: The Dialectics of Modernity on a South African Frontier*. Vol 2. Chicago: University of Chicago Press.

Conrad, D. 1995. 'The Personal Law Question and Hindu Nationalism', in V. Dalmia and H. von Stietencron (eds), *Representing Hinduism: The Construction of Religious Traditions and National Identity*. Thousand Oaks: Sage, pp. 306–37.

Corea, G. 1985a. 'How the New Reproductive Technologies could be Used to Apply the Brothel Model of Social Control over Women', *Women's Studies International Forum* 8(4): 299–305.

———. 1985b. *The Mother Machine: Reproductive Technologies from Artificial Insemination to Artificial Wombs*. London: The Women's Press.

———. 1987. *Man-Made Women: How The New Reproductive Technologies Affect Women*. London: Hutchinson.

Cornwell, J. 1984. *Hard-Earned Lives: Accounts of Health and Illness from East London*. London: Tavistock.

Cussins, C. 1996. 'Ontological Choreography: Agency through Objectification in Infertility Clinics', *Social Studies of Science* 26: 575–610.

———. 1998a. 'Quit Sniveling, Cryo-Baby, We'll Work Out Which One's Your Mama!', in R.E. Davis-Floyd and J. Dumit (eds), *Cyborg Babies: From Techno-Sex to Techno-Tots*. London: Routledge, pp. 40–66.

———. 1998b. 'Producing Reproduction: Techniques of Normalization and Naturalization in Infertility Clinics', in S. Franklin and H. Ragoné (eds), *Reproducing Reproduction: Kinship, Power, and Technological Innovation*. Philadelphia: University of Pennsylvania Press, pp. 66–101.

_______. 2000. 'Fertile Ground: Feminist Theorize Infertility', in F. Van Balen et al. (eds), *Social Science Research on Childlessness in a Global Perspective: Proceedings of the Conference 8-11 November 1999*. Amsterdam: SCO-Kohnstamm Institute, pp. 51–64.

Dalmia, V. and H. von Stietencron. 2010. *The Oxford India Hinduism Reader*. Oxford: Oxford University Press.

Damania, D. 1998. *Counselling for Adoption: The Setting up of an Indian Adoption Programme*. Mumbai: Tata Institute of Social Sciences Monograph Series.

Daniels, K. and E. Haimes (eds). 1998. *International Social Science Perspectives on Donor Insemination*. Cambridge: Cambridge University Press.

Das, V. 1976a. 'Masks and Faces: An Essay on Punjabi Kinship', *Contributions to Indian Sociology* 10(1): 1–30.

_______. 1976b. 'Indian Women: Work, Power and Status', in B.R. Nanda (ed.), *Indian Women: From Purdah to Modernity*. New Delhi: Vikas.

_______. 1995. 'National Honor and Practical Kinship: Unwanted Women and Children', in F.D. Ginsburg and R. Rapp (eds), *Conceiving the New World Order: The Global Politics of Reproduction*. Berkeley: University of California Press, pp. 212–33.

_______. 1999. *Critical Events: An Anthropological Perspective on Contemporary India*, 3rd edn. New Delhi: Oxford University Press.

_______. 2000. 'The Practice of Organ Transplants: Networks, Documents, Translations', in M. Lock et al. (eds), *Living and Working with the New Medical Technologies*. Cambridge: Cambridge University Press, pp. 263–87.

_______. 2001. *Stigma, Contagion, Defect: Issues in the Anthropology of Public Health*. Johns Hopkins University. http://www.stigmaconference.nih.gov/DasPaper.htm

_______. 2004. 'The Signature of the State: The Paradox of Illegibility', in V. Das and D. Poole (eds), *Anthropology in the Margins of the State*. Santa Fe: School of American Research Press, pp. 225–78.

Das Gupta, M., L. Chen and T.N. Krishnan (eds). 1998. *Health, Poverty and Development in India*. Oxford: Oxford University Press.

Davis-Floyd, R.E. 1990. 'The Role of Obstetrical Rituals in the Resolution of Cultural Anomaly', *Social Science and Medicine* 31(2): 175– 89.

_______. 1992. *Birth as an American Rite of Passage*. Berkeley: University of California Press.

_______. 1994. 'The Technocratic Body: American Childbirth as Cultural Expression', *Social Science and Medicine* 38(8): 1125–140.

Davis-Floyd, R.E. and J. Dumit (eds). 1998. *Cyborg Babies: From Techno-Sex to Techno-Tots*. London: Routledge.

Derrida, J. 1998. *Of Grammatology*. Baltimore: Johns Hopkins University Press.

Dey, S. 2015. 'Genital TB Leading to Infertility among 25-30% Women in India', *The Times of India*, 24 March. Retrieved on 24 March 2015 from http://timesofindia.indiatimes.com/india/Genital-TB-leading-to-infertility-among-25-30-women-in-India/articleshow/46669977.cms.

Dhruvarajan, V. 1989. *Hindu Women and the Power of Ideology*. Gramby: Bergin and Garvey.

Doniger, W. 1995. 'Begetting on Margin: Adultery and Surrogate Pseudomarriage in Hinduism', in L. Harlan and P.B. Courtright (eds), *From the Margins of Hindu Marriage: Essays on Gender, Religion, and Culture*. New York: Oxford University Press, pp. 160–83.

_______. 2009. *The Hindus: An Alternative History*. New York: Penguin Publishing Group.

Drummer, T.J.B. and I.G. Cook. 2008. 'Health in China and India: A Cross-Country Comparison in a Context of Rapid Globalization', *Social Science and Medicine* 67(4): 590–605.

Dube, L. 1956. *The Gond Woman*. Ph.D. dissertation, Nagpur University.

_______. 1986. 'Seed and Earth: The Symbolism of Biological Reproduction and Sexual Relations of Production', in E. Leacock and S. Ardener (eds), *Visibility and Power. Essays in on Women in Society and Development*. Delhi: Oxford University Press, pp. 119–53.

_______. 1988. 'On the Construction of Gender: Hindu Girls in Patrilineal India', *Economic and Political Weekly*, 30 April, WS11–19.

_______. 1997. *Women and Kinship: Comparative Perspectives on Gender in South and South-East Asia*. New Delhi: Vistaar.

Duggal, R. and A. Amin. 1989. *Cost of Health Care: A Household Survey in an Indian District*. Mumbai: Foundation for Research in Community Health.

Duggal, R. and N.H. Anita. 1993. 'Health Financing in India: A Review and an Agenda', in P. Berman and M.E. Khan (eds), *Paying for India's Health Care*. New Delhi: Sage, p. 57.

Dumont, L. and D.F. Pocock. 1957. 'For a Sociology of India', *Contributions to Indian Sociology* 1: 7–22.

Dutta, S. 1990. 'Relinquishing the Halo: Portrayal of Mother in Indian Writing in English', *Economic and Political Weekly*, 20-29 October, WS84–93.

Dworkin, A. 1983. *Right Wing Women*. London: The Women's Press.

EPW. 2001. 'Adoption Racket: All-Round Callousness', *Economic and Political Weekly*, 5 May, 1487.

Ercikan, K. 1998. 'Translation Effects in International Assessments', *International Journal of Educational Research* 29: 543–53.

Fahim, H. (ed.). 1982. *Indigenous Anthropology in Non-Western Countries*. Durham: Carolina Academic Press.

Feldman-Savelsberg, P. 1994. 'Plundered Kitchens and Empty Wombs: Fear of Infertility in the Cameroonian Grassfields', *Social Science and Medicine* 39(4): 463–74.

_______. 1999. *Plundered Kitchens, Empty Wombs: Threatened Reproduction and Identity in the Cameroon Grassfields*. Ann Arbor: University Michigan Press.

_______. 2002. 'Is Infertility an Unrecognized Public Health and Population Problem? A View from the Cameroon Grassfields', in M.C. Inhorn and F.

Van Balen (eds), *Infertility around the Globe: New Thinking on Childlessness, Gender, and Reproductive Technologies*. Berkeley: University of California Press, pp. 215–32.

Fine, G.A. 1993. 'Ten Lies of Ethnography: Moral Dilemmas of Field Research', *Journal of Contemporary Ethnography* 22: 267–94.

Firestone, S. 1971. *The Dialectic of Sex*. London: Jonathan Cape.

Franklin, S. 1990. 'Deconstructing "Desperateness": The Social Construction of Infertility in Popular Representations of New Reproductive Technologies', in M. McNeil et al. (eds), *The New Reproductive Technologies*. London: Macmillan, pp. 200–229.

_______. 1997. *Embodied Progress: A Cultural Account of Assisted Conception*. London: Routledge.

_______. 2013. *Biological Relatives: IVF, Stem Cells, and the Future of Kinship*. Durham: Duke University Press.

Franklin, S. and H. Ragoné (eds). 1998. *Reproducing Reproduction: Kinship, Power and Technological Innovation*. Philadelphia: University of Pennsylvania Press.

Fraser, N. 1992. 'Rethinking the Public Sphere: A Contribution to the Critique of Actually Existing Democracy', in C. Calhoun (ed.), *Habermas and the Public Sphere*. Cambridge: MIT Press, pp. 109–42.

Foundation for Research in Community Health. 1993. 'Health Sector Resources: Investment and Expenditure in a District'. Pune.

Friedman, J. 2002. 'Modernity and Other Traditions', in B.M. Knauft (ed.), *Critically Modern: Alternatives, Alterities, Anthropologies*. Bloomington: Indiana University Press, pp. 287–313.

Fruzzetti, L. and A. Ostor. 1976. 'Seed and Earth: A Cultural Analysis of Kinship in a Bengali Town', *Contributions to Indian Sociology* 10(1): 96–131.

Fuller, C. 2003. *The Renewal of Priesthood: Modernity and Traditionalism in a South Indian Temple*. Princeton: Princeton University Press.

Ganesh, K. 1990. 'Mother Who is Not a Mother: In Search of the Great Indian Goddess', *Economic and Political Weekly*, 20-27 October, WS58–64.

Ganguly, S. and S. Unisa. 2010. 'Trends of Infertility and Childlessness in India: Findings from NFHS Data', *ObGyn* 2(2): 131–38.

Gellner, E. 1983. *Nations and Nationalism*. Oxford: Blackwell.

Gentleman, A. 2008. 'India Nurtures Business of Surrogate Motherhood', *The New York Times*, 10 March. Retrieved 6 February 2010 from http://www.nytimes.com/2008/03/10/world/asia/10surrogate.html?_r=1.

George, A., I. Shah and S. Nandraj. 1993. *A Study of Household Health Expenditure in Madhya Pradesh*. Mumbai: Foundation for Research in Community Health.

Gerrits, T. 1997. 'Social and Cultural Aspects of Infertility in Mozambique', *Patient Education and Counselling* 31: 39–48.

Gilbert, G.N. and M. Mulkay. 1984. *Opening Pandora's Box: A Sociological Analysis of Scientific Discourse*. Cambridge: Cambridge University Press.

Ginsburg, F.D. and R. Rapp. 1995. *Conceiving the New World Order: The Global Politics of Reproduction*. Berkeley: University of California Press.

Goffman, E. 1963. *Stigma: Notes on the Management of Spoiled Identity*. New Jersey: Prentice-Hall.

Goldberg, H. 2009. 'The Sex in the Sperm: Male Infertility and Its Challenges to Masculinity in an Israeli-Jewish Context', in M.C. Inhorn, T. Tjørnhøj-Thomsen, H. Goldberg and M. la Cour Mosegaard (eds), *Reconceiving the Second Sex: Men, Masculinity, and Reproduction*. New York: Berghahn Books, pp. 203–25.

Good, B.J. 1997. *Medicine, Rationality and Experience: An Anthropological Perspective*. Cambridge: Cambridge University Press.

Good, A. 2000. 'Power and Fertility: Divine Kinship in South India', in M. Böck and A. Rao (eds), *Culture, Creation, and Procreation: Concepts of Kinship in South Asian Practice*. Oxford: Berghahn Books, pp. 323–53.

Goode, E. 1996. 'The Ethics of Deception in Social Research: A Case Study', *Qualitative Sociology* 19(1): 11–33.

Government of India. 1997. 'Report of the Sub-Committee on Reproductive Health Research Needs Assessment'. Delhi: Ministry of Health and Family Welfare. June.

_______. 2009. 'National Health Accounts India 2004–05 with Provisional Estimates from 2005–06 to 2008–09'. Delhi: Ministry of Health and Family Welfare.

Goyder, J. 1987. *The Silent Minority: Non-Respondents in Sample Surveys*. Cambridge: Polity Press.

Gray, J. 1980. 'Hypergamy, Kinship and Caste amongst the Chattris of Nepal', *Contributions to Indian Sociology* 14: 1–34.

Greer, G. 1984. *Sex and Destiny: The Politics of Human Fertility*. London: Secker and Warburg.

Greil, A.L. 1991. *Not Yet Pregnant: Infertile Couples in Contemporary America*. New Jersey: Rutgers University Press.

_______. 1994. 'Infertile Bodies: Medicalization, Metaphor and Agency'. Annual Meeting of the Eastern Sociological Society. Baltimore.

Gupta, A. and K. Sivaramakrishnan. 2010. *The State in India after Liberalization: Interdisciplinary Perspectives*. New York: Routledge.

Gupta, C. 2001. 'The Icon of Mother in Late Colonial North India: "Bharat Mata", "Matri Bhasha" and "Gau Mata"', *Economic and Political Weekly* 36(45): 4291–99.

Gupta, D. 2000. *Mistaken Modernity: India between Worlds*. New Delhi: Harper Collins.

Gupta, J.A. 2000. *New Reproductive Technologies, Women's Health and Autonomy: Freedom or Dependency?* New Delhi: Sage.

_______. 2006. 'Towards Transnational Feminisms: Some Reflections and Concerns in Relation to the Globalization of Reproductive Technologies', *European Journal of Women's Studies* 13(1): 23–38.

Gupta, N. et al. 2007. 'Genital Tuberculosis in Indian Infertility Patients', *International Journal of Gynecology and Obstetrics* 97(2): 135–38.

Habermas, J. 1989. *The Structural Transformation of the Public Sphere: An Inquiry into a Category of Bourgeois Society*. Cambridge: MIT Press.

Haimes, E., 1993. 'Issues of Gender in Gamete Donation', *Social Science and Medicine* 36(1): 85–93.

Haimes, E. and N. Timms. 1985. *Adoption, Identity and Social Policy: The Search for Distant Relatives*. Gower: Aldershot.

Haimes, E. and R. Williams. 1998. 'Social Constructionism and the New Technologies of Reproduction', in I. Velody and R. Williams (eds), *The Politics of Constructionism*. London: Sage, pp. 132–46.

Handwerker, L. 2002. 'The Politics of Making Modern Babies in China: Reproductive Technologies and the "New" Eugenics', in M.C. Inhorn and F. Van Balen (eds), *Infertility around the Globe: New Thinking on Childlessness, Gender, and Reproductive Technologies*. Berkeley: University of California Press, pp. 298–314.

Haraway, D. 1990. 'A Manifesto for Cyborgs: Science, Technology, and Socialist Feminism in the 1980s', in L.J. Nicholson (ed.), *Feminism/Postmodernism*. London: Routledge, pp. 190–233.

_______. 1991. *Simians, Cyborgs, and Women: The Reinvention of Nature*. New York: Routledge.

_______. 1999. 'Modest_Witness@Second_Millennium', in D. MacKenzie and J. Wajcman (eds), *The Social Shaping of Technology*, 2nd edn. Buckingham: Open University Press, pp. 41–49.

Harlan, L. and P.B. Courtright (eds). 1995. *From the Margins of Hindu Marriage: Essays on Gender, Religion, and Culture*. New York: Oxford University Press.

Hirsch, E. 1993. 'Negotiated Limits: Interviews in South-East England', in J. Edwards et al. (eds), *Technologies of Procreation: Kinship in the Age of Assisted Conception*. Manchester: Manchester University Press, pp. 67–95.

_______. 1999. 'Negotiating Limits: Interviews in South-East England', in J. Edwards et al. (eds), *Technologies of Procreation: Kinship in the Age of Assisted Conception*, 2nd edn. London: Routledge, pp. 91–121.

Hobsbawm, E. and T. Ranger. 1983. *The Invention of Tradition*. Cambridge: Cambridge University Press.

Holstein, J. and J. Gubrium. 1995. *The Active Interview*. Thousand Oaks: Sage.

Howell, S. 2006. *The Kinning of Foreigners: Transnational Adoption in a Global Perspective*. New York: Berghahn Books.

Inden, R. 1992. *Imagining India*. Oxford: Blackwell.

Inden, R.B. and R. Nicholas. 1977. *Kinship in Bengali Culture*. Chicago: University of Chicago Press.

Independent Commission on Health in India. 1997. 'Report'. New Delhi.

ICMR (Indian Council for Medical Research). 1986. 'In Vitro Fertilization and Embryo Transfer: A Collaborative Project between the KEM Hospital and the Institute for Research in Reproduction'. *Annual Report*, pp. 73–75.

_______. 2000. 'Need and Feasibility of Providing Assisted Technologies for Infertility Management in Resource-Poor Settings', *ICMR Bulletin* 3: 6–7.

_______. 2010. 'The Assisted Reproduction Technologies (Regulation) Rules'. Delhi: Ministry of Health and Family Welfare.

RNCOS Business Consulting Services. 2013. *Indian Hospital Services Market Outlook*. Retrieved 30 September 2014 from www.rncos.com/Market-Analysis-Reports/Indian-Hospital-Services-Market-Outlook-IM381.htm.

Ingold, T. 1986. *Evolution and Social Life*. Cambridge: Cambridge University Press.

Inhorn, M.C. 1994a. *Quest for Conception: Gender, Infertility, and Egyptian Medical Traditions*. Philadelphia: University of Pennsylvania Press.

_______. 1994b. 'Interpreting Infertility: Medical Anthropological Perspectives', *Social Science and Medicine* 39(4): 459–61.

_______. 1996a. *Infertility and Patriarchy: The Cultural Politics of Gender and Family Life in Egypt*. Philadelphia: University of Pennsylvania Press.

_______. 1996b. 'Population, Poverty, and Gender Politics: Motherhood Pressures and Marital Crisis in the Lives of Poor Urban Egyptian Women', in M.E. Bonine (ed.), *Population, Poverty, and Politics in Middle East Cities*. Gainesville: University Press of Florida, pp. 186–207.

_______. 2002. 'The "Local" Confronts the "Global": Infertile Bodies and New Reproductive Technologies in Egypt', in M.C. Inhorn and F. Van Balen (eds), *Interpreting Infertility: Childlessness, Gender and Reproductive Technologies in Global Perspective*. Berkeley: University of California Press, pp. 263–82.

_______. 2003. *Local Babies, Global Science: Gender, Religion, and In Vitro Fertilization in Egypt*. New York: Routledge.

_______. 2007. 'Reproductive Disruptions and ARTs in the Muslim Middle East', in M.C. Inhorn (ed.), *Reproductive Disruptions: Gender, Technology, and Biopolitics in the New Millennium*. New York: Berghahn Books, pp. 183–99.

_______. 2012. *The New Arab Man: Emergent Masculinities, Technologies and Islam in the Middle East*. Princeton University Press.

_______. 2015. *Cosmopolitan Conceptions: IVF Sojourns in Global Dubai*. Durham: Duke University Press.

Inhorn, M.C. and A. Bharadwaj. 2007. 'Reproductively Disabled Lives: Infertility, Stigma and Suffering in Egypt and India', in B. Ingstad and S. Reynolds Whyte (eds), *Disability in Local and Global Worlds*. Berkeley: University of California Press, pp. 78–106.

Inhorn, Marcia C. and D. Birenbaum-Carmeli. 2009. 'Male Infertility, Chronicity, and the Plight of Palestinian Men in Israel and Lebanon', in L. Manderson and C. Smith-Morris (eds), *Chronic Conditions, Fluid States: Globalization and the Anthropology of Illness*. New Brunswick: Rutgers University Press, pp. 77–95.

Inhorn, M.C. and K.A. Buss. 1993. 'Infertility, Infection, and Iatrogenesis in Egypt: The Anthropological Epidemiology of Blocked Tubes', *Medical Anthropology* 15(3): 217–44.

_______. 1994. 'Ethnography, Epidemiology, and Infertility in Egypt', *Social Science and Medicine* 39(5): 671–86.

Inhorn, M.C. and P. Patrizio. 2015. 'Infertility Around the Globe: New Thinking on Gender, Reproductive Technologies and Global Movements in the 21st Century', *Human Reproduction Update* 21(4): 411–26.

Inhorn, M.C. and F. Van Balen (eds). 2002. *Infertility around the Globe: New Thinking on Childlessness, Gender, and Reproductive Technologies*. Berkeley: University of California Press.

Irvine, L. 1998. 'Organizational Ethics and Fieldwork Realities: Negotiating Ethical Boundaries in Codependents Anonymous', in S. Gills (ed.), *Doing Ethnographic Research: Fieldwork Settings*. Thousand Oaks: Sage, pp. 167–83.

Iyer, M. 2013. 'Infertility Cure Part of Family Planning Now: Govt Plans Cheap Treatment', *Sunday Times of India*, 11 August. New Delhi.

Jeffery, P., R. Jeffery and A. Lyon. 1989. *Labour Pains and Labour Power: Women and Childbearing in India*. London: Zed Books.

Jeffery, R. 1977. 'Allopathic Medicine in India: A Case of Deprofessionalization?', *Social Science and Medicine* 11: 561–73.

______. 1988. *The Politics of Health in India*. Berkeley: University of California Press.

Jejeebhoy, S.J. 1998. 'Infertility in India, Levels, Patterns and Consequences: Priorities for Social Science Research', *Journal of Family Welfare* 44(3): 15–24.

Jejeebhoy, S., M. Koeing and C. Elias. 2003. *Investigating Reproductive Tract Infections and other Gynaecological Disorders: A Multidisciplinary Research Approach*. Cambridge: Cambridge University Press.

Jones, H.W., J. Cohen, I. Cooke and R. Kempers. 2007. IFFS Surveillance 07. *Fertility and Sterility*; 87(1): 1–67.

Jones, H.W., I. Cooke, R. Kempers, P. Brinsden and D. Saunders. 2010. International Federation of Fertility Societies: Surveillance 2010. www.iffs-reproduction.org/doocuments/IFFS_Surveillance_2010.pdf

Joyee, A.G., S.P. Thyagarajan, E. Reddy Vikram, P. Rajendran and C. Venkatesan. 2007. 'Diagnostic Utility of Serologic Markers for Genital Chlamydial Infection in STD Patients in Chennai, India', *JAPI* 55: 777–80.

Kahn, S.M. 2000. *Reproducing Jews: A Cultural Account of Assisted Conception in Israel*. Durham: Duke University Press.

______. 2002. 'Rabbis and Reproduction: The Uses of New Reproductive Technologies among Ultraorthodox Jews in Israel', in M.C. Inhorn and F. Van Balen (eds), *Interpreting Infertility: Childlessness, Gender and Reproductive Technologies in Global Perspective*. Berkeley: University of California Press, pp. 283–97.

______. 2006. 'Making Technology Familiar: Orthodox Jews and Infertility Support, Advice, and Inspiration', *Culture, Medicine and Psychiatry* 30(4): 467–80.

Kakar, S. 1978. *The Inner World: A Psycho-Analytic Study of Childhood and Society in India*. Delhi: Oxford University Press.

______. 1990. *Intimate Relations: Exploring Indian Sexuality*. Chicago: University of Chicago Press.

_______. 1998. *The Indian Psyche*, 2nd edn. Delhi: Oxford University Press.

Kane, P.V. 1974. *History of Dharmasastra*, Vols 1 and 3. Poona: Bhandarkar Oriental Research Institute.

Kanjilal, B. and S. Mazumdar. 2013. 'Transition in the Indian Healthcare Market', in G. Bloom et al. (eds). *Transforming Health Markets in Asia and Africa*. New York: Routledge, pp. 18–34.

Karve, I. 1968. *Kinship Organisation in India*. London: Asia Publishing House.

Kautilya. 1992. *The Arthashastra*, trans. L.N. Rangrajan. Haryana: Penguin Classics.

Keller, E.F. 1995. *Refiguring Life: Metaphors of Twentieth-Century Biology*. New York: Columbia University Press.

Khare, R.S. 1982. 'From Kanya to Mata: Aspects of the Cultural Language of Kinship in Northern India', in Á. Östör et al. (eds), *Concepts of Person: Kinship, Caste and Marriage in India*, 3rd edn. Delhi: Oxford University Press, pp. 143–71.

King, R. 1999. 'Orientalism and the Modern Myth of "Hinduism"', *Numen* 46(2): 146–85.

Klein, R. (ed.). 1989. *Infertility: Women Speak Out about Their Experiences of Reproductive Medicine*. London: Pandora Press.

Klein, R. and R. Rowland. 1988. 'Women as Test-Sites for Fertility Drugs: Clomiphene Citrate and Hormonal Cocktails', *Reproductive and Genetic Engineering* 1(3): 251–73.

Kleinman, A. 1992. 'Local Moral Worlds of Suffering: An Interpersonal Focus for Ethnographies of Illness Experience', *Qualitative Health Research* 2(2): 127–34.

_______. 1995. *Writing at the Margin: Discourse between Anthropology and Medicine*. Berkeley: University of California Press.

Kleinman, A. et al. 1995. 'The Social Course of Epilepsy: Chronic Illness as Social Experience in Interior China', *Social Science and Medicine* 40(10): 1319–330.

Krishnan, P. 1990. 'In the Idiom of Loss: Ideology of Motherhood in Television Serials', *Economic and Political Weekly*, 20-27 October, WS103–16.

Kuhn, T. 1970. *The Structure of Scientific Revolutions*, 2nd edn. Chicago: University of Chicago Press.

Kumar, D. 2007. 'Prevalence of Female Infertility and its Socio Economic Factors in Tribal Communities of Central India', *Rural and Remote Health* 7(456): 1–5.

Kumar, N. (ed.). 1994. *Women as Subjects: South Asian Histories*. New Delhi: Stree.

Kumar, R. and G. Gautam. 2006. 'Tobacco Chewing and Male Infertility', *Indian Journal of Urology* 22(2): 161–62.

Kushtagi, P. et al. 1991. 'Prevalence of Antibodies to Chlamydia Trachomatis among Infertile Couples', *Journal of Obstetrics and Gynaecology of India* 41: 671–73.

Laborie, F. 1987. 'Looking for Mothers You only Find Fetuses', in P. Spallone and D.L. Steinberg (eds), *Made to Order: The Myth of Reproductive and Genetic Progress*. Oxford: Pergamon Press, pp. 48–57.

Lakshmi, C.S. 1990. 'Mother, Mother-Community and Mother-Politics in Tamil Nadu', *Economic and Political Weekly*, 20-29 October, WS72–82.

Laqueur, T. 1990. *Making Sex: Body and Gender from the Greeks to Freud*. Cambridge: Harvard University Press.

Larsen, U. 1995. 'Differentials in Infertility in Cameroon and Nigeria', *Population Studies* 49(2): 329–46.

_______. 1996. 'Childlessness, Subfertility and Infertility in Tanzania', *Studies in Family Planning* 27(1): 18–28.

Latour, B. 1997. *Science in Action: How to Follow Scientists and Engineers through Society*. Cambridge, MA: Harvard University Press.

Latour, B. 1993. *We Have Never Been Modern*. Cambridge, MA: Harvard University Press.

Latour, B. and S. Woolgar. 1979. *Laboratory Life: The Social Construction of Scientific Facts*. London: Sage Publications.

Leach, E.R. 1976. *Culture and Communication: The Logic by which Symbols are Connected*. London: Cambridge University Press.

Lee, R.M. 1999. *Doing Research on Sensitive Topics*. London: Sage.

Lefebvre, B. 2010. 'Hospital Chains in India: The Coming of Age?', Centre Asie Ifri. Retrieved on 24 November 2012 from https://hal.archives-ouvertes.fr/hal-00687105/document.

Lingam, L. 1990. 'New Reproductive Technologies in India: A Print Media Analysis', *Issues in Reproductive and Genetic Engineering* 3(1): 13–21.

MacCormack, C.P. 1980. 'Nature, Culture and Gender: A Critique', in C.P. MacCormack and M. Strathern (eds), *Nature, Culture and Gender*. Cambridge: Cambridge University Press, pp. 1–24.

MacCormack, C.P. and M. Strathern (eds). 1980. *Nature, Culture and Gender*. Cambridge: Cambridge University Press.

Madan, T.N. 1965. *Family and Kinship: A Study of the Pandits of Rural Kashmir*. Mumbai: Asia Publishing House.

_______. 1976. 'Hindu Women at Home', in B.R. Nanda (ed.), *Indian Women: From Purdah to Modernity*. New Delhi: Vikas.

_______. 1981. 'Ideology of the Householder among the Kashmiri Pandits', *Contributions to Indian Sociology* 15(1/2): 223–50.

_______. 1982. 'The Ideology of the Householder among the Kashmiri Pandits', in Á. Östör et al. (eds), *Concepts of Person: Kinship, Caste and Marriage in India*, 3rd edn. Delhi: Oxford University Press.

Madan, T.N. et al. 2003. *The Hinduism Omnibus*. New Delhi: Oxford University Press.

Mahanta R. et al. 2011. 'Prevalence of Azoospermia Factor (AZF) Deletions in Idiopathic Infertile Males in North-East India', *International Journal of Human Genetics* 11(2): 99–104.

Malpani A. and A. Malpani. 2002. 'Simplifying Assisted Conception Techniques to Make them Universally Available – A View from India', *Human Reproduction* 7(1): 49–50.

Marcus, G.E. 1995. 'Ethnography in/of the World System: The Emergence of Multi-Sited Ethnography', *Annual Review of Anthropology* 24: 95–117.

Martin, E. 1987. *The Woman in the Body: A Cultural Analysis of Reproduction*. Boston: Beacon Press.

________. 1991. 'The Egg and the Sperm', *Signs* 16(3): 48–501.

________. 1994. *Flexible Bodies: Tracing Immunity in American Culture from the Days of Polio to the Age of Aids*. Boston: Beacon Press.

Matthew, P. 2011. 'Letter from the Managing Editor', *The Week*, 3 April, 3.

McKevitt, C. 2000. 'Short Stories about Strokes: Interviews and Narrative Production', *Anthropology and Medicine* 7(1): 79–96.

McNeil, M. et al. (eds). 1990. *The New Reproductive Technologies*. London: Macmillan.

Mehta, R.H. 2010. 'Dr T.C. Anand Kumar – A Doyen in Reproductive Biology', *Indian Journal of Medical Research* 131: 466–67.

Mentor, S. 1998. 'Witches, Nurses, Midwives and Cyborgs: IVF, ART and Complex Agency in the World of Technobirth', in R.E. Davis-Floyd and J. Dumit (eds), *Cyborg Babies: From Techno-Sex to Techno-Tots*. London: Routledge, pp. 67–89.

Merchant, C. 1983. *The Death of Nature: Women, Ecology and the Scientific Revolution*. San Francisco: Harper and Row.

Meyer, J.J. 1971. *Sexual Life in Ancient India*. Delhi: Motilal Banarsidass.

Miall, C.E. 1985. 'Perceptions of Informal Sanctioning and the Stigma of Involuntary Childlessness', *Deviant Behaviour* 6(4): 383–403.

Mills, C.W. 1959. *The Sociological Imagination*. New York: Oxford University Press.

Modell, J. 1994. *Kinship with Strangers: Adoption and Interpretation of Kinship in American Culture*. Berkeley: University of California Press.

Modell, J. 2002. *Sealed and Secret Kinship: The Culture of Policies and Practices in American Adoption*. New York: Berghahn Books.

Modell, J. 1998. 'Rights to the Children: Foster Care and Social Reproduction in Hawaii', in S. Franklin and H. Ragone (eds), *Reproducing Reproduction: Kinship, Power and Technological Innovation*. Philadelphia: University of Pennsylvania Press.

Mogobe, K. 2000. 'Traditional Therapies for Infertility in Botswana: Implications for the Brokerage Role of the Nurse', in F. Van Balen et al. (eds), *Social Science Research on Childlessness in a Global Perspective: Proceedings of the Conference 8-11 November 1999*. Amsterdam: SCO-Kohnstamm Institute, pp. 111–17.

Moscucci, O. 1990. *The Science of Women: Gynaecology and Gender in England 1800-1929*. Cambridge: Cambridge University Press.

Mukherjee, M. 1997. 'Test-Tube Baby's Parents Reveal All: Resurrect Scorned Scientist, Amends Won't Bring Him Back, Rues Doctor's Widow', *The Telegraph*, 21 February, Calcutta.

Mukherjee, R. 2011. 'Strong Does: Govt May Make Pharma Code Mandatory', *Times of India*, 7 June. Retrieved on 16 February 2015 from http://timesofindia.indiatimes.com/business/india-business/Strong-dose-Govt-ay-make-pharma-code-mandatory/articleshow/8753928.cms.

_______. 2014. 'From Jan 1, No Freebies for Docs from Pharma Firms', *Times of India*, 23 December. Retrieved on 16 February 2015 from http://timesofindia.indiatimes.com/business/india-business/From-Jan...cos-can-no-longer-gift-freebies-to-doctors/articleshow/45610957.cms.

Mulgaonkar, V. 2000. 'Treatment-Seeking Behaviour of Childless Couples in the Slums of Mumbai', in F. Van Balen et al. (eds), *Social Science Research on Childlessness in a Global Perspective: Proceedings of the Conference 8-11 November 1999*. Amsterdam: SCO-Kohnstamm Institute, pp. 95–101.

Müller, F.M. 1894. *The Sacred Books of the East: Translated by Various Oriental Scholars and Edited by F. Max Müller*, Vols. 1–49. Oxford: Clarendon Press.

Nadkarni, S. 2010. *Healthcare System is an Industry, Management of the Sick Healthcare System*. Delhi: *Vora Medical Publications*.

Nahar, P. et al. 2000. 'Living with Infertility: Experiences from Urban Slum Populations in Bangladesh', *Reproductive Health Matters* 8(15): 33–44.

Nahar, P. and S. van der Geest. 2014. 'How Women in Bangladesh Confront the Stigma of Childlessness: Agency, Resilience and Resistance', *Medical Anthropology Quarterly* 28(3): 381–98.

Nahman, M. 2008. 'Synecdochic Ricochets: Biosocialities in a Jerusalem IVF Clinic', in S. Gibbon and C. Novas (eds), *Biosocialities, Genetics, and the Social Sciences: Making Biologies and Identities*. London: Routledge, pp. 117–35.

_______. 2013. *Extractions: An Ethnography of Reproductive Tourism*. Basingstoke: Palgrave Macmillan.

Nandan, D. et al. 2001. 'Reproductive Tract Infection in Women of Reproductive Age Group in Sitapur/ Shahjahanpur District of Uttar Pradesh', *Indian Journal of Public Health* 45(1): 8–13.

Nandraj, S. 1994. 'Beyond the Law and the Lord: Quality of Private Health Care', *Economic and Political Weekly* 29(27): 1680–685.

Nandraj, S., V.R. Muraleedharan, R. Baru, V. Qadeer and R. Priya. 2001. *Private Health Sector in India: Review and Annotated Bibliography*. Mumbai: CEHAT.

National Family Health Survey. 1992–1993. *India*. Mumbai: International Institute for Population Sciences.

Neff, D.L. 1994. 'The Social Construction of Infertility: The Case of the Matrilineal Nayars in South India', *Social Science and Medicine* 39(4): 475–85.

Nichter, M. and M. Nichter. 1996. *Anthropology and International Health: Asian Case Studies*, 2nd edn. Amsterdam: Gordon and Breach.

O'Flaherty, W.D. 1980. *Women, Androgynes, and other Mythical Beasts*. Chicago: University of Chicago Press.

O'Flaherty, W.D. and J.D.M. Derrett (eds). 1978. *The Concept of Duty in South Asia*. New Delhi: Vikas.

Obeyesekere, G. 1968. 'Theodicy, Sin and Salvation in a Sociology of Buddhism', in Edmund R. Leach (ed.), *Dialectic in Practical Religion*. London: Cambridge University Press, pp. 7–40.

Ohnuki-Tierney, E. 1984. '1984 Monkey Performances: A Multiple Structure of Meaning and Reflexivity in Japanese Culture', in E. Bruner (ed.), *Text, Play and Story*. Washington, D.C.: American Ethnological Society, pp. 278–314.

Okonofua, F.E. 1996. 'The Case against New Reproductive Technologies in Developing Countries', *British Journal of Obstetrics and Gynaecology* 103(10): 957–62.

Ombelet, W. 2011. 'Global Access to Infertility Care in Developing Countries: A Case of Human Rights, Equity and Social Justice', *Facts, Views and Visions in ObGyn* 3(4): 257–66.

Ombelet W. and R. Campo. 2007. 'Affordable IVF for Developing Countries', *Reproductive BioMedicine Online* 15: 257–65.

Oomman, N. 2000. 'A Decade of Research on Reproductive Tract Infections and Other Gynaecological Morbidity in India: What We Know and What We Don't Know', in R. Ramasubban and S.J. Jejeebhoy (eds), *Women's Reproductive Health in India*. Jaipur: Rawat Publications, pp. 236–79.

Östör, Á. and L. Fruzzetti. 1995. 'Concept of Person: Fifteen Years Later', in Á. Östör et al. (eds), *Concepts of Person: Kinship, Caste and Marriage in India*, 3rd edn. Delhi: Oxford University Press, pp. xv–xxviii.

Oudshoorn, N. 1994. *Beyond the Natural Body: An Archeology of Sex Hormones*. London: Routledge.

_______. 1999. 'The Decline of the One-Size-Fits-All Paradigm, or, How Reproductive Scientists Try to Cope with Postmodernity', in D. MacKenzie and J. Wajcman (eds), *The Social Shaping of Technology*, 2nd edn. Philadelphia: Open University Press, pp. 325–42.

Pande, A. 2010a. '"At Least I am not Sleeping with Anyone": Resisting the Stigma of Commercial Surrogacy in India', *Feminist Studies*, Special Issue on Reproduction and Mothering, 36(2): 292–312.

_______. 2010b. 'Commercial Surrogacy in India: Manufacturing the Perfect "Mother Worker"', *Signs* 35(4): 969–92.

______. 2014. *Wombs in Labor: Transnational Commercial Surrogacy in India*. New York: Columbia University Press.

Pande, M. 2016. 'What the lives of the five virgins of the Ramayan and Mahabharat can teach us: The panch kanyas stand for the timeless struggles for truth and justice by the meek and marginalised'. *Scroll*, March 30. Retrieved on 1st May 2016 from http://scroll.in/article/805344/what-the-lives-of-the-five-virgins-of-the-ramayan-and-mahabharat-can-teach-us

Pandya, S.K. 1995. 'Medical Council of India and the General Medical Council, United Kingdom', *The National Medical Journal of India* 8(3): 136–38.

Panicker, L. 'Population Prescription', *The Times of India*, 31 August 2004.

Parashari, A. et al. 1994. 'Clinical and Aetiological Profile of Reproductive Tract Infections (RTIs) among Women Attending Gynaecology

Out-Patient Department of a Major City Hospital in Delhi', *Journal of Obstetrics and Gynaecology of India* 44(5): 790–97.

Parikh, F.R. et al. 1997. 'Genital Tuberculosis: A Major Pelvic Factor Causing Infertility in Indian Women', *Fertility and Sterility* 67(3): 497–500.

Parsons, Talcott. 1949. *The Structure of Social Action: A Study in Social Theory with Special Reference to a Group of Recent European Writers*, 2nd edn. Glencoe, IL: Free Press.

Pashigian, M.J. 2000. 'Infertility and the Politics of Marriage in Northern Vietnam', in F. Van Balen et al. (eds), *Social Science Research on Childlessness in a Global Perspective: Proceedings of the Conference 8-11 November 1999*. Amsterdam: SCO-Kohnstamm Institute, pp. 129–35.

_______. 2009. 'Inappropriate Relations: The Ban on Surrogacy with In Vitro Fertilization and the Limits of State Renovation in Contemporary Vietnam', in D. Birenbaum-Carmeli and M.C. Inhorn (eds), *Assisting Reproduction, Testing Genes: Global Encounters with the New Biotechnologies*. New York: Berghahn Books, pp. 164–88.

Patel, T. 1994. *Fertility Behaviour: Population and Society in a Rajasthan Village*. Delhi: Oxford University Press.

Patnaik, P. 2014. 'Neo-liberalism and Democracy', *Economic and Political Weekly* 49(15): 39–44.

Pearce, T.O. 1999. 'She Will not be Listened to in Public: Perceptions among the Yoruba of Infertility and Childlessness in Women', *Reproductive Health Matters* 7(13): 69–79.

Pennington, B.K. 2005. *Was Hinduism Invented? Britons, Indians, and Colonial Construction of Religion*. New York: Oxford University Press.

Pfeffer, N. 1987. 'Artificial Insemination, In-Vitro Fertilization and the Stigma of Infertility', in M. Stanworth (ed.), *Reproductive Technologies: Gender, Motherhood and Medicine*. Cambridge: Polity Press, pp. 81–97.

_______. 1992. 'From Private Patients to Privatization', in M. Stacey (ed.), *Changing Human Reproduction: Social Science Perspectives*. London: Sage, pp. 48–74.

_______. 1993. *The Stork and the Syringe: A Political History of Reproductive Medicine*. Cambridge: Polity Press.

Phadke, A. 1993. *Private Health Sector*. Mumbai: Foundation for Research in Community Health.

Piercy, M. 1979. *Women on the Edge of Time*. London: Women's Press.

Prakash, G. 1999. *Another Reason: Science and the Imagination of Modern India*. Princeton: Princeton University Press.

Pratap, R.K. 2011. 'IVF Baby Boom'. *Outlook Business*, October. Retrieved on 12 January 2013 from http://www.outlookbusiness.com/printarticle.aspx?278530.

Price, F. 1993. 'Beyond Expectation: Clinical Practices and Clinical Concerns', in J. Edwards et al. (eds), *Technologies of Procreation: Kinship in the Age of Assisted Conception*. Manchester: Manchester University Press, pp. 29–52.

______. 1999. 'Solutions for Life and Growth? Collaborative Conceptions in Reproductive Medicine', in J. Edwards et al. (eds), *Technologies of Procreation: Kinship in the Age of Assisted Conception*, 2nd edn. London: Routledge, pp. 53–59.

Qadeer, I. 2009. 'Social and Ethical Basis of Legislation on Surrogacy: Need for Debate', *Indian Journal of Medical Ethics* 6(1): 28–32.

______. 2010. 'The ART of Marketing Babies', *Indian Journal of Medial Ethics* 7(4): 209–15.

______. 2011. 'The Challenge of Building Rural Health Services', *Indian Journal of Medical Research* 134(5): 591–93.

Rabinow, P. 1992. 'Artificiality and Enlightenment: From Sociobiology to Biosociality', in J. Crary and S. Kwinter (eds), *Incorporations*. New York: Zone, pp. 234–52.

Radcliffe-Brown, A.R. 1940. 'On Joking Relationships', *Africa* 13(3): 195–210.

______. 1949. 'A Further Note on Joking Relationships', *Africa* 19(2): 133–40.

Ragoné, H. 1994. *Surrogate Motherhood: Conception in the Heart*. Boulder: Westview Press.

Ragoné, H. and F.W. Twine. 2000. *Ideologies and Technologies of Motherhood: Race, Class, Sexuality, Nationalism*. New York: Routledge.

Ram, U. 2006. *Childlessness and Its Consequences in India: Levels, Patterns and Differentials*. Mumbai: Department of Public Health and Mortality Studies International Institute for Population Sciences. Retrieved on 30 August 2014 from http://www.iipsindia.org/pdf/Childlessness%20in%20India.pdf.

Ramanujan, A.K. 1989. 'Is There an Indian Way of Thinking? An Informal Essay', *Contributions to Indian Sociology* 23(1): 41–58.

Ramasubban, R. and B. Rishyasringa. 1998. '"Ashaktapana" (Weakness) and Reproductive Health in a Slum Population in Mumbai, India', in C.M. Obermeyer (ed.), *Cultural Perspectives in Reproductive Health*. Oxford: Oxford University Press, pp. 13–37.

Rao, C. 1990. 'An Ill-Conceived Move: Research Rivalry Leads to Winding Up of Test-Tube Baby Project', *The Week*, 4 November.

Rao, N.B. et al. 1993. 'The Planning Process and Government Health Expenditure Patterns in India in the Early 1980s', in P. Berman and M.E. Khan (eds), *Paying for India's Health Care*. New Delhi: Sage, pp. 91–120.

Raymond, J. 1993. *Women as Wombs*. San Francisco: Harper San Francisco.

Reddy, D.S. 2011. 'Hindutva: Formative Assertions', *Religious Compass* 5(8): 439–51.

Reddy, P.A. 2004. *Problems of Widows in India*. New Delhi: Sarup and Sons.

Relman, A. 1987. 'Sounding Board: The Changing Climate of Medical Practice', *New England Journal of Medicine* 316(6): 333–42.

Rich, A. 1995. *Of Woman Born: Motherhood as Experience and Institution*, 2nd edn. New York: W.W. Norton & Company.

Riessman, C.K. 1996. 'Book Reviews and Notices of Shalini Bharat's *Child Adoption in India: Trends and Emerging Issues: A Study of Adoption Agencies'. Contributions to Indian Sociology* 30(1): 168–69.

Riessman, C.K. 2000. 'Stigma and Everyday Resistance Practices: Childless Women in South India', *Gender and Society* 14(1): 111–35.

_______. 2002. 'Positioning Gender Identity in Narratives of Infertility: South Indian Women's Lives in Context', in M.C. Inhorn and F. Van Balen (eds), *Infertility around the Globe: New Thinking on Childlessness, Gender, and Reproductive Technologies*. Berkeley: University of California Press, pp. 152–70.

Roberts, E.F.S. 2006. 'God's Laboratory: Religious Rationalities and Modernity in Ecuadorian In Vitro Fertilization', *Culture, Medicine, and Psychiatry* 30(4): 507–36.

_______. 2007. 'Extra Embryos: The Ethics of Cyropreservation in Ecuador and Elsewhere', *American Ethnologist* 34(1): 181–99.

_______. 2009. 'The Traffic between Women: Female Alliance and Familial Egg Donation in Ecuador', in D. Birenbaum-Carmeli and M.C. Inhorn (eds), *Assisting Reproduction, Testing Genes: Global Encounters with the New Biotechnologies*. New York: Berghahn Books, pp. 113–43.

_______. 2012. *God's Laboratory: Assisted Reproduction in the Andes*. Berkeley: University of California Press.

Robertson, G. et al. 1996. *FutureNatural: Nature, Science, Culture*. London: Routledge.

Rosaldo, M.Z. and L. Lamphere (eds). 1974. *Women, Culture, and Society*. Stanford: Stanford University Press.

Rothman, B.K. 1982. *In Labor: Women and Power in the Birthplace*. New York: Norton.

Roy, S. 2007. *Beyond Belief: India and the Politics of Postcolonial Nationalism*. Durham: Duke University Press.

Rozati, R., P.P. Reddy, P. Reddanna and R. Mujtaba. 2002. 'Role of Environmental Estrogens in the Deterioration of Male Factor Fertility', *Fertility and Sterility* 78(6): 1187–194.

Rudrappa, S. 2012. 'India's Reproductive Assembly Line', *Context* 1(2): 22–27.

SAMA. 2007. 'Assisted Reproductive Technologies in India: Implications for Women', *Economic and Political Weekly* 42(23): 2184–89.

_______. 2010. 'Unraveling the Fertility Industry: Challenges and Strategies for Movement Building'. Delhi: SAMA Publication.

_______. 2012. 'Birthing a Market: A Study on Commercial Surrogacy'. Delhi: SAMA Publication.

Sandelowski, M. 1990. 'Failures of Volition: Female Agency and Infertility in Historical Perspective', *Signs* 15: 475–99.

_______. 1991. 'Compelled to Try: The Never Enough Quality of Conceptive Technology', *Medical Anthropology Quarterly* 5(1): 29–47.

Sangari, K. 1993. 'Consent, Agency and Rhetorics of Incitement', *Economic and Political Weekly*, 1 May, 867–82.

Saravanan, L. 2014. 'HC Urges Pre-marital Potency Test', *Times of India*, 28 August. Retrieved on 9 September 2015 from http://timesofindia.indiatimes.com/city/madurai/HC-urges-pre-marital-potency-test/articleshow/41055991.cms.

Sarojini, N., M. Vrinda and A. Shenoi. 2011. 'Globalisation of Birth Markets: A Case Study of Assisted Reproductive Technologies in India', *Globalization and Health* 7(27). http://globalizationandhealth.biomedcentral.com/articles/10.1186/1744-8603-7-27.

Scheper-Hughes, N. 2000. 'The Global Traffic in Human Organs', *Current Anthropology* 41(2): 191–224.

_______. 2002. 'The Ends of the Body: Commodity Fetishism and the Global Traffic in Organs', *SAIS Review* 22(1): 61–80.

Schmidt, M. and L.J. Moore. 1998. 'Constructing a "Good Catch", Picking a Winner: The Development of Technosemen and the Deconstruction of the Monolithic Male', in R.E. Davis Floyd and J. Dumit (eds), *Cyborg Babies: From Techno-Sex to Techno-Tots*. London: Routledge, pp. 21–39.

Scott, R. 1978. *The Making of Blind Men*. New York: Russell Sage.

Sengupta, A. and S. Nundy. 2005. 'The Private Health Sector in India', *British Medical Journal* 331: 1157–158.

Serres, M. 2007. *The Parasite*. University of Minnesota Press.

Shah, A.M. 1998. *The Family in India: Critical Essays*. New Delhi: Orient Longman.

Shah, U. and R. Mohanty. 2010. 'Private Sector in Indian Healthcare Delivery: Consumer Perspective and Government Policies to Promote Private Sector', *Information Management and Business Review* 1(2): 79–87.

Sharma, J. 2006. *Hindutva: Exploring the Idea of Hindu Nationalism*. Delhi: Penguin India.

Silverman, D. 1993. *Interpreting Qualitative Data: Methods for Analysing Talk, Text and Interaction*. London: Sage.

_______. 2000. *Doing Qualitative Research: A Practical Handbook*. London: Sage.

Simpson, R. 2004. 'Acting Ethically, Responding Culturally: Framing the New Reproductive and Genetic Technologies in Sri Lanka', *The Asia Pacific Journal of Anthropology* 5(3): 227–43.

Singer, M. 1972. *When a Great Tradition Modernizes*. New York: Praeger.

Singh, K. et al. 2005. 'Mutation C677T in the Methylenetetrahydrofolate Reductase Gene Associated with Male Infertility in an Indian Population', *International Journal of Andrology* 28(2): 115–19.

Sinha, C. 2007. 'Images of Motherhood: The Hindu Code Bill Discourse', *Economic and Political Weekly*, 27 October, 49–57.

Skramstad, H. 2000. 'Are Foster Children a Solution for Infertile Gambian Women?', in F. Van Balen et al. (eds), *Social Science Research on Childlessness in a Global Perspective: Proceedings of the Conference 8–11 November 1999*. Amsterdam: SCO-Kohnstamm Institute, pp. 15–27.

Smerdon, U.R. 2009. 'Crossing Bodies, Crossing Borders: International Surrogacy between the United States and India', *Cumberland Law Review* 39(1): 15–85.

Sontheimer, G.D. 1977. *The Joint Hindu Family: Its Evolution as a Legal Institution*. New Delhi: Munshiram Manoharlal.

Sontheimer, G.D. and H. Kulke (eds). 1991. *Hinduism Reconsidered*. New Delhi: Manohar.

Soules, M.R. 1985. 'The In-Vitro Fertilization Pregnancy Rate: Let's be Honest with One Another', *Fertility and Sterility* 43(4): 511–13.

Spallone, P. 1989. *Beyond Conception: The New Politics of Reproduction*. London: Macmillan.

Spallone, P. and D.L. Steinberg (eds). 1987. *Made to Order: The Myth of Reproductive and Genetic Progress*. Oxford: Pergamon Press.

Srinivas, M.N. 1989. *The Cohesive Role of Sanskritization and other Essays*. Delhi: Oxford University Press.

_______. 1997. 'Practicing Social Anthropology in India', *Annual Review of Anthropology* 26: 1–24.

Stanworth, M. 1987a. 'Reproductive Technologies and the Deconstruction of Motherhood', in M. Stanworth (ed.), *Reproductive Technologies: Gender, Motherhood and Medicine*. Cambridge: Polity Press, pp. 10–35.

_______. 1987b. *Reproductive Technologies: Gender, Motherhood and Medicine*. Cambridge: Polity Press.

Stark, R. 1985. 'Lay Workers in Primary Health Care: Victims in the Process of Social Transformation', *Social Science and Medicine* 20: 269–75.

Steinberg, D.L. 1990. 'The Depersonalisation of Women through the Administration of In Vitro Fertilization', in M. McNeil et al. (eds), *The New Reproductive Technologies*. London: Macmillan, pp. 74–122.

Strathern, M. 1992a. *After Nature: English Kinship in the Late Twentieth Century*. Cambridge: Cambridge University Press.

_______. 1992b. *Reproducing the Future: Anthropology, Kinship and the New Reproductive Technologies*. New York: Routledge.

_______. 1998. 'Surrogates and Substitutes: New Practices for Old?', in J. Good and I. Velody (eds), *The Politics of Postmodernity*. Cambridge: Cambridge University Press, pp. 182–209.

_______. 1999. 'A Question of Context', in J. Edwards et al. (eds), *Technologies of Procreation: Kinship in the Age of Assisted Conception*, 2nd edn. London: Routledge, pp. 9–28.

Sundby, J. 1997. 'Infertility in the Gambia: Traditional and Modern Health Care', *Patient Education and Counselling* 31(1): 29–37.

_______. 2002. 'Infertility and Health Care in Countries with Less Resources: Case Studies from Sub-Saharan Africa', in M.C. Inhorn and F. Van Balen (eds), *Infertility around the Globe: New Thinking on Childlessness, Gender, and Reproductive Technologies*. Berkeley: University of California Press, pp. 247–60.

Sundby, J. and A. Jacobus. 2001 'Health and Traditional Care for Infertility in the Gambia and Zimbabwe', in T. Boerma and Z. Mgalla (eds), *Women and Infertility in Sub-Saharan Africa: A Multi-Disciplinary Perspective.* Amsterdam: KIT Publishers, pp. 257–68.

Sunder Rajan, K. 2007. 'Experimental Values: Indian Clinical Trials and Surplus Health', *New Left Review* 45: 67–88.

______. 2008. 'Biocapital as an Emergent Form of Life: Speculations on the Figure of the Experimental Subject', in S. Gibbon and C. Novas (eds), *Biosocialities, Genetics and the Social Sciences: Making Biologies and Identities.* London: Routledge, pp. 157–87.

Sunder Rajan, R. 1993. *Real and Imagined Women: Gender, Culture and Postcolonialism.* London: Routledge.

______. 2001. *Real and Imagined Women: Gender, Culture and Postcolonialism,* 2nd edn. London: Routledge.

Sunitha, L.F. and R. Ajil Babu. 2013. 'Role of FDI in India's Health Care Sector: Major Issues and Challenges', *International Journal of Humanities and Social Science Invention* 2(5): 37–40.

Sutherland, G.H. 1990. 'Bija (Seed) and Ksetra (Field): Male Surrogacy or Niyoga in the Mhabharata', *Contributions to Indian Sociology* 24(1): 77–103.

Sutherland, S.J.M. 1991. *Bridging Worlds: Studies on Women in South Asia.* Delhi: Oxford University Press.

Tarlo, E. 2003. *Unsettling Memories: Narratives of the Emergency in Delhi*. Berkeley: University of California Press Berkeley.

Teman, E. 2010. *Birthing the Mother: The Surrogate Body and the Pregnant Self.* Berkeley: University of California Press.

Thankappan, K.R. et al. 1987. *Health and Development in Rural Kerala*. Thiruvanthapuram: KSSP.

Thapar, R. 1989. 'Imagined Religious Communities? Ancient History and the Modern Search for a Hindu Identity', *Modern Asian Studies* 23(2): 209–31.

Thomas, S. 2013. 'Give Indian Parents First Preference in Child Adoptions: HC', *Times of India,* 15 November. Retrieved on 30 August 2014 from http://timesofindia.indiatimes.com/india/Give-Indian-parents-first-preference-in-child-adoption-HC/articleshow/25782693.cms.

Thompson, C. 2001. 'Strategic Naturalizing: Kinship in an Infertility Clinic', in S. Franklin and S. McKinnon (eds), *Relative Values: Reconfiguring Kinship Studies*. Durham: Duke University Press, pp. 175–202.

______. 2005. *Making Parents: The Ontological Choreography of Reproductive Technologies*. Cambridge: MIT Press.

Thompson, E.P. 1971. 'The Moral Economy of the English Crowd in the Eighteenth Century', *Past and Present* 50(1): 76–136.

Tikku, A. 2013. 'ICMR has not Delayed Surrogacy Law: RS Sharma', *Hindustan Times,* 25 March. Retrieved on 30 September 2014 from http://www.hindustantimes.com/comment/interviewsnews/icmr-has-not-delayed-surrogacy-law-rs-sharma/article1-1031633.aspx.

Tremayne, S. 2006. 'Not all Muslims are Luddites', *Anthropology Today* 22: 1–2.

_______. 2009. 'Law, Ethics, and Donor Technologies in Shia Iran', in D. Birenbaum-Carmeli and M.C. Inhorn (eds), *Assisting Reproduction, Testing Genes: Global Encounters with New Biotechnologies*. New York: Berghahn Books, pp. 144–63.

Tully, M. 1996. *The Heart of India*. London: Penguin Books.

Uberoi, P. 1993. *Family, Kinship and Marriage in India*. Delhi: Oxford University Press.

_______. 1996. 'Hindu Marriage Law and the Judicial Construction of Sexuality', in R. Kapur (ed.), *Feminist Terrains in Legal Domains: Interdisciplinary Essays on Women and Law in India*. New Delhi: Kali for Women, pp. 184–209.

Unisa, S. 1999. 'Childlessness in Andhra Pradesh, India: Treatment-Seeking and Consequences', *Reproductive Health Matters* 7(13): 54–64.

Unnithan-Kumar, M. 2001. 'Emotion, Agency and Access to Healthcare: Women's Experiences of Reproduction in Jaipur', in S. Tremayne (ed.), *Managing Reproductive Life: Cross-Cultural Themes in Fertility and Sexuality*. Oxford: Berghahn, pp. 25–52.

_______. 2004 'Conception Technologies, Local Healers and Negotiations around Childbearing in Rajasthan', in M. Unnithan-Kumar (ed.), *Reproductive Agency, Medicine and the State: Cultural Transformations in Childbearing*. Oxford: Berghahn Books, pp. 59–83.

_______. 2010. 'Learning from Infertility: Gender, Health Inequities and Faith Healers in Women's Experiences of Disrupted Reproduction in Rajasthan', *Journal of South Asian History and Culture* 1(2): 315–27.

_______. 2013. 'Thinking through Surrogacy Legislation in India: Reflections on Relational Consent and the Rights of Infertile Women', *Journal of Legal Anthropology* 1(3): 287–313.

Van Balen F. and T. Gerrits. 2001. 'Quality of Infertility Care in Poor-Resource Areas and the Introduction of New Reproductive Technologies', *Human Reproduction* 16(2): 215–19.

Van Maanen, J. 1988. *Tales of the Field: On Writing Ethnography*. Chicago: University of Chicago Press.

Vayena, E., J.P. Rowe and H.B. Peterson. 2002. 'Assisted Reproductive Technology in Developing Countries: Why Should We Care?', *Fertility and Sterility* 78(1): 13–15.

Vemuri, M.D. and D. Manohar. 1986. 'Childlessness in India', *Biology and Biology* 3(4): 163–66.

Venkatesan, J. 2011. 'Private Practice by Government Doctors no Criminal Offense: Court', *The Hindu*, 1 May 2011. Retrieved on 18 February 2014 from http://www.thehindu.com/sci-tech/health/policy-and-issues/private-practice-by-government-doctors-no-criminal-offence-court/article1981589.ece.

Venkatratnam, R. 1973. *Medical Sociology in an Indian Setting*. New Delhi: Macmillan.

_______. 1987. 'Health System and the Polity: A Note on Indian Scene', in S.K. Lal and A. Chandani (eds), *Medical Care: Readings in Medical Sociology*. New Delhi: Jainsons Publications, pp. 16–27.

Vishwanathan, H. and J.E. Rohde. 1990. *Diarrhoea in Rural India: A Nation-wide Study of Mothers and Practitioners*. New Delhi: Vision Books.

Viswanath, K. and P. Kirbat. 1998. 'The Campaign of the Women's Movement Against New Contraceptive Technologies', Working Paper No. 18. Social Science and Immunization, Delhi: Centre for Development Economics.

Vloeberghs, V., G. Verheyen and H. Tournaye. 2013. 'Intracytoplasmic Spermatid Injection and In Vitro Maturation: Fact or Fiction?', *Clinics* 68(Suppl 1): 151–56.

Von Stietencron, H. 1991. 'Hinduism: On the Proper Use of a Deceptive Term', in G.D. Sontheimer and H. Kulke (eds), *Hinduism Reconsidered*. New Delhi: Manohar, pp. 11–28.

Vora, K. 2009. 'Indian Transnational Surrogacy and the Commodification of Vital Energy', *Subjectivities* 28: 266–78.

Waitzkin, H. 1991. *The Politics of Medical Encounters: How Patients and Doctors Deal with Social Problems*. New Haven: Yale University Press.

Widge A. and J. Cleland. 2009. 'The Public Sector's Role in Infertility Management in India', *Health Policy and Planning* 24(2): 108–15.

Whiteford, L.M. and L. Gonzalez. 1995. 'Stigma: The Hidden Burden of Infertility', *Social Science and Medicine* 40(1): 27–36.

World Health Organisation. 2014. 'Trends in Maternal Mortality: 1990 to 2013: Estimates by WHO, UNICEF, UNFPA, World Bank and the United Nations Population Division'. Geneva.

Yesudian, C.A.K. 1990. *A Study of Health Services Utilization and Expenditure*. Mumbai: Tata Institute of Social Sciences.

Index

Fertility, Reproduction and Sexuality

General Editors:

Soraya Tremayne, Founding Director, Fertility and Reproduction Studies Group and Research Associate, Institute of Social and Cultural Anthropology, University of Oxford.

Marcia C. Inhorn, William K. Lanman, Jr., Professor of Anthropology and International Affairs, Yale University.

Philip Kreager, Director, Fertility and Reproduction Studies Group and Research Associate, Institute of Social and Cultural Anthropology and Institute of Human Sciences, University of Oxford.

Volume 1
Managing Reproductive Life: Cross-Cultural Themes in Fertility and Sexuality
Edited by Soraya Tremayne

Volume 2
Modern Babylon? Prostituting Children in Thailand
Heather Montgomery

Volume 3
Reproductive Agency, Medicine and the State: Cultural Transformations in Childbearing
Edited by Maya Unnithan-Kumar

Volume 4
A New Look at Thai AIDS: Perspectives from the Margin
Graham Fordham

Volume 5
Breast Feeding and Sexuality: Behaviour, Beliefs and Taboos among the Gogo Mothers in Tanzania
Mara Mabilia

Volume 6
Ageing without Children: European and Asian Perspectives on Elderly Access to Support Networks
Edited by Philip Kreager and Elisabeth Schröder-Butterfill

Volume 7
Nameless Relations: Anonymity, Melanesia and Reproductive Gift Exchange between British Ova Donors and Recipients
Monica Konrad

Volume 8
Population, Reproduction and Fertility in Melanesia
Edited by Stanley J. Ulijaszek

Volume 9
Conceiving Kinship: Assisted Conception, Procreation and Family in Southern Europe
Monica M. E. Bonaccorso

Volume 10
Where There Is No Midwife: Birth and Loss in Rural India
Sarah Pinto

Volume 11
Reproductive Disruptions: Gender, Technology, and Biopolitics in the New Millennium
Edited by Marcia C. Inhorn

Volume 12
Reconceiving the Second Sex: Men, Masculinity, and Reproduction
Edited by Marcia C. Inhorn, Tine Tjørnhøj-Thomsen, Helene Goldberg and Maruska la Cour Mosegaard

Volume 13
Transgressive Sex: Subversion and Control in Erotic Encounters
Edited by Hastings Donnan and Fiona Magowan

Volume 14
European Kinship in the Age of Biotechnology
Edited by Jeanette Edwards and Carles Salazar

Volume 15
Kinship and Beyond: The Genealogical Model Reconsidered
Edited by Sandra Bamford and James Leach

Volume 16
Islam and New Kinship: Reproductive Technology and the Shariah in Lebanon
Morgan Clarke

Volume 17
Childbirth, Midwifery and Concepts of Time
Edited by Christine McCourt

Volume 18
Assisting Reproduction, Testing Genes: Global Encounters with the New Biotechnologies
Edited by Daphna Birenbaum-Carmeli and Marcia C. Inhorn

Volume 19
Kin, Gene, Community: Reproductive Technologies among Jewish Israelis
Edited by Daphna Birenbaum-Carmeli and Yoram S. Carmeli

Volume 20
Abortion in Asia: Local Dilemmas, Global Politics
Edited by Andrea Whittaker

Volume 21
Unsafe Motherhood: Mayan Maternal Mortality and Subjectivity in Post-War Guatemala
Nicole S. Berry

Volume 22
Fatness and the Maternal Body: Women's Experiences of Corporeality and the Shaping of Social Policy
Edited by Maya Unnithan-Kumar and Soraya Tremayne

Volume 23
Islam and Assisted Reproductive Technologies: Sunni and Shia Perspectives
Edited by Marcia C. Inhorn and Soraya Tremayne

Volume 24
Militant Lactivism? Attachment Parenting and Intensive Motherhood in the UK and France
Charlotte Faircloth

Volume 25
Pregnancy in Practice: Expectation and Experience in the Contemporary US
Sallie Han

Volume 26
Nighttime Breastfeeding: An American Cultural Dilemma
Cecília Tomori

Volume 27
Globalized Fatherhood
Edited by Marcia C. Inhorn, Wendy Chavkin and José-Alberto Navarro

Volume 28
Cousin Marriages: Between Tradition, Genetic Risk and Cultural Change
Edited by Alison Shaw and Aviad Raz

Volume 29
Achieving Procreation: Childlessness and IVF in Turkey
Merve Demircioğlu Göknar

Volume 30
Thai *in Vitro*: Gender, Culture and Assisted Reproduction
Andrea Whittaker

Volume 31
Assisted Reproductive Technologies in the Third Phase: Global Encounters and Emerging Moral Worlds
Edited by Kate Hampshire and Bob Simpson

Volume 32
Parenthood between Generations: Transforming Reproductive Cultures
Edited by Siân Pooley and Kaveri Qureshi

Volume 33
Patient-Centred IVF: Bioethics and Care in a Dutch Clinic
Trudie Gerrits

Volume 34
Conceptions: Infertility and Procreative Technologies in India
Aditya Bharadwaj